Nephrology

D1296859

Contributors

Ronald J. Falk, MD, FACP, Book Editor [1]
Doc J. Thurston Professor of Medicine
Director, University of North Carolina Kidney Center
Chief of Nephrology and Hypertension
The University of North Carolina at Chapel Hill
Chapel Hill, North Carolina

Virginia U. Collier, MD, FACP, Associate Editor [2]
Vice Chairman
Director of Education
Chief, Section of General Internal Medicine
Department of Medicine
Christiana Care Health System
Newark, Delaware

Hanna E. Abboud, MD, FACP [1]
Jay H. Stein Professor of Medicine
Chief, Division of Nephrology
The University of Texas Health Science Center at San Antonio
San Antonio, Texas

Phyllis August, MD, MPH [1]
Ralph A. Baer Professor of Medical Research
Professor of Medicine in Obstetrics and Gynecology and Public Health
Division of Nephrology and Hypertension
Weill Medical College of Cornell University
New York, New York

Juan Carlos Ayus, MD, FACP [1]
Professor of Medicine
Director of Dialysis Service
Texas Diabetes Institute at University of Texas Health
 Science Center at San Antonio
San Antonio, Texas

Gerald A. Hladik, MD [1]
Associate Professor of Medicine
Division of Nephrology and Hypertension
The University of North Carolina at Chapel Hill
Chapel Hill, North Carolina

Michelle Whittier Krause, MD, MPH [1]
Assistant Professor of Medicine
Division of Nephrology
University of Arkansas for Medical Sciences
Little Rock, Arkansas

Co-Editors-in-Chief

Patrick C. Alguire, MD, FACP [1]
Director, Education and Career Development
American College of Physicians
Philadelphia, Pennsylvania

Paul E. Epstein, MD, FACP [1]
Clinical Professor of Medicine
University of Pennsylvania School of Medicine
Philadelphia, Pennsylvania

ACP Staff

Sean McKinney, Director, Self-Assessment Programs [1]
Charles Rossi, Managing Editor [1]
Amanda Neiley, Staff Editor [1]

Disclosure of Relationships with any Proprietary Entity that Provides Health Care Goods or Services, with the Exception of Non-Profit or Government Organizations, and Non–Health Care–Related Companies

Virginia U. Collier, MD, FACP
Stock Options/Holdings
Celgene, Pfizer, Merck, Schering-Plough, Abbott, Johnson & Johnson, Medtronic, McKesson, Amgen

AMERICAN COLLEGE OF PHYSICIANS

MKSAP®14

MEDICAL KNOWLEDGE *Self-Assessment Program®*

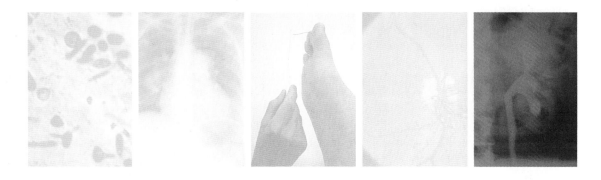

Nephrology

Principal Staff

Senior Vice President, Medical Education and Publishing
Steven Weinberger, MD, FACP

Vice President, Medical Education and Publishing
D. Theresa Kanya, MBA

Director, Self-Assessment Programs
Sean McKinney

Managing Editor
Charles Rossi

Senior Staff Editors
Charlotte Fierman
Becky Krumm
Ellen McDonald, PhD, ELS
Margaret Wells

Staff Editor
Amanda Neiley

Production Administrator
Sheila O'Steen

Program Administrator
Valerie Dangovetsky

Editorial Coordinators
Katie Idell
Karen Williams

Developed by the American College of Physicians

Acknowledgements

The American College of Physicians (ACP) gratefully acknowledges the special contributions to the development and production of the 14th edition of the Medical Knowledge Self-Assessment Program® of Scott Thomas Hurd (systems analyst/developer), Ricki Jo Kauffman (senior systems analyst/developer), and Michael Ripca (graphics technical design administrator). The CD-ROM and Online versions are developed within the Electronic Product Development department by Steven Spadt (Director) and Christopher Forrest, John McKnight, Sean O'Donnell, and Elijah Odumosu (software developers). Computer scoring and reporting are being done by ACT, Iowa City, Iowa. The College also wishes to acknowledge that many other persons, too numerous to mention, have contributed to the production of this program. Without their dedicated efforts, this program would not have been possible.

Continuing Medical Education

The American College of Physicians is accredited by the Accreditation Council for Continuing Medical Education (ACCME) to provide continuing medical education for physicians.

The American College of Physicians designates this educational activity for a maximum of 150 *AMA PRA Category 1 Credits™*. Physicians should only claim credit commensurate with the extent of their participation in the activity.

The American Medical Association has determined that physicians not licensed in the United States who participate in this CME activity are eligible for *AMA PRA Category 1 Credit™*.

Credit is available from December 29, 2006 to July 31, 2009.

Learning Objectives

The learning objectives of the Medical Knowledge Self-Assessment Program are to assess the current state of your knowledge in clinical medicine, update your knowledge in key areas of internal medicine, apply new clinical problem-solving skills to improve the health of your patients, compare your performance on the self-assessment tests with that of your peers, and pursue in-depth study using critically reviewed evidence-based references.

Target Audience

- General internists and primary care physicians
- Subspecialists who need to remain up-to-date in internal medicine
- Residents preparing for the certifying examination in internal medicine
- Physicians participating in maintenance of certification in internal medicine (recertification)

Educational Disclaimer

The editors and publisher of Medical Knowledge Self-Assessment Program 14 recognize that the development of new material offers many opportunities for error. Despite our best efforts, some errors may persist in print. Drug dosage schedules are, we believe, accurate and in accordance with current standards. Readers are advised, however, to ensure that the recommended dosages in MKSAP 14 concur with the information provided in the product information material. This is especially important in cases of new, infrequently used, or highly toxic drugs.

The primary purpose of MKSAP 14 is educational. Information presented, as well as publications, technologies, products, and/or services discussed, are intended to inform subscribers about the knowledge, techniques, and experiences of the contributors. A diversity of professional opinion exists, and the views of the contributors are their own and not those of the ACP. The ACP disclaims any and all liability for damages and claims, which may result from the use of information, publications, technologies, products, and/or services discussed in MKSAP 14.

Publisher's Information

ISBN: 1-930513-78-X

Printed in the United States of America.

For order information in US or Canada call 800-523-1546, extension 2600, all other countries call 215-351-2600. Fax inquiries to 215-351-2799, or email to custserv@acponline.org.

DISCLOSURE

It is the policy of the American College of Physicians (ACP) to ensure balance, independence, objectivity, and scientific rigor in all its educational activities. To this end, and consistent with the policies of the ACP and the Accreditation Council for Continuing Medical Education (ACCME), contributors to all ACP continuing medical education activities are required to disclose all financial relationships they have with proprietary entities producing health care goods or services, with the exception of non-for-profit or government organizations and non–health care–related companies. Contributors are required to use only generic names in the discussion of therapeutic options and are required to identify any unapproved or investigative use of commercial products or devices. If trade-name products manufactured by companies with whom they have relationships are discussed, contributors are asked to provide evidence-based citations in support of the discussion. The information is reviewed by the committee responsible for producing this text and by a separate group of outside physician reviewers. If necessary, adjustments to topics or contributors' roles in content development are made to balance the discussion. Further, all readers of this text are asked to evaluate the content for evidence of commercial bias so that future decisions about content and contributors can be made in light of this information.

Contributors' disclosure information can be found at the beginning of this book.

Table of Contents

Nephrology

CLINICAL EVALUATION OF KIDNEY FUNCTION

An estimated 20 million people in the United States have chronic kidney disease. The clinical evaluation of kidney function includes the estimation of the glomerular filtration rate (GFR), interpretation of the urinalysis and radiographic imaging of the genitourinary tract, and examination of histology by kidney biopsy. Identification of kidney disease is important, because early treatment may delay or prevent progression to kidney failure.

Estimation of the Glomerular Filtration Rate

The GFR is defined as the volume of water filtered from the plasma per unit of time. The estimation of the GFR ideally requires a substance that is freely filtered by the glomerulus, not reabsorbed or secreted in the tubules; is excreted only by the kidney; and is measurable in the plasma under steady-state conditions. The GFR in healthy patients ranges from 120 mL/min per 1.73 m² to 130 mL/min per 1.73 m² for men and 100 mL/min per 1.73 m² to 110 mL/min per 1.73 m² for women.

Historically, the clearance of inulin, an oligosaccharide, was considered the gold standard for estimation of the GFR. However, the inulin clearance is no longer routinely used to estimate the GFR, because of the expense and complexity of administering this agent in the clinical setting. The creatinine clearance; serum levels of creatinine, blood urea nitrogen (BUN), and cystatin C; and radionuclide scanning can be used to estimate the GFR.

Creatinine and Creatinine Clearance

Creatinine is converted from creatine, a naturally occurring amino acid that is predominantly found in skeletal muscle and released into the bloodstream at a constant rate. Creatinine is freely filtered in the glomerulus, excreted by the kidney, and readily measured in the plasma. As the plasma creatinine level increases, the GFR exponentially decreases. For example, an increase in the plasma creatinine level from 1 mg/dL to 2 mg/dL correlates with a 50% decrease in the GFR.

There are several limitations in using creatinine levels to estimate the GFR. Patients with conditions associated with a decrease in muscle mass, such as liver disease, malnutrition, and advanced age, may have low or normal creatinine levels despite underlying kidney disease. A total of 15% to 20% of creatinine in the bloodstream is not filtered in the glomerulus but is secreted by the renal tubules into the urine, resulting in an overestimation of the GFR. In addition, medications such as cimetidine and trimethoprim inhibit the tubular secretion of creatinine, causing an increase in the plasma creatinine level.

Because of the limitations of using the creatinine level to evaluate kidney function, the National Kidney Foundation Kidney Disease Outcomes Quality Initiative guidelines recommend using the creatinine clearance to estimate the GFR instead of the creatinine level alone (www.kidney.org/professionals/kdoqi/guidelines_ckd/p5_lab_g4.htm). The creatinine clearance is calculated using a 24-hour urine collection or mathematical equations. The following equation is used to calculate clearance of a substance from plasma:

$$\text{Creatinine Clearance} = \frac{\text{Urine Creatinine Level} \times \text{Urine Volume}}{\text{Plasma Creatinine Level}}$$

Mathematical equations for creatinine clearance generally are preferred over 24-hour urine collections to estimate the GFR. Timed urine collections are cumbersome and often inaccurate due to collection of either too much or too little urine. The accuracy of a 24-hour urine collection is assessed by measuring the total creatinine in the urine compared with the expected levels of creatinine secretion (20 to 25 mg/kg per 24 h in men; 15 to 20 mg/kg per 24 h in women).

The Cockcroft–Gault and Modification of Diet in Renal Disease (MDRD) equations for creatinine clearance adjust for factors that affect the creatinine level, such as body weight, ethnicity, sex, and age. However, conditions associated with reduced muscle mass limit the ability of these formulas to estimate the GFR. In addition, the MDRD equations were developed to estimate the GFR in patients with chronic kidney disease and are less accurate in patients who are healthy, have acute renal failure, or have a kidney transplant (1). Equations to estimate the GFR are still being modified and their precision improved. Timed urine collection or radionuclide scanning is recommended to estimate the GFR in healthy patients, such as those undergoing evaluation for kidney transplant donation.

There is no consensus regarding the optimal method of estimating the GFR in patients with acute renal failure in non–steady-state conditions. Some experts suggest that a daily rate of increase in the plasma creatinine level of 1 mg/dL to 1.5 mg/dL characterizes an anephric state and complete GFR loss. A daily rate of increase in the creatinine level >1.5 mg/dL usually is associated with increased production of creatinine, which occurs in rhabdomyolysis. Conversely, a daily rate of increase in the creatinine level <1 mg/dL suggests a degree of residual kidney function, but the precise estimation of the GFR in this setting is not known.

Blood Urea Nitrogen

Use of other markers to evaluate kidney function, such as the BUN and cystatin C levels, has been variously successful. BUN is derived from protein waste products metabolized by the liver, secreted into the bloodstream, and freely filtered by the glomerulus. The proximal tubules reabsorb approximately 40% to 50% of the filtered BUN.

The BUN and creatinine levels are often measured simultaneously to evaluate kidney function. The normal BUN–creatinine ratio is 10 to 15:1. In patients with conditions that decrease kidney perfusion, such as hypovolemia or congestive heart failure, reabsorption of the BUN in the proximal tubules increases and the BUN–creatinine ratio disproportionately increases to >20:1.

High-protein diets, catabolic states, and gastrointestinal bleeding also cause elevations in the BUN level and may not reflect underlying kidney disease. Conversely, conditions such as liver failure and malnutrition may cause a decreased BUN level because of associated decreased urea production and inadequate protein intake, respectively. In these settings, the ability of the BUN level to detect abnormalities in kidney function is limited.

Cystatin C

Cystatin C is a low-molecular-weight protein in the cysteine protease family that all nucleated cells release into the bloodstream at a constant rate. Unlike creatinine, cystatin C is produced independently of age, sex, muscle mass, and body weight. The glomerulus freely filters cystatin C, and the proximal tubular cells then completely reabsorb and metabolize this protein. Therefore, cystatin C is immeasurable in the urine.

In healthy patients, levels of cystatin C range from 0.54 mg/L to 1.21 mg/L, which is slightly lower than creatinine levels in healthy patients. Thyroid disorders and the use of dexamethasone have been associated with increases in the level of cystatin C. These factors limit the ability of this protein to estimate the GFR.

Several small studies have shown that the correlation between cystatin C and 1/cystatin C is more useful than creatinine and 1/creatinine alone in estimating the GFR (2). However, the cystatin C level is used only sporadically in the clinical setting to estimate the GFR. Whether it will replace the creatinine level or creatinine clearance in the evaluation of kidney function is unknown.

Radionuclide Scanning

Imaging studies used to estimate the GFR include ^{125}I-iothalamate, iohexol, or technetium-99m diethylenetetraminepentaacetic acid (DTPA) radionuclide scanning. In a subgroup of the MDRD study cohort, the same patient underwent GFR estimation on two separate occasions,

once using inulin clearance and once using ^{125}I-iothalamate radionuclide scanning (3). The estimated GFR using these two methods was nearly identical. Therefore, because of the limitations associated with using the inulin clearance, ^{125}I-iothalamate radionuclide scanning is the gold standard for estimation of the GFR. However, radionuclide scanning is associated with several limitations in evaluating kidney function that prevent its widespread use for this purpose.

KEY POINTS

- The glomerular filtration rate in healthy patients ranges from 120 to 130 mL/min per 1.73 m^2 for men and 100 to 110 mL/min per 1.73 m^2 for women.
- Guidelines recommend using the creatinine clearance instead of the creatinine level alone to estimate the glomerular filtration rate.
- Mathematical equations to estimate creatinine clearance generally are preferred over 24-hour urine collections.
- Timed urine collection or radionuclide scanning is recommended to estimate the glomerular filtration rate in healthy patients.
- The normal blood urea nitrogen–creatinine ratio is 10 to 15:1.
- High-protein diets, catabolic states, gastrointestinal bleeding, liver failure, and malnutrition affect the blood urea nitrogen level and limit its use in the evaluation of kidney function.
- In healthy patients, levels of cystatin C range from 0.54 mg/L to 1.21 mg/L.
- Thyroid disorders and dexamethasone use may limit the usefulness of cystatin C in estimating the glomerular filtration rate.
- ^{125}I-iothalamate radionuclide scanning is the gold standard for estimation of the glomerular filtration rate in clinical settings.

Interpretation of the Urinalysis

The urinalysis is invaluable in the assessment of kidney function. This study involves interpretation of the dipstick urinalysis and analysis of the microscopic urine sediment. Microscopic assessment is an important and inexpensive study required to identify and quantify the presence of leukocytes, erythrocytes, renal tubular casts, and crystals in the urine as an initial step in the evaluation of kidney function.

Pyuria

Pyuria is characterized by an increase in the leukocytes in the urine >5 leukocytes/hpf. Genitourinary tract infections primarily cause this condition, especially when urinalysis reveals bacteria.

Sterile pyuria is characterized by leukocytes in the urine without associated bacterial infections. Inflammatory disorders of the kidney, such as acute interstitial nephritis due to antibiotic or nonsteroidal anti-inflammatory drug use, often are associated with sterile pyuria, as well as eosinophiluria revealed on Wright's or Hansel's stain. However, eosinophiluria is relatively nonspecific and may be present in other conditions associated with kidney inflammation, including atheroembolic disease, postinfectious glomerulonephritis, rapidly progressive glomerulonephritis, and pyelonephritis. Less common causes of sterile pyuria include chronic tubulointerstitial disorders, such as hypertensive nephrosclerosis and analgesic nephropathy; *Mycobacterium* or viral infections of the genitourinary tract; kidney transplant rejection; and genitourinary tract malignancies.

Asymptomatic Hematuria and Recurrent Gross Hematuria

The presence of hematuria and/or proteinuria on dipstick urinalysis is commonly associated with abnormalities in kidney function. Hematuria is defined as the presence of >3 erythrocytes/hpf on a centrifuged urine sediment sample on more that two occasions. Hematuria is a common finding that occurs in 1% to 3% of all patients and may affect up to 10% of men.

Dipstick urinalysis is very sensitive for detecting small amounts of blood in the urine, generally as low as 1 to 3 erythrocytes/hpf. In rhabdomyolysis, myoglobin classically causes a false-positive result for blood on the dipstick urinalysis, but no intact erythrocytes are visible in the urine sediment. Similarly, other substances, including the pigment in beets and phenazopyridine, rifampin, and chloroquine, may cause a false-positive result for blood on dipstick urinalysis without associated erythrocytes visible on urine microscopy. Hematuria may be either isolated or persistent on repeat urinalyses. Isolated hematuria is typically benign and most likely secondary to infections, trauma, exercise, or menstruation.

One of the most important initial steps in the evaluation of microscopic hematuria is microscopic analysis of the urine sediment to assess erythrocyte morphology, which distinguishes between glomerular and nonglomerular hematuria of the urinary tract. Monomorphic or intact erythrocytes characterize nonglomerular hematuria, and helical CT scanning of the urinary tract without intravenous contrast is used to diagnose this condition.

If an abnormality is discovered, referral for appropriate therapy is recommended. If no abnormality is revealed, three morning urine samples should be evaluated for malignancy. In patients <50 years of age without significant risk factors for bladder malignancy (such as cigarette smoking, analgesic abuse, benzene exposure, or a history of voiding abnormalities), no further evaluation is required. Cystoscopy is indicated for patients with risk factors for malignancy.

TABLE 1 Different Measurements of Proteinuria
Microalbuminuria
30–300 mg of albumin/24 h
20–200 ug/min of creatinine
30–300 ug/mg of creatinine
Albuminuria
24-Hour collection
<30 mg/24 h
<20 ug/g creatinine/min
Spot albumin–creatinine ratio
<30 mg/g of creatinine
Proteinuria
24-Hour collection
<150 mg/24 h
Spot protein–creatinine ratio
<200 mg/g of creatinine

A separate clinical evaluation is indicated for microscopic hematuria due to glomerular disorders. Glomerular bleeding is associated with dysmorphic erythrocytes on urinalysis. These cells, particularly acanthocytes, are nicknamed "Mickey Mouse cells" because of the presence of multiple bullae and are a consequence of physical damage to the erythrocytes as they traverse the nephron. Coexistent proteinuria and hematuria and the presence of casts (particularly erythrocyte casts) confirm a diagnosis of glomerulonephritis.

The most common causes of asymptomatic glomerular hematuria without evidence of proteinuria or glomerular abnormality are thin basement membrane disease and IgA nephropathy. These conditions exemplify the structural basis of hematuria. The thinning of the basement membrane most likely allows erythrocytes to escape into the urine. In IgA nephropathy, the proliferation of mesangial cells disturbs the glomerular capillary wall as it faces the mesangium (the site of the perimesangial basement membrane). This disturbance results in hematuria. Glomerular disorders are discussed in the Glomerular Diseases section.

Proteinuria

The identification and quantification of proteinuria is important in the evaluation of kidney function, because a higher amount of proteinuria is considered an adverse risk factor for the progression of chronic kidney disease. Urinary proteins are comprised of high-molecular-weight albumin, low-molecular-weight immunoglobulins, and Tamm–Horsfall proteins that the renal tubular cells secrete.

Various measurements can be used to identify proteinuria (**Table 1**). Dipstick urinalysis detects only albumin and does not reveal conditions such as multiple myeloma. However, adding sulfosalicylic acid to the urine precipitates all proteins, including urinary light chains or Bence–Jones proteins. Moreover, dipstick urinalysis is relatively insensitive for albuminuria, requiring >30 mg/dL (300 mg/24 h) of urinary albumin for detection.

Conditions such as early diabetic nephropathy or hypertensive nephrosclerosis may be associated with microalbuminuria, which is a more sensitive and earlier marker for kidney disease. In the National Health and Nutrition Examination Survey, 10.6% of patients had microalbuminuria and 1.1% had albuminuria on a single urine sample. Almost two thirds of these patients had repeat protein abnormalities on subsequent studies, which suggests underlying chronic kidney disease.

When evaluating proteinuria using dipstick urinalysis, quantification using a random protein–creatinine ratio is recommended instead of a 24-hour urine collection. For example, a urine protein–creatinine ratio of 3.5 mg/g correlates to a 24-hour urine total protein of 3.5 g.

The amount of protein excreted in the urine may help determine the underlying kidney disorder. A total of 1% to 3% of adolescents and young adults may have orthostatic proteinuria, a benign condition characterized by increased proteinuria during the day with normal nocturnal protein excretion. In affected patients, a split 12-hour urine collection during the day and an enforced 12-hour collection in the recumbent position at night reveals that all of the proteinuria occurs during the time of physical activity and that proteinuria is virtually absent during recumbency. The cause of this physiologic event remains uncertain, but 40 to 50 years of follow-up in patients with orthostatic proteinuria reveals no evidence of kidney dysfunction (4).

Transient proteinuria develops in hospitalized patients with febrile illnesses or major traumatic stresses. Urinary protein levels in this setting typically decrease as the underlying disease remits.

Isolated proteinuria in the absence of an orthostatic relationship is defined as fixed or persistent proteinuria. Some patients who have urinary protein levels <500 mg/24 h may show no evidence of kidney dysfunction for decades. However, some affected patients progress to more worrisome proteinuria; the conditions that affect these patients are described in the Glomerular Diseases section.

The nephrotic syndrome is characterized by a urinary protein level >3.5 g/24 h and develops in diabetic nephropathy, focal segmental glomerulosclerosis, membranous glomerulopathy, amyloidosis, and minimal change disease. Proteinuria of <1 g/24 h to 2 g/24 h associated with chronic kidney disease and a urine sediment that is bland (lacks formed elements on microscopic examination) characterizes tubulointerstitial disorders, such as hypertensive nephrosclerosis and analgesic nephropathy.

KEY POINTS

- The presence of hematuria and/or proteinuria on dipstick urinalysis is commonly associated with abnormalities in kidney function.
- Analysis of three morning urine samples is indicated for patients with persistent hematuria with no abnormalities revealed on microscopic analysis of the urine sediment.
- Risk factors for bladder malignancy include cigarette smoking, analgesic abuse, benzene exposure, and a history of voiding abnormalities.
- Coexistent proteinuria and hematuria and the presence of erythrocyte casts confirm a diagnosis of glomerulonephritis.
- Thin basement membrane disease and IgA nephropathy most commonly cause asymptomatic glomerular hematuria without evidence of proteinuria or glomerular abnormality.
- Microalbuminuria is a sensitive and early marker for kidney disease.
- Orthostatic proteinuria usually is not associated with kidney dysfunction.
- Proteinuria of <1 g/24 h to 2 g/24 h associated with chronic kidney disease and a bland urine sediment characterizes tubulointerstitial disorders.

Imaging Studies

Imaging studies of the genitourinary tract reveal vital data in the clinical evaluation of kidney function. Radionuclide scanning is used to estimate the GFR as well as determine the anatomic structures of the genitourinary tract and assess for urinary tract obstruction.

Cystic lesions in the kidney are one of the most common abnormalities revealed on imaging studies and increase with age. Overwhelmingly, they are considered simple and generally do not require further evaluation. Complex cysts or mass lesions may be associated with malignancy; evaluation of these conditions should include ultrasonography, CT, or MRI.

Ultrasonography often is used to differentiate between simple and complex lesions and to determine changes in cyst characteristics in serial follow-up examinations. Abdominal CT scanning with contrast differentiates neoplastic lesions from benign cystic structures in the kidney but is contraindicated in patients at risk for contrast-associated acute renal failure; abdominal MRI is the procedure of choice in these patients.

Referral for nephrectomy generally is indicated for complex cystic or mass lesions in the kidney that raise suspicion for malignancy. Factors that suggest possible malignancy include enhancement after contrast administration, a diameter >3 cm, areas of necrosis, or marginal irregularities. Kidney biopsy of cystic or mass lesions is contraindicated, because malignant tumors may metastasize via the biopsy tract to other areas in the abdomen.

KEY POINTS

- Simple cystic lesions in the kidney generally do not require further evaluation.
- Complex cysts or mass lesions in the kidney may be associated with a risk for malignancy.
- Ultrasonography differentiates between simple and complex renal lesions and determines changes in renal cyst characteristics in serial follow-up examinations.
- Abdominal CT scanning with contrast differentiates neoplastic lesions from benign cystic structures in the kidney.
- In patients at risk for contrast-associated acute renal failure, abdominal MRI should be performed instead of abdominal CT scanning with contrast.
- Referral for nephrectomy generally is indicated for complex cystic or mass lesions in the kidney that raise suspicion for malignancy.
- Kidney biopsy of cystic or mass lesions is contraindicated, because malignant tumors may metastasize via the biopsy tract to other areas in the abdomen.

Kidney Biopsy

Clinical judgment alone may not sufficiently help to differentiate the pattern of glomerular injury. In this setting, kidney biopsy frequently is needed to determine the diagnosis, indicate the cause, predict the natural history and prognosis of the injury, and direct treatment.

Kidney biopsy is indicated for patients with kidney disease when less-invasive diagnostic studies cannot determine the cause of the condition and clinical signs and symptoms suggest that a pathologic evaluation may be diagnostic (for example, in patients with concomitant hematuria and proteinuria). Kidney biopsies are commonly performed as diagnostic studies in adults with the nephrotic syndrome or glomerulonephritis with no obvious postinfectious glomerular disease, children with corticosteroid-resistant nephrotic syndrome, and all patients with acute renal failure of unclear cause.

Kidney biopsies also provide information about the severity and potential reversibility of glomerular damage. For example, patients with lupus nephritis or antineutrophil cytoplasmic antibody–associated glomerulonephritis typically require immunomodulating drugs associated with substantial risk, including infections, leukopenia, hemorrhagic cystitis, secondary malignancies, and death. A finding of widespread

glomerular and tubular interstitial scarring suggests little possibility of reversing the glomerular damage; therefore, the risks of treatment may outweigh the benefits. Similarly, kidney biopsy may reveal a much less or more aggressive glomerular injury than clinical judgment alone could have predicted.

Contraindications to percutaneous kidney biopsy include a solitary kidney, an uncooperative patient, hemorrhagic tendencies, uncontrolled severe hypertension, cystic kidneys, hydronephrosis, or multiple renal artery aneurysms. Multiple masses within the kidney, including cysts, abscesses, or kidney neoplasms, are additional contraindications.

In patients with contraindications to percutaneous kidney biopsy, an open-wedge kidney biopsy is advocated as a safer procedure when a diagnosis is imperative. Complications of kidney biopsy using real-time ultrasonography or CT guidance are infrequent. After the biopsy, many patients develop small, typically minimally consequential perirenal hematomas revealed on ultrasonography. Gross hematuria develops in <10% of patients, and arteriovenous fistulas occur in <1%. Less than 1% of patients develop hemorrhage requiring intervention with interventional radiology or surgery, and death occurs in <0.1%.

Kidney biopsy typically is performed with real-time ultrasonography or CT-guided localization of the kidney using a spring-loaded, disposable "gun" device. The biopsied tissue is processed for light, immunofluorescence, and electron microscopy in order to fully evaluate the nature of the glomerular and tubulointerstitial injury.

KEY POINTS

- Kidney biopsy is indicated for patients with kidney disease when less-invasive diagnostic studies are inconclusive and clinical signs and symptoms suggest that a pathologic evaluation may be diagnostic.
- Kidney biopsy helps to determine the severity and potential reversibility of glomerular damage.
- Contraindications to percutaneous kidney biopsy include a solitary kidney, an uncooperative patient, hemorrhagic tendencies, uncontrolled severe hypertension, cystic kidneys, hydronephrosis, or multiple renal artery aneurysms.
- Kidney biopsy typically is performed with real-time ultrasonography or CT-guided localization of the kidney.

References

1. **Poggio ED, Wang X, Greene T, Van Lente F, Hall PM.** Performance of the modification of diet in renal disease and Cockcroft-Gault equations in the estimation of GFR in health and in chronic kidney disease. J Am Soc Nephrol. 2005;16:459-66. [PMID: 15615823]
2. **Rule AD, Bergstralh EJ, Slezak JM, Bergert J, Larson TS.** Glomerular filtration rate estimated by cystatin C among different clinical presentations. Kidney Int. 2006;69:399-405. [PMID: 16408133]

3. **Klahr S, Levey AS, Beck GJ, Caggiula AW, Hunsicker L, Kusek JW, et al.** The effects of dietary protein restriction and blood-pressure control on the progression of chronic renal disease. Modification of Diet in Renal Disease Study Group. N Engl J Med. 1994;330:877-84. [PMID: 8114857]

4. **Rytand DA, Spreiter S.** Prognosis in postural (orthostatic) proteinuria: forty to fifty-year follow-up of six patients after diagnosis by Thomas Addis. N Engl J Med. 1981;305:618-21. [PMID: 7266586]

FLUID AND ELECTROLYTES

RECENT ADVANCE

- Exercise-induced hyponatremia and marathon runners

Sodium is mainly confined to the extracellular space, and sodium intake and excretion determine the extracellular fluid volume. The renin–angiotensin–aldosterone system and atrial natriuretic peptide regulate volume status and influence sodium excretion without affecting the serum sodium concentration.

The serum sodium concentration generally reflects the extracellular fluid tonicity. Changes in the sodium concentration usually reflect disturbances in water balance, not gain or loss of sodium. Arginine vasopressin regulates water balance. The result of the arginine vasopressin system is to maintain a constant plasma osmolality through osmoreceptors in the brain that affect vasopressin excretion, which affects urinary concentration via aquaporin in the collecting tubules of the kidneys.

The renin–angiotensin–aldosterone system and the arginine vasopressin system act independently except in volume depletion, in which sodium (through renin–angiotensin–aldosterone) and water (through arginine vasopressin) conservation are simultaneously activated to maintain plasma volume and tissue perfusion. When plasma volume is severely compromised, the conservation of constant plasma osmolality is overridden by conservation of sodium.

To maintain water balance, the thirst mechanism must be intact, and the kidneys must be able to vary urinary concentration. Arginine vasopressin is the most important hormone involved in water balance. When arginine vasopressin activity is absent (as in diabetes insipidus), urinary concentration is very low (50–80 mosm/kg H_2O). Conversely, when arginine vasopressin activity is maximal, urinary concentration may increase to 1200 mosm/kg H_2O. Plasma osmolality generally remains within a narrow range because of the wide range of urine concentrations and the powerful stimulus of the thirst mechanism.

In hyponatremia and hypernatremia, calculating electrolyte-free water intake and output is helpful if accurate intake and output data can be obtained and the sodium and potassium concentrations of the fluid can be measured (1).

Calculation of electrolyte-free water helps to assess water need and water balance. The amount of electrolyte-free water in a body fluid (such as urine, sweat, or nasogastric aspirate) is calculated by the following formula:

$$[1 - (\text{Fluid } [Na^+] + \text{Fluid } [K^+])/(\text{Plasma } [Na^+] + \text{Plasma } [K^+])] \times \text{Volume of Fluid (mL)}$$

The resulting value represents the volume of fluid required to dilute the electrolytes in the fluid to the same tonicity as the electrolytes in the serum. The remainder of the fluid contains the nonelectrolyte osmoles.

If the urine sodium plus potassium value is equal to the serum sodium plus potassium value, urine output will not affect the serum sodium because the urine and serum electrolytes are isotonic. However, if the urine sodium plus potassium value is less than their combined serum value, the excreted electrolyte-free water as calculated above is a positive value. If this water is not replaced, a water deficit and thus hypernatremia will develop. Conversely, if the urine sodium plus potassium value is greater than the serum value, the calculated urinary electrolyte-free water is a negative value. If this water is not excreted (or electrolytes replaced), hyponatremia develops.

KEY POINTS

- **The serum sodium concentration generally reflects the extracellular fluid tonicity.**
- **Changes in the sodium concentration usually reflect disturbances in water balance, not gain or loss of sodium.**
- **Water balance determines the serum sodium concentration, and arginine vasopressin regulates water balance.**
- **To maintain water balance, the thirst mechanism must be intact, and the kidneys must be able to vary urinary concentration.**

Hyponatremia

Pathogenesis

Hyponatremia is characterized by a serum sodium concentration <135 meq/L. The kidneys' ability to dilute the urine and thus excrete free water is the primary defense against the development of hyponatremia. Excess ingestion of water is rarely the sole cause of hyponatremia, because a typical adult with normal renal function can excrete a massive free water load (15 L/d) without diluting the serum. Free water intake in the setting of an underlying condition that impairs free water excretion is needed for hyponatremia to develop (**Table 2**) (See also Reference 1).

Diagnosis

In patients with hyponatremia, exclusion of hyperosmolar hyponatremia is initially indicated (**Figure 1**). The presence of an osmotically active substance that is confined to the extracellular fluid (usually glucose or mannitol) osmotically

TABLE 2 States of Impaired Water Excretion

Appropriate ADH Release
Normovolemic states of ADH excess
Postoperative state
Pain
Nausea
States of effective circulating volume depletion
CHF
Cirrhosis
Diuretics
Inappropriate ADH Release
SIADH
Cortisol deficiency
Hypothyroidism

ADH = antidiuretic hormone; CHF = congestive heart failure; SIADH = syndrome of inappropriate antidiuretic hormone secretion.

removes water from the intracellular space and dilutes the serum sodium concentration. To assess for a dysnatremia in this setting, add 1.6 meq/L for every 100 mg/dL increment of serum glucose above 100 mg/dL to correct the serum sodium.

High glucose levels in hyperglycemia may mask dangerous hypernatremia. For example, the serum sodium in a patient with a serum glucose level of 550 mg/dL and a serum sodium concentration of 128 meq/L can be corrected as follows:

$$(550 \text{ mg/dL} - 100 \text{ mg/dL})/(100 \text{ mg/dL}) \times 1.6 \text{ meq/L}$$
$$= 4.5 \times 1.6 \text{ meq/L} = 7.2 \text{ meq/L}$$

Therefore, the corrected serum sodium in this patient is 135 meq/L.

Pseudohyponatremia also must be excluded. Hyperproteinemia and hyperlipidemia may cause spuriously low serum sodium concentrations if the samples are diluted before measurement, unless a potentiometric method of measurement is used.

Clinical Manifestations

As plasma tonicity decreases, symptoms occur because of osmotic swelling of the brain. Manifestations of this condition are varied. Patients may be asymptomatic, as occurs in chronic heart failure or cirrhosis. Early signs of symptomatic hypoosmolality may be very nonspecific, such as nausea, vomiting, and headaches (hyponatremic encephalopathy). Worsening of brain swelling then causes decreased mental status and seizures. If this condition is not resolved, coma, respiratory arrest, and death may result (2).

Diuretic- and exercise-induced hyponatremia may cause atypical manifestations of hyponatremia. Diuretic-induced hyponatremia most commonly occurs in patients taking thi-

azide diuretics. Elderly women with low body mass indices who tend to increase fluid intake after initiation of therapy with these agents are often affected. Because fluid intake is increased and water excretion is impaired secondary to thiazide diuretics, these patients are susceptible to developing symptomatic hyponatremia (3). Therefore, it is important to weigh patients before initiating diuretic therapy and 48 hours later. If a patient's weight is still the same or has increased, electrolyte levels should be measured. Common manifestations of this condition in the elderly include confusion and falls.

Recently, exercise-induced hyponatremia has been recognized as a common complication that affects 15% to 20% of marathon participants. Hyponatremia is secondary to increased fluid consumption of hypotonic fluids in the presence of nonosmotic release of arginine vasopressin, which is common in marathon runners and may further impair renal water excretion. The clinical manifestations include noncardiogenic pulmonary edema due to increased intracranial pressure secondary to cerebral edema. Nausea, vomiting, seizures, and respiratory arrest may occur if this condition is not treated aggressively (4).

Most cases of symptomatic hyponatremia occur in the postoperative setting, during diuretic therapy, during oxytocin treatment, and in compulsive water drinking.

Risk Factors for Hyponatremic Encephalopathy

Menstruant women, children, and patients with hypoxia are at high risk for hyponatremia, have higher risk for poor outcomes compared with the general population, and require prompt medical attention (5, 6). Menstruant women are more susceptible to the development of symptomatic hyponatremia because they have differences in osmoregulation compared with the general population. Children have higher brain size to cranial vault size ratios compared with adults and therefore become symptomatic more quickly and cannot tolerate as much cerebral edema. Hypoxia impairs the body's adaptive responses to hyponatremia and leads to worse neurologic outcomes; this condition should be corrected early in the disease course to maximize the likelihood of a good neurologic outcome.

Prevention

Hospitalized patients have numerous stimuli for arginine vasopressin production. Therefore, these patients should be considered at risk for developing hyponatremia. The most common factor resulting in hospital-acquired hyponatremia is the administration of hypotonic intravenous fluids to patients with a compromised ability to maintain water balance. In high-risk patients (such as postoperative patients who usually have increased vasopressin levels secondary to pain, nausea, and narcotics), preventive measures should include use of isotonic saline rather than hypotonic fluids. The postoperative state of impaired water excretion, during which the use of

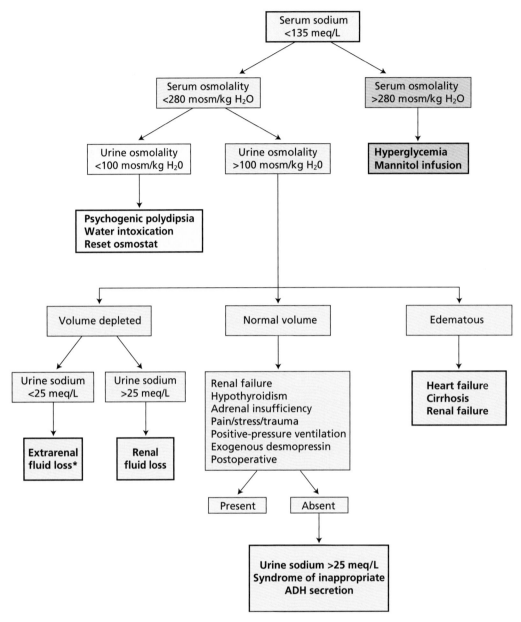

FIGURE 1.
Diagnostic approach to hyponatremia.

ADH = antidiuretic hormone

*For example, gastrointestinal.

hypotonic fluids may cause severe iatrogenic hyponatremia, merits immediate therapy with hypertonic saline.

Maintenance of water balance may also be compromised in patients with effective circulating volume depletion (cirrhosis and heart failure), gastrointestinal fluid losses, renal failure (acute and chronic), inappropriate antidiuretic hormone secretion, cortisol deficiency, and hypothyroidism and in those who use diuretics (especially thiazides) (7).

Treatment

Early treatment of symptomatic hyponatremia is indicated to prevent severe neurologic sequelae. Rapid treatment with infusion of hypertonic saline with or without a loop diuretic (to prevent volume overload) is indicated when symptoms of hyponatremic encephalopathy are present (**Figure 2**). This treatment must occur in an intensive care unit setting with close monitoring and follow-up.

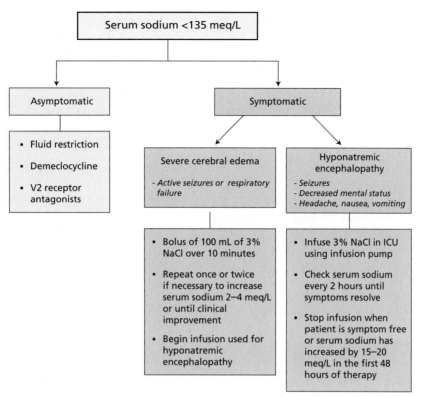

FIGURE 2.
Treatment of hyponatremia.
High-risk groups for poor outcome: Young women and children.

ICU = intensive care unit; V2 = type 2 vasopressin

Aggressive therapy with hypertonic saline should be initiated in all patients with hyponatremic encephalopathy, regardless of the underlying cause of the disorder. This therapy is appropriate only for symptomatic patients (Figure 2) (see also Reference 1) (8). Mortality is high in symptomatic patients who have concomitant hypoxia or who receive delayed treatment.

KEY POINTS

- Hyponatremia is characterized by a serum sodium concentration <135 meq/L.
- In patients with hyponatremia, exclusion of hyperosmolar hyponatremia is initially indicated.
- High glucose levels in hyperglycemia may mask hypernatremia.
- As plasma tonicity decreases, osmotic swelling of the brain causes symptoms.
- Diuretic- and exercise-induced hyponatremia may cause atypical manifestations of hyponatremia.
- Hospitalized patients have numerous stimuli for arginine vasopressin production.
- Aggressive hypertonic saline therapy should be initiated in all symptomatic patients with hyponatremic encephalopathy, regardless of the underlying cause of the disorder.

Hypernatremia

Hypernatremia is characterized by a serum sodium concentration >145 meq/L. Because thirst is a potent stimulus and a powerful protective mechanism, restricted access to water is nearly always necessary for this condition to develop. If the thirst mechanism is intact and water is accessible, the development of hypernatremia is rare regardless of other factors. Hypernatremia may occur in various clinical settings, including debilitation by an acute or chronic condition; neurologic impairment, such as dementia; a moribund state; and use of mechanical ventilation.

Hypernatremia commonly occurs in the intensive care unit, mostly in patients who are intubated or have altered mental status and therefore have restricted access to fluids. Additional factors in this setting that may contribute to hypernatremia include significant renal water losses caused by solute diuresis (mainly urea) in patients on high-protein feeds or in a hypercatabolic state, excess hypertonic sodium bicarbonate administration, renal concentrating defects, and gastrointestinal fluid losses (especially associated with nasogastric suction and lactulose administration). Many patients with hypernatremia have a combination of impaired water access and significant ongoing free water losses (**Table 3**) (see also Reference 1). The defenses against the development of hypernatremia are the thirst mechanism and urinary concentrating ability to minimize water losses in the urine.

TABLE 3 Common Causes of Hypernatremia
Solute diuresis secondary to tube feedings or hyperalimentation
Nasogastric suction
Nonketotic hyperosmolar coma
Diabetes insipidus
Impaired water intake (usually occurs in dementia)

TABLE 4 Treatment of Hypernatremia
Replete intravascular volume with colloid solution, isotonic saline, or plasma.
Estimate water deficit. Replace deficit over 48–72 hours, aiming for a correction of 1 mosm/L/h. In severe hypernatremia (>170 meq/L), serum sodium should not be corrected to <150 meq/L in the first 48–72 hours. Replacement of ongoing water losses are given in addition to the deficit.
Hypotonic fluid should be used. Usual replacement fluid is 77 meq/L (0.5% normal saline). Glucose-containing solutions should be avoided, and an oral route of administration should be used.
Monitor plasma electrolytes every 2 hours until the patient is neurologically stable.

Central Diabetes Insipidus

Early identification of central diabetes insipidus (CDI) is important, because specific therapy is indicated. Insufficient arginine vasopressin secretion causes this condition, which presents as polyuria secondary to water diuresis. Severe hypernatremia may rapidly develop in a patient with restricted fluid access.

Common causes of CDI include head injury, brain neoplasm, pituitary surgery, central nervous system infection, and cerebral hemorrhage and/or infarct. Patients with CDI conserve sodium appropriately and therefore typically do not develop clinical volume depletion. CDI should be suspected if urine is not maximally concentrated in the presence of hypernatremia. However, urinary concentration may be difficult to interpret, because significant polyuria and subclinical renal disease may impair urinary concentrating ability independent of arginine vasopressin action.

In CDI, the plasma osmolality typically exceeds the urine osmolality. Administration of the type 2 vasopressin (V2) receptor agonist desmopressin (dDAVP) helps to differentiate CDI from nephrogenic diabetes insipidus; a 50% increase in urine osmolality after dDAVP administration strongly suggests CDI. Subcutaneous or intranasal dDAVP is the preferred treatment for this condition. Water intake should be adjusted appropriately to avoid precipitating significant hyponatremia.

Diagnosis

To discover the underlying disorders in a patient with hypernatremia, investigation into water intake and water losses is indicated. A precise history focusing on fluid intake is needed to determine if the patient has impaired access to fluids or an abnormal thirst mechanism or is not receiving sufficient free water in enteral or parenteral form.

Water losses in the urine and from the gastrointestinal tract (diarrhea and nasogastric suction) and insensible losses (fever, sepsis, massive diaphoresis, burns) should be calculated or estimated, if accurate measurements are unavailable. Measurement of the urine osmolality and electrolyte levels is indicated to assess urinary concentrating ability and to calculate the free water losses in the urine. Free water loss in the urine is calculated using the following formula:

$$(1 - \text{Urine } [Na^+] + \text{Urine } [K^+]/\text{Plasma } [Na^+] + \text{Plasma } [K^+]) \times \text{Urinary Output (expressed as an hourly rate)}$$

Failure to significantly increase urine osmolality in patients with hypernatremia may indicate a renal concentrating defect. However, other causes of a renal concentrating defect, such as loop diuretic use, renal failure, and preceding polyuria, should be excluded before suspicion for nephrogenic diabetes insipidus is raised.

Clinical Manifestations

Because cell membranes are permeable to water, hypernatremia causes an efflux of fluid from the intracellular space to the extracellular space in order to maintain osmotic equilibrium across the cell membranes. Cerebral dehydration with cell shrinkage ensues.

Central nervous system depression causes the primary clinical manifestations of this condition. Affected patients develop decreased mental status, confusion, abnormal speech, and obtundation with stupor or coma in severe cases. Rhabdomyolysis also may complicate severe hypernatremia.

Mortality

The mortality rate of patients with hypernatremia ranges between 40% and 70%. Patients with end-stage liver disease are at high risk for complications from hypernatremia such as cerebral demyelination and have a high morbidity and mortality. In particular, patients with hepatic encephalopathy frequently have hypernatremia from osmotic diarrhea due to oral administration of lactulose.

Treatment

Treatment of hypernatremia is directed at maintaining a normal circulatory volume while correcting the serum sodium with free water replacement (**Table 4**). First, the current free water deficit should be assessed using the following formula:

$$\text{Plasma } [Na^+] - 140/140 \times \text{Total Body Water (L)}$$

Where: Total body water = 0.5 × weight (kg) in women or 0.6 × weight (kg) in men.

This value represents the amount of water of replacement needed to obtain a serum sodium concentration of 140 meq/L. Any ongoing losses should not be addressed at this point but are accounted for in the replacement fluids to achieve the goals of correction.

In patients with volume depletion, fluid resuscitation with normal saline or colloid should precede correction of the water deficit. Oral hydration is preferable to parenteral hydration and is indicated when possible. Serial measurement of electrolytes, every 2 hours, is recommended until the patient is neurologically stable.

In the absence of hypernatremic encephalopathy, the serum sodium should not be corrected more quickly than 1 meq/h or 15 meq/24 h. In severe cases (serum sodium >170 meq/L), sodium should not be corrected to <150 meq/L in the first 48 to 72 hours. Patients with documented acute hypernatremia can be corrected more quickly (see also Reference 1).

KEY POINTS

- Hypernatremia is characterized by a serum sodium concentration >145 meq/L.
- Restricted access to water is nearly always necessary for the development of hypernatremia.
- Insufficient arginine vasopressin secretion causes central diabetes insipidus, which presents as polyuria secondary to water diuresis.
- Subcutaneous or intranasal desmopressin is the preferred treatment for central diabetes insipidus.
- Investigation into water intake and water losses helps to discover the underlying disorders in hypernatremia.
- Hypernatremia causes cerebral dehydration with cell shrinkage.
- Patients with liver disease are at high risk for cerebral demyelination when hypernatremia develops.
- The goal of hypernatremia treatment is maintaining a normal circulatory volume while correcting the serum sodium with free water replacement.
- In the absence of hypernatremic encephalopathy, the serum sodium typically should not be corrected more quickly than 1 meq/h or 15 meq/24 h.

Potassium Homeostasis

The kidneys have the principal role in regulating potassium balance. In the steady state, urinary potassium excretion varies with changes in dietary or parenteral intake (typically 120 meq/24 h to 140 meq/24 h). Under normal circumstances, trivial amounts of potassium are excreted through the sweat and gastrointestinal tract (<15 meq/24 h). Ninety percent of the filtered load of potassium is reabsorbed in the proximal tubule and loop of Henle, and 10% is delivered to the distal tubule.

The physiologic regulation of urinary potassium excretion occurs through reabsorption and secretion in the distal tubule and collecting duct. The main determinants of potassium

excretion are distal delivery of fluid to these segments of the nephron and the action of aldosterone.

Maintenance of potassium balance is possible in patients with volume depletion or volume excess, despite changes in sodium excretion. In states of volume excess, distal delivery of solute is increased, aldosterone (and thus potassium secretion) is suppressed, and overall potassium excretion is not changed. Conversely, in states of volume depletion, delivery of fluid to the distal tubule is decreased, but aldosterone action and potassium secretion are increased; therefore, potassium excretion is unchanged in this setting, as well.

The effect of aldosterone can be estimated by calculating the transtubular potassium concentration gradient (TTKG) using the following formula:

$$\text{Urinary } [K^+] \times \text{Plasma Osmolality/Plasma } [K^+] \times \text{Urinary Osmolality}$$

The TTKG typically is 8 to 9. A TTKG <7 in a patient with hyperkalemia suggests a decreased effect of aldosterone. A TTKG >7 suggests adequate mineralocorticoid activity, whereas a TTKG <4 suggests deficient mineralocorticoid activity.

Potassium is located primarily in the intracellular compartment. Therefore, alterations of serum potassium concentrations may be caused by shifting of potassium from one compartment to another or absolute excesses or deficiencies of total body potassium. Serum potassium values alone cannot be used to assess total body potassium.

A disassociation of total potassium stores and serum potassium levels commonly occurs in diabetic ketoacidosis. Patients with this condition typically have decreased food intake and frequently are vomiting, which decreases potassium intake. Hyperglycemia simultaneously causes copious urine output, and potassium is continually lost in the urine. Therefore, total body potassium is decreased. However, serum potassium levels are typically elevated in diabetic ketoacidosis. In this setting, metabolic acidosis, insulin deficiency, and hyperglycemia cause shifting of potassium from the intracellular compartment to the extracellular fluid, which masks the total body potassium deficit.

Hypokalemia is very common in patients with HIV and is caused by chronic diarrhea (often from opportunistic infections), nausea, and vomiting; low enteral intake may worsen these conditions. Hyperkalemia also commonly occurs in the setting of HIV nephropathy and renal failure, as a side effect of trimethoprim or pentamidine therapy (which reduces potassium secretion), or with adrenal insufficiency, which commonly occurs in HIV (9).

Hyperkalemia
Pathophysiology
Hyperkalemia occurs as a result of shifts in potassium from the intracellular compartment to the extracellular fluid or through total body potassium excess (**Table 5**). In clinical practice, total body potassium excess always suggests a deficiency in

TABLE 5 Causes of Hyperkalemia

Assess for Increased Potassium Intake

Low-sodium salt substitutes and potassium supplements

Assess for Shift of Potassium from Intracellular Fluid to Extracellular Fluid

Metabolic acidosis

Tissue necrosis (rhabdomyolysis, bowel infarction, tumor lysis) or depolarization

Insulin deficiency

β_2-Blockade

Assess for Reduced Potassium Excretion in Urine

Renal failure

Low aldosterone action (drugs, particularly heparin, cyclosporine, tacrolimus, ARBs, ACEIs)

Decreased distal nephron flow rate

ARBs = angiotensin receptor blockers; ACEIs = angiotensin-converting enzyme inhibitors

TABLE 6 Medications That Cause Hyperkalemia

Drugs That Interfere with Potassium Excretion

Interfere with renin–angiotensin–aldosterone axis:

ACEIs, ARBs, aldosterone blockers, heparin (decrease aldosterone synthesis), β-blockers (decrease renin release), NSAIDs, COX-2 inhibitors

Interfere with tubular potassium handling:

Potassium-sparing diuretics (amiloride, triamterene), trimethoprim, calcineurin inhibitors (cyclosporine, tacrolimus), pentamidine

Drugs That Shift Potassium from Intracellular to Extracellular Fluid

β_2-Blockers, depolarizing paralytics (such as succinylcholine), digitalis

ACEIs = angiotensin-converting enzyme inhibitors; ARBs = angiotensin receptor blockers; NSAIDs = nonsteroidal anti-inflammatory drugs; COX-2 = cyclooxygenase-2

TABLE 7 Risk Factors for Hyperkalemia

ESRD

Postsurgery* status

Post–cardiac catheterization status

Post–IV-contrasted radiographic study status

Administration of nephrotoxic antibiotics[†]

Adrenal insufficiency

Type 4 RTA[‡]

Crush injury

Tissue trauma in surgery

Diabetes

Massive blood transfusion

ESRD = end-stage renal disease; RTA = renal tubular acidosis

* Especially after cardiac or vascular surgery.

[†] Particularly aminoglycosides.

[‡] Usually presents in diabetes mellitus.

renal potassium excretion, as the kidneys are primarily responsible for maintaining potassium excretion and can significantly increase potassium excretion. Therefore, in patients with normal renal function, it is difficult to overcome the kidneys' ability to increase urinary potassium excretion by increasing potassium intake, except in patients with a massive potassium load (rhabdomyolysis, tumor lysis syndrome).

Chronic renal failure usually does not cause hyperkalemia without other mitigating factors until the glomerular filtration rate decreases to <15 mL/min. These factors particularly include use of medications characterized as risk factors for development of hyperkalemia (**Table 6**). Hyperkalemia commonly complicates acute renal failure and is less tolerated in the acute compared with the chronic setting (which usually develops in patients with end-stage renal disease). In addition to use of certain medications, there are various risk factors for the development of hyperkalemia (**Table 7**).

Treatment

Evaluation of hyperkalemia involves differentiating life-threatening hyperkalemia from less urgent presentations and verifying the diagnosis. Absolute levels of potassium cannot reliably determine if a life-threatening condition exists. Therefore, electrocardiography is indicated to assess the effect of elevated potassium concentrations on the cardiac membrane (**Figure 3**). Initially, serial electrocardiograms should be performed in patients with electrocardiographic changes until the electrocardiographic abnormalities have resolved. The plasma potassium concentration should also be measured to exclude hemolysis.

Management strategies differ depending upon the presence or absence of electrocardiographic changes (Figure 3).

Close follow-up with serial measurement of electrolytes is indicated in the acute setting. Agents causing hyperkalemia such as NSAIDs or spironolactone often have long half-lives and their effect may persist for up to 2 weeks. The effects of these medications often are additive. Therefore, combinations of potassium-sparing diuretics, angiotensin-converting enzyme inhibitors, angiotensin receptor blockers, and NSAIDs may cause serious hyperkalemia.

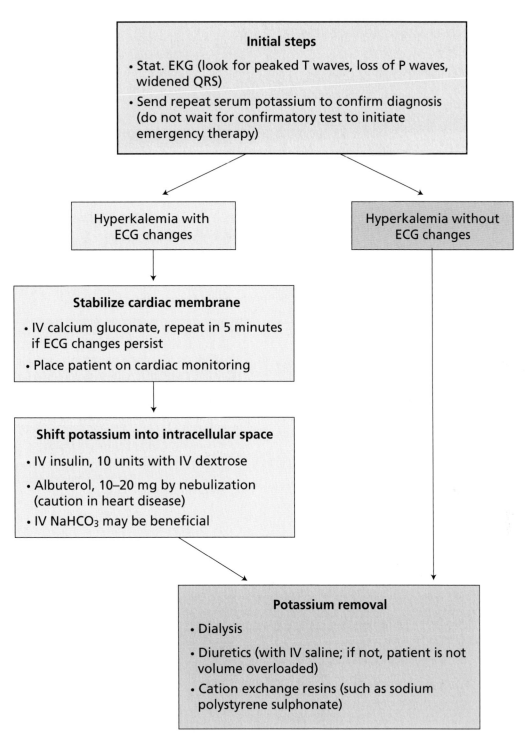

FIGURE 3.
Treatment of hyperkalemia.

ECG = electrocardiogram; IV = intravenous

Chronic hyperkalemia usually occurs because of chronic renal failure with or without angiotensin-converting enzyme inhibitor or angiotensin receptor blocker therapy. In this setting, increasing sodium intake and restricting dietary potassium may decrease serum potassium concentrations.

Prognosis and Follow-up
Serial potassium measurement is mandatory to assess treatment response. If managed properly, hyperkalemia almost always is associated with a successful outcome and good long-term prognosis (10).

TABLE 8 Common Causes of Hypokalemia

Potassium Shift into Cells

Alkalosis, recovery from diabetic ketoacidosis, β₂-agonists, insulin

Gastrointestinal Potassium Losses

Vomiting, nasogastric suction, diarrhea

Renal Potassium Losses

Diuretics, hypomagnesemia, hyperaldosteronism, drugs (amphotericin B, cisplatin), proximal (type 2) and distal (type 1) RTA

Decreased Potassium Intake

RTA = renal tubular acidosis

TABLE 9 Hypokalemia

Clinical Manifestations

Arrhythmias*
Muscle weakness
Ileus
Muscle cramps
Increased renal ammonia production†
Rhabdomyolysis

Risk Factors

Diuretic use
Diarrhea
Vomiting
Nasogastric suction
Insulin
β-Agonist use

* Particularly in patients using digitalis or with heart disease.

† Predisposes patients to hepatic encephalopathy.

Hypokalemia
Pathophysiology

Hypokalemia occurs through shifting from extracellular fluid to intracellular fluid or through total body potassium depletion via urinary or gastrointestinal losses (**Table 8**). Shifting of potassium into the intracellular compartment occurs under physiologic conditions in response to insulin secretion. Without shifting, the serum potassium concentration could become dangerously high after a meal.

β₂-Adrenergic stimulation also leads to cellular uptake of potassium. This stimulation is clinically significant because β₂-agonists are useful in transiently treating hyperkalemia and may potentially lead to hypokalemia in certain clinical settings.

The physiologic response to hypokalemia is to reduce urinary potassium losses. Because Western diets provide adequate potassium and the body is able to conserve potassium, inadequate potassium intake alone rarely causes hypokalemia. Once intracellular shifting is excluded, sources of potassium loss (almost always renal or gastrointestinal) should be evaluated. There are various clinical manifestations and risk factors for hypokalemia (**Table 9**).

Treatment

Potassium chloride repletes total body potassium. For severe hypokalemia, intravenous potassium chloride, 10 meq/h, is indicated. Hypomagnesemia should be corrected, if present. Total body potassium deficits are typically large (200–300 mmol for a serum potassium concentration of 3 meq/L); therefore, repeat replacement doses may be warranted. Serial potassium measurement is mandatory to assess response to treatment (see also Reference 10).

KEY POINTS

- Maintenance of potassium balance is possible in patients with volume depletion or volume excess, despite changes in sodium excretion.
- Hypokalemia is common in patients with HIV.
- Hyperkalemia occurs through shifting from the intracellular compartment to the extracellular fluid or through total body potassium excess.
- Chronic renal failure usually does not cause hyperkalemia without other mitigating factors until the glomerular filtration rate decreases to <15 mL/min.
- Evaluation of hyperkalemia involves differentiating life-threatening hyperkalemia from less urgent presentations through electrocardiography.
- Removal of offending agents; diuretics; and intravenous saline and cation exchange resins usually manage hyperkalemia not associated with changes on electrocardiography.
- In renal failure, emergency hemodialysis often is needed for treatment of hyperkalemia.
- In chronic hyperkalemia, increasing sodium intake and restricting dietary potassium may decrease serum potassium concentrations.
- The body's compensatory response to hypokalemia is to reduce urinary potassium losses.
- Because Western diets provide adequate potassium and the body is able to conserve potassium, inadequate potassium intake alone rarely causes hypokalemia.
- Once intracellular shifting is excluded, sources of potassium loss (almost always renal or gastrointestinal) should be evaluated.

TABLE 10 Causes of Hypophosphatemia
Decreased Phosphate Absorption, GI Phosphate Losses
Alcoholism/poor nutrition
Diarrhea
GI tract surgery
Ingestion of phosphate-binding medications or antacids
TPN preparations with inadequate phosphorus
Vitamin D deficiency
Use of corticosteroids
Shifting of Phosphate from Extracellular Space
Refeeding syndrome
Respiratory alkalosis
Hungry bone syndrome
High-grade lymphoma, acute leukemia
Administration of glucagon, epinephrine
Increased Renal Losses of Phosphate
Hyperparathyroidism
Fanconi's syndrome (proximal tubular dysfunction seen in several diseases, particularly multiple myeloma)
Diuretics, particularly carbonic anhydrase inhibitors
Acute volume expansion
Amphotericin B
Oncogenic osteomalacia
Hypophosphatemic rickets (X linked and AD)

GI = gastrointestinal; TPN = total parenteral nutrition; AD = autosomal dominant

TABLE 11 Hypophosphatemia
Clinical Manifestations
Muscle weakness*
Rhabdomyolysis
Hypotension
Arrhythmias
Hypoventilation
Irritability
Seizures
Coma
Hemolytic anemia
Osteomalacia[†]
Risk Factors
Alcoholism
Critical illness
Nasogastric suction
Malnutrition
Extensive bowel resection
Parathyroid surgery
Renal transplant
Malignancy
Low sun exposure
Diuretic use

* Particularly large muscle groups, including proximal muscle groups in the extremities.

[†] Occurs in the chronic setting.

Phosphorus Homeostasis

Phosphate is primarily excreted through the kidneys and is reabsorbed mainly in the proximal tubule. The primary hormonal factors regulating phosphorus balance are parathyroid hormone, which decreases phosphorus reabsorption and thus promotes renal phosphate excretion, and calcitriol $(1,25[OH]_2D)$, which stimulates phosphate absorption in the gut.

Typically, 5% to 20% of the filtered phosphorus load is excreted. However, this percentage may be decreased significantly in states of phosphate depletion. Phosphorus absorption occurs through the gastrointestinal tract and may be inadequate in malnourished patients.

Hypophosphatemia
Pathophysiology

Hypophosphatemia most often occurs as a multifactorial disease; contributing factors include decreased phosphate intake, acid–base disturbances, and renal phosphate losses (**Table 10**). This condition commonly develops in patients with alcoholism and in hospitalized patients. Usually, the diagnosis is evident from the history. However, if the diagnosis is uncertain, renal phosphate losses can be assessed by calculating the fractional excretion of phosphorus in order to determine if the losses are renal or gastrointestinal in origin using the following formula:

$$\text{Fractional Excretion of Phosphorus} = \text{Urinary Phosphorus} \times \text{Plasma Creatinine}/\text{Plasma Phosphorus} \times \text{Urinary Creatinine}$$

The fractional excretion of phosphorus should be measured when serum phosphorus is low. If renal phosphate–conserving mechanisms are intact, this value should be <5% in a phosphate-depleted state.

There are various clinical manifestations and risk factors for hypophosphatemia (**Table 11**).

Treatment

In asymptomatic patients, oral phosphorus replacement administered as a sodium or potassium salt is indicated. Parenteral therapy with either of these agents is indicated for symptomatic patients or those whose phosphorus level is <1 mg/dL. Parenteral phosphate is generally ordered in mmol (1 mmol of phosphate = 31 mg of phosphorus), and every mmol of phosphate administered contains 1 meq of sodium

TABLE 12 Causes of Hypocalcemia
Hypoparathyroidism/pseudohypoparathyroidism
Hyperphosphatemia
Hypomagnesemia
Vitamin D deficiency
Dietary deficit
Reduced sun exposure
Decreased 25–hydroxylation of vitamin D (liver disease, alcoholism)
Decreased vitamin D-sensitive rickets type 1 (1-α hydroxylase deficiency) and type 2 (receptor deficiency)
Renal failure (reduced 1-hydroxylation of 25-hydroxyvitamin D)
Osteoblastic metastases (prostate, breast)
Saponification in severe pancreatitis
Citrate load (blood transfusion)

TABLE 13 Risk Factors for Hypocalcemia
Parathyroid surgery
Neck irradiation
Renal transplantation in patients with tertiary hyperparathyroidism
Malignancy
Alcoholism
Low sun exposure
Malnutrition

(sodium phosphate) or 1 meq of potassium (potassium phosphate).

Judicious phosphate replacement is indicated for patients with renal failure. In patients with severe deficiency and those who are symptomatic, serial serum phosphorus measurement is indicated to assess response to therapy (11).

KEY POINTS

- **Hypophosphatemia commonly develops in patients with alcoholism and in hospitalized patients.**
- **To determine if phosphate losses have a renal or gastrointestinal origin, calculate the fractional excretion of phosphorus.**
- **In asymptomatic hypophosphatemia, oral phosphorus replacement administered as a sodium or potassium salt is indicated.**
- **In patients with symptomatic hypophosphatemia or those with phosphorus levels <1 mg/dL, parenteral therapy with sodium or potassium salt is indicated.**

Calcium Homeostasis

The serum calcium level is tightly regulated. Intracellular calcium levels are very low, and calcium is stored in the bone. Intestinal absorption, which is regulated by vitamin D and urinary excretion, maintains calcium balance, whereas parathyroid hormone regulates the synthesis of vitamin D, urinary reabsorption, and calcium reabsorption. Plasma calcium is typically measured as total calcium in mg/dL. A reduction in plasma albumin of 1 g/L decreases the serum total calcium by 0.8 mg/dL.

Hypocalcemia
Pathophysiology
Hypocalcemia is caused by efflux of calcium out of the extracellular space or by decreased entry of calcium into the extracellular space (**Table 12**). Under normal circumstances, homeostatic mechanisms can maintain serum calcium levels despite low calcium intake.

Decreased calcium absorption and decreased calcium mobilization from bone stores can occur in conditions such as hypoparathyroidism and vitamin D deficiency. Increased calcium removal from the serum occurs in osteoblastic metastatic disease and in severe pancreatitis through saponification of fats (Table 12).

Clinical manifestations of hypocalcemia include tetany (Chvostek's and Trousseau's signs) and altered mental status. There are various risk factors for this condition (**Table 13**).

Treatment
Calcium chloride or intravenous calcium gluconate is indicated for acute symptomatic hypocalcemia. In symptomatic hypocalcemia, the ionized calcium determines disease severity; therefore, alterations in protein binding of calcium may aggravate or precipitate this condition. Alkalemia increases the affinity of albumin for calcium by altering the net charge of the protein to a more positive state and therefore decreases the ionized calcium. Acute increases in total albumin also may decrease ionized calcium.

Hypercalcemia
Pathophysiology
Entrance of calcium into the intravascular space in excess of renal excretion causes hypercalcemia (**Table 14**). Intestinal absorption and bone reabsorption cause calcium influx into the intravascular space.

Hypercalcemia is most commonly caused by alterations in the hormonal stimulation of calcium absorption from the gut and bone reabsorption due to primary hyperparathyroidism,

TABLE 14 Causes of Hypercalcemia

Excess Calcium Influx into Vascular Space
Primary hyperparathyroidism (usually adenoma or gland hyperplasia; parathyroid malignancy is rare)
Malignancy (multiple myeloma, carcinomas through production of PTH-related peptide, osteosarcomas)
Immobilization
Granulomatous disease (increased vitamin D production)
Sarcoidosis
Tuberculosis
Paget's disease
Milk-alkali syndrome
Vitamin D intoxication
Hyperparathyroidism (stimulation of osteoclasts)
Decreased Calcium Excretion
Primary hyperparathyroidism
Thiazide diuretics
Familial hypocalciuric hypercalcemia

PTH = parathyroid hormone

TABLE 15 Clinical Manifestations of Hypercalcemia

Lethargy
Confusion
Coma
Nausea
Constipation
Polyuria
Hypertension
Volume depletion
Nephrolithiasis
Nephrogenic diabetes insipidus

malignancy, and granulomatous diseases. Hypercalcemia also may be caused by decreased renal excretion, which occurs in primary hyperparathyroidism and thiazide diuretic use. Because of protein binding, the total calcium level must be corrected for serum albumin.

Hypercalcemia has various clinical manifestations, including a decrease in neuromuscular excitability that causes decreased muscular tone (**Table 15**). Risk factors for this condition include malignancy and use of thiazide diuretics or use of vitamin D sterols.

Treatment

Acute treatment of symptomatic hypercalcemia includes normal saline to replete volume and intravenous furosemide to increase renal calcium excretion. Bisphosphonates are indicated for hypercalcemia of malignancy to decrease calcium reabsorption from the bone; however, monitoring for hypocalcemia is indicated for patients using these agents, particularly in the setting of renal failure. Adjunctive therapy for hypercalcemia may include calcitonin, although this agent usually has a short-term effect and tachyphylaxis may develop (12).

KEY POINTS

- Risk factors for hypercalcemia include malignancy and use of thiazide diuretics or use of vitamin D sterols.
- Acute treatment of symptomatic hypercalcemia includes volume repletion; intravenous furosemide; bisphosphonates; and calcitonin, if needed.

References

1. **Achinger SG, Moritz ML, Ayus JC.** Dysnatremias: Why are patients still dying? South Med J. 2006 Apr;99(4):353-62; quiz 363-4. [PMID: 16634244]

2. **Moritz ML, Ayus JC.** The pathophysiology and treatment of hyponatraemic encephalopathy: an update [Editorial]. Nephrol Dial Transplant. 2003;18:2486-91. [PMID: 14605269]

3. **Ayus JC, Arieff AI.** Chronic hyponatremic encephalopathy in postmenopausal women: association of therapies with morbidity and mortality. JAMA. 1999;281:2299-304. [PMID: 10386554]

4. **Ayus JC, Arieff AI.** Noncardiogenic Pulmonary Edema in Marathon Runners. Ann Intern Med. 2000;133:1011. [PMID: 11119411]

5. **Ayus JC, Wheeler JM, Arieff AI.** Postoperative hyponatremic encephalopathy in menstruant women. Ann Intern Med. 1992;117:891-7. [PMID: 1443949]

6. **Ayus JC, Armstrong D, Arieff AI.** Hyponatremia with hypoxia: effects on brain adaptation, perfusion, and histology in rodents. Kidney Int. 2006;69:1319-25. [PMID: 16614721]

7. **Moritz ML, Ayus JC.** Prevention of hospital-acquired hyponatremia: a case for using isotonic saline. Pediatrics. 2003;111:227-30. [PMID: 12563043]

8. **Ayus JC, Krothapalli RK, Arieff AI.** Treatment of symptomatic hyponatremia and its relation to brain damage. A prospective study. N Engl J Med. 1987;317:1190-5. [PMID: 3309659]

9. **Giebisch G.** Renal potassium transport: mechanisms and regulation. Am J Physiol. 1998;274:F817-33. [PMID: 9612319]

10. **Gennari FJ.** Disorders of potassium homeostasis. Hypokalemia and hyperkalemia. Crit Care Clin. 2002;18:273-88, vi. [PMID: 12053834]

11. **Weisinger JR, Bellorin-Font E.** Magnesium and phosphorus. Lancet. 1998;352:391-6. [PMID: 9717944]

12. **Lafferty FW.** Differential diagnosis of hypercalcemia. J Bone Miner Res. 1991;6 Suppl 2:S51-9; discussion S61. [PMID: 1763670]

ACID–BASE DISORDERS

Evaluation of all acid–base disorders begins by determining which acid–base disorder(s) are present, the cause of each disorder, and whether there is adequate compensation.

The following are four basic parameters used to determine acid–base status:

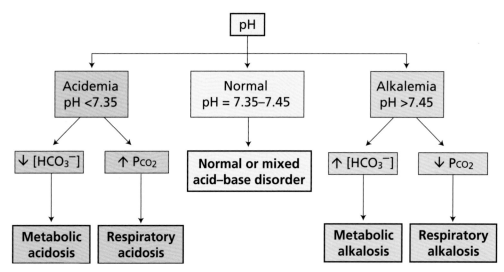

FIGURE 4.
General approach to acid–base disorders.

1) Arterial pH: The negative logarithm of the concentration of H$^+$. The physiologic range is 7.38 to 7.44.

2) Arterial PCO_2: Indicates the volatile acid and generally reflects the respiratory response or contribution to the acid–base disorder. Normal range is 35 mm Hg to 45 mm Hg.

3) Serum bicarbonate (HCO$_3^-$) or total carbon dioxide (CO$_2$): Indicates the level of fixed acids present. Normal value is 24 meq/L.

4) Anion gap: The difference between the concentrations of the measured cations and the measured anions in the plasma. The anion gap is an indirect index of the presence of "extra anions." These anions may be endogenous substances normally found at low levels, such as lactate, or exogenous substances, such as salicylates.

The values of these parameters determine the approach to acid–base disorders (**Figure 4**).

The anion gap can be calculated using the following formula:

$$[Na^+] - ([Cl^-] + [HCO_3^-])$$

Metabolic acidosis can be subdivided into anion gap and non–anion gap metabolic acidosis based on the value of the anion gap. Generally, metabolic acidosis is caused either by the loss of bicarbonate (renal or gastrointestinal) or by the gain of acid associated with an unmeasured anion.

The normal range of the anion gap is wide. When interpreting an anion gap, other causes for an increase in acid as well as hypoalbuminemia, or the presence of cationic proteins (myeloma), should be considered. For every 1 mg/dL decrease in the plasma albumin concentration, the anion gap decreases by approximately 2 meq/L to 5 meq/L.

KEY POINTS

- Metabolic acidosis is caused by renal or gastrointestinal loss of bicarbonate or the gain of acid associated with an unmeasured anion.
- When interpreting an anion gap, other causes for an increase in acid as well as hypoalbuminemia, or the presence of cationic proteins, should be considered.

Carbon Dioxide–Bicarbonate Buffer System and Mechanisms for Acid–Base Compensation

The buffering of acids and excretion of the daily acid load allow the body to maintain a pH within a narrow range close to neutrality. Intra- and extracellular buffers decrease the intensity of acute disturbances in acid–base equilibrium. The excretion of the daily acid load occurs through the respiratory excretion of volatile acid (carbon dioxide) and the renal excretion of fixed acid.

The buffering capacity is approximately 1 mmol of H$^+$. The overall buffering system is complex; clinically, the most important system is the carbon dioxide–bicarbonate system. Through the interconversion of bicarbonate, carbonic acid, and carbon dioxide, fixed and volatile acids can be buffered until they are excreted through the urine or respiration. The kidneys reabsorb all the filtered load of bicarbonate in order to avoid losing base and regenerate one "new" HCO$_3^-$ for every H$^+$ excreted in the urine.

To reabsorb bicarbonate, the corresponding H$^+$ generated in this process must be excreted in the urine. The renal

TABLE 16 Compensations for Acid–Base Disorders

Metabolic Acidosis

Every 1 mmol/L decrease in HCO_3^- → 1 mm Hg decrease in Pco_2

Expected Pco_2 = 1.5 (HCO_3^-) + 8 +/– 2

Pco_2 should approach last two digits of pH

Metabolic Alkalosis

Every 1 mmol/L increase in HCO_3^- → 0.7 mm Hg increase in Pco_2

Respiratory Acidosis

Acute: 10 mm Hg increase in Pco_2 → 1 mmol/L increase in HCO_3^-

Chronic: 10 mm Hg increase in Pco_2 → 4 mmol/L increase in HCO_3^-

Respiratory Alkalosis

Acute: Every 10 mm Hg decrease in Pco_2 → 2 mmol/L decrease in HCO_3^-

Chronic: Every 10 mm Hg decrease in Pco_2 → 4 mmol/L decrease in HCO_3^-

secretion of H^+ is tenfold greater in the proximal tubule (approximately 4000 mmol/d) compared with the distal tubule (approximately 400 mmol/d). However, the distal tubule maintains a higher luminal–intracellular H^+ gradient than the proximal tubule (500:1).

Urinary excretion of H^+ (and, therefore, the generation of a new HCO_3^-) occurs through titratable (mostly phosphates) and nontitratable (ammonium) acids. The excretion of titratable acid has a definite limit and depends on the filtered load of PO_4^{2-}. However, the renal capacity to generate ammonia and to excrete acid as ammonium under normal conditions is practically unlimited. Essentially, ammonia–ammonium acts as a urinary buffer system that allows the elimination of one H^+ for nearly every ammonia produced without generating an excessively acidic urine. Chronic metabolic acidosis stimulates the renal production of ammonia, which reaches its maximum production at 3 to 7 days.

The urinary anion gap may be used to indirectly estimate the amount of ammonium in the urine and can be calculated using the following formula:

$$[Na^+] + [K^+] - [Cl^-]$$

Because ammonium is not a measured cation, the presence of significant amounts of ammonia causes an abundance of chloride relative to measured cations. Therefore, a highly negative urinary anion gap suggests that there is a high amount of ammonium in the urine and that the renal response to metabolic acidosis is intact. Conversely, an anion that is near positive or positive suggests that there is little or no ammonium in the urine, which is reflected by a paucity of chloride in the urine relative to the concentration of measured

cations. One caveat is that the presence of unmeasured anions in the urine (such as β-hydroxybutyrate) rarely may falsely depress the urinary anion gap.

Mechanisms of Compensation

The three main compensatory mechanisms that defend the body against acid–base disturbances are the buffering systems, respiratory compensation, and renal compensation (**Table 16**). The buffering systems and respiratory compensation are very rapid, whereas renal compensation may take days to become fully effective. The principal buffer is the bicarbonate system.

Respiration eliminates the carbon dioxide generated by the metabolism of nutrients. The kidneys effect fine adjustments of acid–base equilibrium and elimination of non-volatile (or fixed) acids. Therefore, this system uses two routes of elimination of bicarbonate.

KEY POINTS

- The buffering of acids and excretion of the daily acid load allow the body to maintain a narrow pH range close to neutrality.
- The urinary anion gap helps to assess the amount of ammonium in the urine.
- A highly negative urinary anion gap suggests that there is a high amount of ammonium in the urine and that the renal response to metabolic acidosis is intact.
- An anion that is near 0 or positive suggests that there is little or no ammonium in the urine, which indicates a paucity of chloride in the urine relative to the concentration of measured cations.
- The three main compensatory mechanisms that defend the body against acid–base disturbances are the buffering systems, respiratory compensation, and renal compensation.

Anion Gap Metabolic Acidosis

Metabolic acidosis associated with an elevated anion gap develops when acids associated with an unmeasured anion (the conjugate base of the acid, such as lactate) are produced or exogenously gained (**Figure 5**). By far the most common causes of anion gap metabolic acidosis are lactic acidosis and diabetic ketoacidosis.

Treatment

The key to treatment of anion gap metabolic acidosis is reversing pathogenesis of the endogenous acid production and eliminating excess acid. Use of bicarbonate replacement therapy remains controversial in the setting of anion gap acidosis (especially lactic acidosis). This therapy can act as a bridge until homeostatic mechanisms begin to reverse the condition

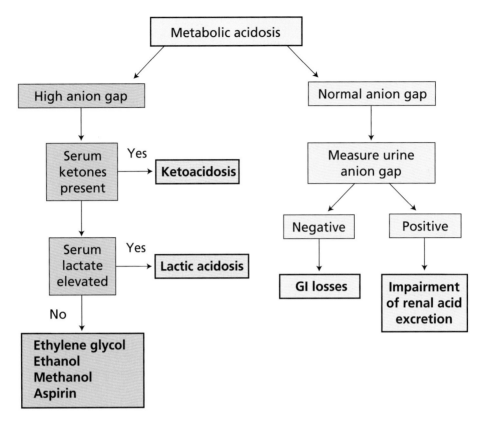

FIGURE 5.
Diagnostic approach to metabolic acidosis.

GI = gastrointestinal

through the formation of bicarbonate via metabolism of the endogenous bases, such as lactate and ketone bodies.

Bicarbonate replacement therapy, if used, should be reserved for patients with a pH <7.10. These endogenous bases are the unmeasured anions that constitute the anion gap and represent "potential bicarbonate." In patients with metabolic acidosis who remain acidic despite maximal respiratory response, administration of bicarbonate is indicated to prevent worsening of the acidemia.

Hemodialysis rapidly corrects acidosis and may be particularly useful in patients with renal failure.

Causes of Anion Gap Acidosis

Diabetic Ketoacidosis

During times of normal enteral intake, insulin is secreted and mediates the metabolism of carbohydrates and the storage of fat. In the fasting state, insulin secretion decreases. In diabetic ketoacidosis, an insulin deficit leads to altered cellular metabolism in which glucose utilization is impaired. This deficiency causes liberation of fatty acids and increased H^+ production. In addition to abnormal ketoacid production, diabetic ketoacidosis is typically associated with a deficit of free water and a decrease in circulatory volume and potassium. Although total body potassium stores are decreased, the

serum potassium concentration is frequently elevated on presentation due to the effects of insulin deficiency and hyperglycemia on potassium distribution. A normal sodium concentration in the presence of hyperglycemia also is abnormal and indicates hypernatremia.

The treatment of diabetic ketoacidosis includes reexpansion of the extracellular fluid volume, administration of insulin to halt acid production, and correction of potassium and phosphorus deficits with close monitoring of plasma electrolytes.

Lactic Acidosis

Lactic acidosis is classified into two types. Type A lactic acidosis is caused by hypoxia and excess formation of lactic acid and constitutes the majority of lactic acidosis cases. Lactate formation occurs in hypoxic tissues undergoing anaerobic metabolism. This disorder develops in the following conditions: ischemia (particularly of the bowel or limb), sepsis, hypotension, and profound anemia. Type A lactic acidosis often is extremely serious, usually due to the severity of the underlying condition.

Type B lactic acidosis is caused by failure of the liver to metabolize lactate and to regenerate a bicarbonate. This condition occurs in severe liver disease and in conditions that interfere with liver metabolism.

Ethylene Glycol or Methanol Intoxication

The osmolal gap can be calculated using the following formula:

$$(\text{Measured Serum Osmolality}) - (\text{Calculated Serum Osmolality})$$

where the calculated serum osmolality is obtained as follows:

$$2 \times [Na^+] \, (meq/L) + \text{Blood Urea Nitrogen} \, (mg/dL)/2.8 + \text{Glucose} \, (mg/dL) /18$$

The osmolal gap is normally approximately 10 mosm/kg H_2O. An elevated osmolal gap suggests the presence of an unmeasured osmole and is most commonly caused by ethanol. The osmolal gap also helps to quantify the level of ethylene glycol or methanol, although direct measurement of these toxins is indicated.

KEY POINTS

- The most common causes of anion gap metabolic acidosis are lactic acidosis or diabetic ketoacidosis.
- The key to treatment of anion gap metabolic acidosis is reversing the condition that led to excess acid production.
- Treatment of diabetic ketoacidosis includes reexpansion of the extracellular fluid volume, administration of insulin to halt acid production, and correction of potassium and phosphorus deficits.
- In diabetic ketoacidosis, the potassium concentration may initially be elevated despite total body potassium depletion.
- A normal sodium concentration in the presence of hyperglycemia indicates hypernatremia.
- The osmolal gap suggests the presence of an unmeasured osmole, such as ethanol (which is most common), ethanol glycol, or methanol.

Non–Anion Gap Acidosis

Non–anion gap (hyperchloremic) acidosis is characterized by a primary decrease in the serum bicarbonate associated with an increase in the serum chloride. The decrease in the serum bicarbonate occurs because of renal or extrarenal (gastrointestinal) losses (**Table 17**).

Treatment

Bicarbonate therapy is generally indicated in non–anion gap acidosis, whereas correction of the underlying cause is the primary concern in anion gap acidosis. Oral bicarbonate (or oral citrate solutions) is the preferred agent for chronic therapy for non–anion gap acidosis. For acute presentations, especially in patients with concomitant impaired respiratory function, intravenous bicarbonate therapy is indicated.

TABLE 17 Causes of Non–Anion Gap Metabolic Acidosis

Extrarenal Source
Gastrointestinal disorders:
Diarrhea
Pancreatic and biliary fistulas
Laxatives, cholestyramine
Ureterointestinal diversions (ileal conduit)
Exogenous acids administration
NH_4Cl
HCl
Amino acids (particularly L-arginine or L-lysine)
Renal Source
Proximal (type 2) tubular acidosis
Distal (type 1) tubular acidosis
Defective ammoniagenesis
Renal failure
Hypoaldosteronism
Hyperkalemia
Acetazolamide

Causes of Non–Anion Gap Metabolic Acidosis

Diarrhea

Severe diarrhea causes non–anion gap metabolic acidosis with volume depletion and usually is accompanied by hypokalemia. In extreme cases, circulatory collapse may occur, which may result in an anion gap component by inducing a lactic acidosis through tissue hypoperfusion. Patients who chronically abuse laxatives are susceptible to developing metabolic acidosis with hypokalemia. However, these patients also often abuse diuretics and frequently have an associated metabolic alkalosis. Measurement of the urinary anion gap is indicated to determine if the acidosis is from a renal or nonrenal source.

Ureterointestinal Diversions

The accumulation of urine in the colon leads to reabsorption of chloride and water by the intestine. The absorption of chloride can induce secretion of bicarbonate into the intestine. In addition, urease-positive bacteria can metabolize the urea in the urine to form ammonium, which, when absorbed, leads to liberation of excess acid after it is converted to ammonia and hydrogen ions in the liver. The presence of chronic pyelonephritis in the diverted kidney is common, and a superimposed distal renal tubular acidosis (RTA) may occur.

Renal Tubular Acidosis

Proximal (type 2) RTA is caused by a decrease in proximal bicarbonate reabsorption, whereas the primary defect in distal (type 1) RTA is an impairment of distal acidification. The preferred bicarbonate salt in hypokalemic RTA is potassium bicarbonate or potassium citrate. The principal difference in treatment of these conditions is that a higher dose of bicarbonate usually is indicated in type 2 RTA.

Type 4 RTA is a clinical syndrome caused by a lack of aldosterone effect on the kidney. This condition may develop because of a lack of aldosterone production or a defect in action of aldosterone. Type 4 RTA is frequently associated with the following factors: diabetes; advanced age; AIDS; interstitial nephritis; obstructive uropathy; post–renal transplant status; and use of angiotensin-converting enzyme inhibitors, heparin (which impairs aldosterone production), and cyclosporine (which decreases aldosterone secretion).

Type 4 RTA typically leads to a non–anion gap metabolic acidosis and hyperkalemia and is therefore usually readily distinguished from type 1 RTA. The defect in acidification in type 4 RTA is less than that in type 1 RTA; consequently, affected patients have an appropriately low urinary pH (usually 5.5).

The clinical presentation of type 4 RTA resembles that of primary adrenal insufficiency with deficient aldosterone production or with the use of potassium-sparing diuretics, such as spironolactone, amiloride, and triamterene. Trimethoprim (and trimethoprim–sulfamethoxazole) and pentamidine close sodium channels in the distal nephron and may cause a similar clinical presentation.

The associated hyperkalemia can be treated with diuretics, sodium bicarbonate, or sodium citrate solutions. Hyperkalemia itself inhibits renal ammonia production; therefore, treatment of the hyperkalemia may enhance renal acid excretion. Salt intake should not be restricted, because distal delivery of solute is important to maintain potassium excretion. In refractory cases, fludrocortisone can be used to enhance potassium excretion. However, sodium retention may occur and frank pulmonary edema may be a complication, particularly in patients with poor cardiac function.

Renal Failure

The capacity of the kidneys to excrete ammonia and organic acids is maintained until kidney function declines to below approximately a glomerular filtration rate of 20 mL/min. The resulting acidosis is of a mixed type and generally but not universally is associated with an elevated anion gap. It is important to treat chronic metabolic acidosis, as bone demineralization may occur with time. The goal of treatment is to maintain normal acid–base status.

KEY POINTS

- Bicarbonate therapy is generally indicated in non–anion gap acidosis.
- Correction of the underlying cause is the primary concern in anion gap acidosis.
- Severe diarrhea causes non–anion gap metabolic acidosis with volume depletion and usually is accompanied by hypokalemia.

TABLE 18 Causes of Alkalosis Generation

Excessive Alkaline Load

| Bicarbonate infusion, hemodialysis |
| CaCO$_3$ supplements |
| Oral citrate solutions |
| Parenteral nutrition (acetate, glutamate) |

Loss of Hydrogen Ions

| GI losses |
| Vomiting, nasogastric suction |
| Renal losses |
| Diuretics |
| Excessive mineralocorticoids |

Metabolic Alkalosis

Metabolic alkalosis is characterized by a primary elevation in the serum bicarbonate. This condition is a common complication in hospitalized patients and may cause serious complications. Generally, metabolic alkalosis is accompanied by hypochloremia, such that the decrease in chloride offsets the incremental increase in bicarbonate. Alterations in the renal handling of bicarbonate must occur to maintain the alkalosis. In the absence of these alterations, the kidneys would simply excrete the bicarbonate load.

Pathophysiology

All metabolic alkaloses are caused by excessive bicarbonate intake or loss of H$^+$ (**Table 18**). In order to maintain the alkalosis, renal bicarbonate excretion must be impaired. This impairment occurs in the setting of depleted chloride or effective circulatory volume, excessive mineralocorticoid activity, or severe renal insufficiency (**Table 19**).

Vomiting, nasogastric suction, and diuretics are the most frequent causes of metabolic alkalosis. Hypokalemia in the presence of vomiting and nasogastric suction is not caused by gastrointestinal losses because the stomach contents are not rich in potassium but rather by renal losses due to potassium bicarbonate excretion and secondary hyperaldosteronism. In these settings, the urinary chloride (not the urinary sodium, which is obligated to accompany the bicarbonate losses in the urine) reflects the effective blood volume. Similar to the loss of gastric secretions, diuretic-induced depletion of the extracellular volume also stimulates aldosterone secretion. This aldosterone secretion stimulates reabsorption of sodium in the distal tubule, coupled with secretion of potassium and H$^+$, and generates urine that is paradoxically acidic.

Renal and Extrarenal Compensation

Immediately after generation of a metabolic alkalosis, buffering systems in the extracellular and intracellular space begin to

TABLE 19 Classification of Metabolic Alkalosis by Chloride Handling

Chloride Sensitive (Urine Cl <20 meq/L)
Gastrointestinal acid losses
Nasogastric suction, vomiting
Congenital Cl losses in stool
Rectal adenoma
Renal acid losses
Penicillins, citrate
Postdiuretic
Posthypercapneic
Chloride Resistant (Urine Cl >40 meq/L)
Hypertensive
Renovascular hypertension
Primary hyperaldosteronism
Cushing's syndrome
Liddle's syndrome
Glycyrrhizic acid
Normotensive
Diuretics
Bartter's and Gitelman's syndromes
Severe potassium depletion
Hypercalcemia and hypoparathyroidism
Administration of alkali

TABLE 20 Treatment of Metabolic Alkalosis

Chloride Sensitive
IV normal saline volume expansion
Discontinue diuretics if possible
H_2 blockers of proton pump inhibitors in cases of nasogastric suction and vomiting
Chloride Resistant
Spironolactone or amiloride
Replace potassium if deficient
Extreme Alkalosis
Hemodialysis
NH_4Cl or HCl also can be used
IV = intravenous

In all patients with low urinary chloride, normal saline is indicated to expand the extracellular space. Saline-resistant metabolic alkalosis is rare and may require more specific therapy (**Table 20**).

Treatment of Metabolic Alkalosis

H_2 blockers and proton pump inhibitors may help to decrease losses of H^+ in patients with prolonged gastric aspiration or chronic vomiting. Potassium chloride is almost always indicated in hypokalemia, although potassium concentrations may increase as the alkalosis is corrected. In very severe metabolic alkalosis (pH >7.6), hemodialysis is the preferred treatment, and use of acidic solutions is rarely indicated.

KEY POINTS

- Metabolic alkalosis is characterized by a primary elevation in the serum bicarbonate.
- Metabolic alkalosis is accompanied by hypochloremia, such that the decrease in chloride offsets the incremental increase in bicarbonate.
- All metabolic alkaloses are caused by excessive bicarbonate intake or loss of H^+.
- Vomiting, nasogastric suction, and diuretics are the most frequent causes of metabolic alkalosis.
- Renal compensation for metabolic alkalosis involves increased renal excretion of bicarbonate.
- In all patients with low urinary chloride, normal saline is indicated to expand the extracellular space.
- H_2 blockers and proton pump inhibitors may help to decrease losses of H^+ in patients with prolonged gastric aspiration or chronic vomiting.
- Potassium chloride is almost always indicated in hypokalemia, although potassium concentrations may increase as the alkalosis is corrected.
- In very severe metabolic alkalosis (pH >7.6), hemodialysis is the preferred treatment.

decrease the effects of the alkaline load. The capacity of the extracellular space to buffer bases is approximately double the capacity of the intracellular space. Respiratory compensation for a metabolic alkalosis involves respiratory suppression, and the P_{CO_2} increases (Table 16).

In the absence of counterregulatory mechanisms such as volume depletion, the kidney responds to metabolic alkalosis through increased renal excretion of bicarbonate. This mechanism involves the proximal tubule and requires adequate extracellular volume. In patients with normal renal function and normal extracellular fluid volume, increasing the serum bicarbonate concentration 2 meq/L to 3 meq/L above the normal value is virtually impossible because the kidneys can easily excrete the excess bicarbonate by decreasing the amount of the filtered load of bicarbonate that is reabsorbed. The secretion of bicarbonate in the distal tubule occurs through the exchange of chloride/bicarbonate in the type B intercalated cells in the collecting tubule.

Severe depletion of chloride theoretically inhibits this exchange and therefore inhibits bicarbonate secretion. Potassium depletion or contraction of the extracellular space also impedes the secretion of bicarbonate into the urine. Finally, hyperaldosteronism secondary to contraction of the extracellular space (as occurs with diuretic therapy) stimulates the tubular secretion of potassium and H^+, producing an acidic urine that also helps to maintain the alkalosis.

Respiratory Acid–Base Disorders

At basal conditions, through endogenous metabolism, between 12,000 mmol/d and 15,000 mmol/d of carbon dioxide is generated. This carbon dioxide enters the plasma and forms carbonic acid, which subsequently dissociates to bicarbonate and H^+. The majority of the carbon dioxide generated is transported to the lungs in the form of bicarbonate without a significant change in blood pH, as bicarbonate acts as the principal extracellular buffer. The H^+ generated is exchanged across the erythrocyte membrane and passes into the plasma. When the bicarbonate reaches the alveoli, the process is reversed; bicarbonate combines with H^+, and carbon dioxide is excreted in respiration.

Carbon dioxide is considered the principal stimulus for respiration, which is activated by minor elevations in the P_{CO_2}. Hypoxia is a minor stimulus for respiration and is effective when the P_{O_2} is 50 mm Hg to 55 mm Hg. In addition, the relationship between the P_{O_2} and alveolar ventilation is altered in the presence of high P_{CO_2}. When a sufficiently severe pulmonary disease is present, hypoxia stimulates ventilation at higher levels of P_{O_2} (between 70 mm Hg and 90 mm Hg).

Respiratory Acidosis

Respiratory acidosis is produced by any process with primary retention of carbon dioxide. The increase in the carbon dioxide decreases the pH by formation of carbonic acid. The principal compensatory mechanisms against acidosis are buffering and renal compensation.

In respiratory acidosis, there is minimal extracellular buffering capacity (bicarbonate cannot act as a buffer for carbonic acid). Therefore, intracellular buffers (hemoglobin and other proteins) are the only protection against acute rises in P_{CO_2}. In the erythrocytes, H^+ is buffered by hemoglobin, then bicarbonate is exchanged with chloride. In other cell types, the H^+ is buffered by other intracellular proteins. The buffering response of carbon dioxide occurs within 10 to 15 minutes of an elevation of P_{CO_2}.

Renal compensatory response occurs in chronic respiratory acidosis. Persistent hypercapnia stimulates the secretion of protons at the level of the distal nephron. The urinary pH decreases, and excretion of urinary ammonium, titratable acid, and chloride is enhanced. Consequently, the reabsorption of bicarbonate throughout the nephron is enhanced.

The renal response is initiated with an acute increase in P_{CO_2}, but the compensation is not complete until 3 to 4 days later. Regulation and maintenance of the pH in acute respiratory acidosis is mostly much less effective compared with the chronic setting.

In addition to the counteractive measures mentioned above, an increase in effective alveolar ventilation is required to eliminate excess carbon dioxide to reestablish equilibrium. If the increase in ventilation occurs in the acute period of the compensation, the decrease in P_{CO_2} reestablishes the equilibrium. However, if the hypercapnia is sustained and the renal response has been initiated, bicarbonaturia accompanies the return of the P_{CO_2} to normal. This condition can only occur if the chloride intake is sufficient to replace the deficit that developed during the renal compensation to the chronic respiratory acidosis (a period of negative chloride balance). If chloride is not available, the bicarbonate will remain elevated (posthypercapnic metabolic alkalosis).

In patients with intrinsic lung disease, hypercapnia is a late finding. Hypoxemia in earlier stages of disease can induce hyperventilation and can retard the development of hypercapnia.

In chronic respiratory acidosis, the respiratory centers are less sensitive to carbon dioxide; therefore, hypoxemia becomes the primary stimulus for the respiratory drive (**Table 21**).

Clinical Presentation

Separating the symptoms of hypercapnia from the symptoms of the accompanying hypoxemia is difficult. Acute respiratory acidosis can produce headaches, confusion, irritability, anxiety, and insomnia. Symptoms can progress to asterixis, delirium, and somnolence. These symptoms may be accompanied by papilledema, tachycardia, diaphoresis, and hypotension.

The severity of the symptoms correlates more closely with the rapidity of the development of the disturbance than the P_{CO_2} level. This correlation exists because acute respiratory acidosis causes a much greater disturbance in intracellular pH of the nervous system than chronic respiratory acidosis.

Chronic respiratory acidosis commonly is associated with cor pulmonale and peripheral edema. Occasionally, arrhythmias also may occur.

Diagnosis

Arterial blood gas studies are used to diagnose respiratory acidosis. In acute hypercapnia, the bicarbonate level typically ranges from 24 meq/L to 30 meq/L. Lesser values indicate superimposed metabolic alterations.

The alveolar–arterial oxygen gradient is increased in intrinsic lung disease and is normal in hypoventilation (caused by a decreased respiratory drive or a neuromuscular condition).

Treatment

Treatment of respiratory acidosis should focus on treating the underlying disorder. In patients with acute respiratory acidosis and hypoxemia, supplemental oxygen may be administered. However, to treat the hypercapnia, an increase in effective alveolar ventilation through reversal of the underlying cause or endotracheal intubation and mechanical ventilation is indicated.

The use of serum bicarbonate in respiratory acidosis in the absence of concurrent metabolic acidosis is potentially harmful. Use of this agent in acute respiratory acidosis may cause acute pulmonary edema, metabolic alkalosis, and augmented

TABLE 21 Causes of Respiratory Acidosis

Airway Obstruction

Foreign body, aspiration

Obstructive sleep apnea

Laryngospasm or bronchospasm

Neuromuscular Disorders of Respiration

Acute

  Myasthenia gravis

  Hypokalemic periodic paralysis

  Guillain–Barré syndrome

  Botulism, tetanus, drugs

  Hypokalemia, hypophosphatemia

  Cervical spinal injury

Chronic

  Morbid obesity (Pickwickian syndrome)

  Myxedema

  Polio, multiple sclerosis, ALS

Central Respiratory Depression

Acute

  Drugs (opiates, sedatives), anesthetics

  Oxygen administration in acute hypercapnia

  Central sleep apnea

  Brain trauma or stroke

  Bulbar poliomyelitis

Respiratory Disorders

Acute

  Severe pulmonary edema

  Asthma or pneumonia

  ARDS

Chronic

  COPD

  Pulmonary fibrosis

  Chronic pneumonitis

Mechanical Ventilation

ALS = amyotrophic lateral sclerosis; ARDS = acute respiratory distress syndrome; COPD = chronic obstructive pulmonary disease

TABLE 22 Causes of Respiratory Alkalosis

Hypoxia

High altitude

CHF

Severe VQ mismatch

Lung Diseases

Pulmonary fibrosis

Pulmonary edema

Pneumonia

Pulmonary embolism

Drugs

Salicylates

Progesterone

Nicotine

Direct Stimulation of Respiratory Drive

Psychogenic hyperventilation

Cirrhosis

Gram-negative sepsis

Pregnancy (progesterone)

Excessive mechanical ventilation

Neurologic disorders: ACV, pontine tumors

CHF = congestive heart failure; VQ = ventilation-perfusion; ACV = acyclovir

The P_{CO_2} should be decreased gradually. Rapid correction may cause alkalosis and an increase in the cerebrospinal fluid pH, because carbon dioxide rapidly equilibrates across the blood–cerebrospinal fluid barrier. In this setting, serious neurologic problems, including seizures and death, may occur.

Respiratory Alkalosis
Pathophysiology
Respiratory alkalosis occurs because of a primary decrease in the P_{CO_2} (**Table 22**). Primary increases in ventilation decrease P_{CO_2} and subsequently reduce carbonic acid levels. The buffering system and renal compensation attempt to maintain plasma pH in this setting.

During an acute respiratory alkalosis, proteins, phosphates, and hemoglobin liberate H^+, which reacts with bicarbonate to form carbonic acid. At the erythrocyte level, a shift of chloride to the extracellular compartment occurs, as bicarbonate and cations enter in exchange for protons. Alkalemia also increases lactate production. Overall, this buffering system minimally reduces plasma pH, accounting for a 2 meq/L decrease in bicarbonate for every 10 mm Hg decrease in the P_{CO_2}.

Persistent respiratory alkalosis results in a renal response, decreasing the secretion of H^+. This renal compensation

carbon dioxide production and increased P_{CO_2} in patients with inadequate respiratory reserve.

In chronic respiratory acidosis, the arterial pH is close to normal due to renal compensation. The primary objective of treatment in this setting is to maintain adequate oxygenation and, if possible, increase effective alveolar ventilation. Specific treatment varies according to the underlying causes of the disorder. Excessive exogenous oxygen and sedatives generally are not indicated, because these treatments can depress the respiratory drive. Mechanical ventilation is indicated when there is an acute exacerbation of chronic hypercapnia.

causes a decrease in the proximal reabsorption of bicarbonate and a decrease in the excretion of titratable acids and of ammonium. The response is maximal at 3 to 4 days.

Clinical Presentation

Respiratory alkalosis may cause an alteration in consciousness, perioral paresthesias, muscle spasms, and cardiac arrhythmias. This condition also may cause a decrease in bicarbonate and an increase in chloride. In addition, alkalemia stimulates glycolysis, which causes phosphate to shift from the extracellular space into the intracellular compartment as glucose-6-phosphate forms. The concentration of ionized calcium may also decrease because of increased albumin and calcium binding.

Diagnosis

Arterial blood gas studies are used to diagnose respiratory alkalosis. An elevation in the pH due to a decrease in the P_{CO_2} and, depending on the degree of compensation, a decrease in the bicarbonate characterize this condition.

Treatment

The underlying cause for respiratory alkalosis should always be pursued (Table 22). In psychogenic hyperventilation, rebreathing air using a bag increases the systemic P_{CO_2}. This method also may help to rapidly reduce the pH in patients with mixed, severe alkalosis, characterized by a pH of 7.7.

KEY POINTS

- An increase in effective alveolar ventilation is necessary in respiratory acidosis in order to eliminate excess carbon dioxide and reestablish equilibrium.
- The severity of the symptoms in respiratory acidosis correlates more closely with the rapidity of the development of the disturbance than with the P_{CO_2} level.
- Chronic respiratory acidosis commonly is associated with cor pulmonale and peripheral edema.
- The primary objective of treatment of respiratory acidosis is to maintain adequate oxygenation and, if possible, to increase effective alveolar ventilation.
- The buffering system and renal compensation minimally reduces plasma pH in respiratory alkalosis.
- Persistent respiratory alkalosis causes a compensatory renal response.
- Respiratory alkalosis may cause alterations in consciousness, perioral paresthesias, muscle spasms, and cardiac arrhythmias.

Mixed Acid–Base Disorders

In patients with a known primary acid–base disturbance, a mixed acid–base disorder should always be suspected if the pH is normal or the "compensation" has surpassed the normal pH. For example, a pH of 7.47 in a patient with metabolic acidosis indicates the presence of an accompanying respiratory alkalosis.

Metabolic and Respiratory Acidosis

Mixed metabolic and respiratory acidosis occurs when the respiratory compensation is insufficient for the degree of decrease in bicarbonate. The most extreme manifestations of this condition occur in patients with cardiopulmonary arrest, when both a decrease in bicarbonate levels (due to lactic acidosis) and retention of carbon dioxide (due to respiratory arrest) occur. Mixed metabolic and respiratory acidosis also affects patients with a primary metabolic acidosis and concomitant lung disease that impairs the ability to increase the ventilatory rate to appropriately decrease the P_{CO_2}, as well as those that have chronic respiratory acidosis without bicarbonate elevation. The presence of an anion gap despite normal serum bicarbonate levels should raise suspicion for this condition.

Two forms of metabolic acidosis can coexist. For example, profound diarrhea (causing a non–anion gap acidosis) may cause circulatory collapse (leading to lactic acidosis). The Δ anion gap–Δ HCO_3^- is used to diagnose this type of mixed disorder (see Δ Anion Gap–Δ HCO_3^- below).

Metabolic and Respiratory Alkalosis

Acidemia can be tolerated to a greater extent than alkalemia. For example, a pH of 7.2 is well tolerated, whereas a pH >7.6 is associated with significant mortality. Therefore, mixed metabolic and respiratory alkalosis is very serious. This condition typically occurs in patients on mechanical ventilation, in whom respiration cannot be decreased in response to a metabolic alkalosis due to diuretic use, administration of bicarbonate solutions, or massive transfusions (citrate load).

Respiratory Alkalosis and Metabolic Acidosis

Salicylate intoxication classically causes mixed metabolic acidosis and respiratory alkalosis, because salicylates cause anion gap metabolic acidosis and directly stimulate respiration. A more common cause of respiratory alkalosis and metabolic acidosis is gram-negative sepsis, which can stimulate the respiratory drive (respiratory alkalosis) and, if it progresses, may cause circulatory collapse (lactic acidosis).

Metabolic Acidosis and Metabolic Alkalosis

Mixed metabolic acidosis and metabolic alkalosis occurs commonly in diabetic ketoacidosis. In this setting, ketoacid production leads to a metabolic acidosis and the accompanying vomiting typically leads to a metabolic alkalosis. The Δ anion gap–Δ HCO_3^- relationship is helpful in diagnosing this condition (see Δ Anion Gap–Δ HCO_3^- below).

Δ Anion Gap–Δ HCO_3^-

In patients with metabolic acidosis, the Δ–Δ is used to infer the presence of either a superimposed non–anion gap metabolic acidosis or a metabolic alkalosis. The Δ anion gap–Δ HCO_3^- is calculated using the following formula, in which it is assumed that there is a 1:1 relationship between the unmeasured anions and "potential bicarbonate":

$$\Delta \text{ Anion Gap} - \Delta \text{ } HCO_3^-$$

where the Δ anion gap is calculated as follows:

Anion Gap – Non–Anion Gap (usually 12 meq/L)

and the Δ HCO_3^- is calculated as follows:

$$24 - [HCO_3^-]$$

If the Δ anion gap–Δ HCO_3^- is 0, only an anion gap metabolic acidosis is present, because the decrease in the bicarbonate equally matches the increase in the anion gap. Therefore, an unmeasured anion is present for every 1 meq/L decrease in the bicarbonate.

If the Δ anion gap–Δ HCO_3^- is >0, a concomitant metabolic alkalosis is present, because the change in bicarbonate is exceeded by the change in the anion gap. Therefore, the final bicarbonate level is higher than it should be if only a metabolic acidosis existed.

If the Δ anion gap–Δ HCO_3^- is <0, a concomitant non–anion gap metabolic acidosis is present, because the change in bicarbonate is greater than the change in the anion gap. Therefore, the anion gap component cannot fully explain the decrease in the bicarbonate.

Because of the wide range of the anion gap under normal circumstances, the values obtained when calculating the Δ anion gap–Δ HCO_3^- should be interpreted cautiously (1, 2, 3).

KEY POINTS

- In patients with a known primary acid–base disturbance, a mixed acid–base disorder should always be suspected if the pH is normal or the "compensation" has surpassed the normal pH.
- Mixed metabolic and respiratory acidosis occurs when the respiratory compensation is insufficient for the degree of decrease in bicarbonate.
- The presence of an increased anion gap despite normal serum bicarbonate levels should raise suspicion for mixed metabolic and respiratory acidosis.
- Non–anion gap metabolic acidosis and anion gap metabolic acidosis can coexist.
- Gram-negative sepsis is a common cause of respiratory alkalosis and metabolic acidosis.
- Mixed metabolic acidosis and metabolic alkalosis occurs commonly in diabetic ketoacidosis.
- In patients with metabolic acidosis, the Δ anion gap–Δ HCO_3^- is used to infer the presence of either a superimposed non–anion gap metabolic acidosis or a metabolic alkalosis.
- If the Δ anion gap–Δ HCO_3^- is 0, only an anion gap metabolic acidosis is present.
- If the Δ anion gap–Δ HCO_3^- is >0, an anion gap metabolic acidosis and a metabolic alkalosis is present.
- If the Δ anion gap–Δ HCO_3^- is <0, an anion gap metabolic acidosis and a non–anion gap metabolic acidosis is present.

References

1. **Halperin ML, Jungas RL.** Metabolic production and renal disposal of hydrogen ions. Kidney Int. 1983;24:709-13. [PMID: 6674669]
2. **Bushinsky DA, Coe FL, Katzenberg C, Szidon JP, Parks JH.** Arterial PCO2 in chronic metabolic acidosis. Kidney Int. 1982;22:311-4. [PMID: 6816981]
3. **Palmer BF, Alpern RJ.** Metabolic alkalosis. J Am Soc Nephrol. 1997;8:1462-9. [PMID: 9294840]

HYPERTENSION

RECENT ADVANCES

- Insulin resistance and hypertension
- ACE inhibitor use and diabetes
- Benefits of ambulatory blood pressure monitoring

Epidemiology

The most recent U.S. National Health and Nutrition Examination Survey determined that the prevalence rate of hypertension, characterized as blood pressure >140/90 mm Hg, is 31.3%. This rate represents an increase of approximately 30% since the last survey was performed between 1988 and 1994 (1). The prevalence of hypertension is higher in black patients and older individuals, particularly women. A total of 74% of patients >80 years of age have hypertension (2).

Hypertension is an important modifiable risk factor for stroke, myocardial infarction, renal failure, congestive heart failure, progressive atherosclerosis, and dementia. Since 1972, morbidity and mortality due to stroke, coronary heart disease, and heart failure have substantially decreased. However, suboptimal blood pressure control is the leading attributable risk factor for death worldwide.

Systolic pressure predicts cardiovascular events better than diastolic pressure. Isolated systolic hypertension, which is prevalent in older patients, is particularly hazardous. Systolic pressure increases with age in most individuals, but diastolic pressure increases until about age 50 years and then stabilizes or decreases with age.

A continuous, graded relationship exists between blood pressure and cardiovascular disease. The level and duration of hypertension and the presence of coexisting cardiovascular risk factors determine a patient's outcome. Treatment of hypertension clearly reduces stroke, coronary artery disease, congestive heart failure, and all-cause cardiovascular morbidity and mortality. However, only 59% of patients with hypertension are treated and only 34% have a blood pressure ≤140/90 mm Hg.

TABLE 23 Classification of Blood Pressure for Adults Age 18 Years and Older

Category	Systolic (mm Hg)		Diastolic (mm Hg)
Normal	<120	and	<80
Prehypertension*	120–139	or	80–89
Stage 1 hypertension	140–159	or	90–99
Stage 2 hypertension	≥160	or	≥100

*Guidelines from other societies, such as the British Hypertension Society and the World Health Organization/International Society of Hypertension, classify a systolic blood pressure of 120–139 mm Hg or a diastolic blood pressure of 80–89 mm Hg as high normal.

Modified with permission from the Joint National Committee on Prevention, Detection, Evaluation, and Treatment of High Blood Pressure.

Definition and Classification

Because of the linear relationship between blood pressure and vascular risk, the definition of hypertension is somewhat arbitrary. This definition is based on thresholds for which there is evidence that the benefits of lowering blood pressure outweigh the potential risks of treatment. Therefore, the level of blood pressure associated with minimal vascular risk characterizes optimal or normal blood pressure.

The most recent National High Blood Pressure Education Program guidelines by the seventh Joint National Committee on Prevention, Detection, Evaluation, and Treatment of High Blood Pressure (JNC 7) define normal blood pressure as <120/80 mm Hg (3). A systolic pressure of 120 to 139 mm Hg or a diastolic pressure of 80 to 89 mm Hg is characterized as "prehypertension," because even this range is associated with a clear increase in risk (4) (**Table 23**). This guideline differentiates between stage 1 (systolic pressure, 140–159 mm Hg; diastolic pressure, 90–99 mm Hg) and stage 2 (blood pressure ≥160/100 mm Hg) hypertension and recommends both lifestyle modification and pharmacotherapy for all patients with stage 2 or higher hypertension.

The JNC 7 classification of blood pressure categories differs from other societies. The British Hypertension Society, the European Guidelines on Hypertension, and the World Health Organization/International Society of Hypertension define optimal blood pressure as <120 mm Hg systolic and <80 mm Hg diastolic blood pressure. Normal is considered <130 mm Hg systolic and <85 mm Hg diastolic. Those with systolic pressure 130 to 139 mm Hg or diastolic pressure 85 to 89 mm Hg are considered to have "high-normal blood pressure" rather than "prehypertension." These guidelines agree with JNC 7 that high-normal blood pressure is associated with increased cardiovascular risk; however, they refrain from giving these individuals a disease label and emphasize, as does JNC 7, that lifestyle modification is appropriate for people with high-normal blood pressure to reduce their likelihood of developing hypertension and the need for drug therapy (5, 6). These guidelines also distinguish among three grades of hypertension and define isolated systolic hypertension as grade 1 (systolic pressure, 140–159 mm Hg) or grade 2 (systolic pressure ≥160 mm Hg).

Approximately 90% of patients with hypertension have primary or essential hypertension. The remainder have elevated blood pressure secondary to an underlying renal or endocrine condition. Essential hypertension represents a dysregulation of various renal, hormonal, and cellular processes in conjunction with environmental factors, such as diet and level of activity.

Pathophysiology

Genetics of Hypertension

Essential hypertension is a prototype of a polygenic, heterogeneous disorder. This condition is hereditary, and twin studies and segregation analyses have shown that between one third and one half of the variability of blood pressure is heritable. However, discovering genes that contribute to complex disorders such as essential hypertension is difficult. Most genes that help to regulate blood pressure exert only modest effects, and different genetic or environmental contexts strongly influence these effects.

Common genes with large effects on blood pressure have not yet been identified, despite several studies describing the results of whole-genome scanning. Strategies used to identify important genes involved in the pathogenesis of essential hypertension include linkage analysis and candidate gene approaches.

TABLE 24 Low-Renin, Hypertensive Syndromes Associated with Specific Genetic Mutations

Disorder	Inheritance/Mutation	Clinical Features	Treatment
Liddle's syndrome	AD; gain of function of epithelial sodium channel	Elevated BP, hypokalemic metabolic alkalosis, low renin, low aldosterone	Thiazides, triamterene
Corticosteroid-remediable hyperaldosteronism	AD; chimeric gene containing promoter-regulatory region of 11 β-hydroxylase and structural region of aldosterone synthase resulting in regulation of aldosterone secretion by ACTH	Elevated BP, hypokalemic metabolic alkalosis, low renin, high aldosterone	Aldosterone blockade, corticosteroids
Apparent mineralocorticoid excess	Autosomal recessive; mutation in renal isoform of 11 β-hydroxysteroid dehydrogenase resulting in activation of mineralocorticoid receptor by cortisol (acquired form caused by excess licorice ingestion)	Elevated BP, younger age at presentation, hypokalemic metabolic alkalosis, low renin, low aldosterone	Thiazides, aldosterone blockade
Type 2 pseudohypo-aldosteronism (Gordon's syndrome)	AD; mutations in WNK kinases 1 and 4	Elevated BP, hyperkalemia, hyperchloremic metabolic acidosis, low renin, low aldosterone	Thiazides
Mineralocorticoid receptor activation	Mutation at codon 819 in mineralocorticoid receptor	Elevated BP, younger age, low renin, low aldosterone, mineralocorticoid receptor activation by steroids such as progesterone; exacerbation in pregnancy	Thiazides

BP = blood pressure; AD = autosomal dominant; ACTH = adrenocorticotropic hormone

Genes involved in the following have been studied using the candidate gene method: renal sodium handling, the renin–angiotensin system (angiotensin-converting enzyme [ACE] gene, angiotensinogen gene), G protein signaling, the cytoskeleton protein α-adducin, endothelial cell products, and adrenoreceptor subtypes. Although none of these genes have been shown to have a major effect on blood pressure variability, several studies have shown a modest effect of polymorphisms in these genes on blood pressure.

In the last decade, significant progress has occurred in the identification of genes responsible for several monogenic forms of hypertension. These conditions tend to present early in life, often with severe (stage 2) hypertension, but variable penetrance also may occur. These disorders are very rare, and the causative mutations do not explain the phenotype of essential hypertension. However, their discovery has led to a greater understanding of the physiology of elevated blood pressure. Moreover, almost all of these mutations cause alterations in renal sodium handling, thus reaffirming the kidney's importance in the pathogenesis of hypertension (**Table 24**). In addition to these low-renin, salt-sensitive hypertensive syndromes, at least five different mutations are known to be associated with pheochromocytoma (7).

The Kidney in Essential Hypertension

Impaired renal sodium excretion characterizes essential hypertension. There are multiple causes of impaired renal sodium excretion in essential hypertension, including genetic alterations in proteins involved in sodium transport, obesity,

and various metabolic and neurohormonal factors that regulate adrenergic tone and endothelial function. Stimulation of the renal sympathetic nerves and activation of the renin–angiotensin system also contribute to sodium retention, and both pathways contribute to the pathogenesis of essential hypertension.

Insulin Resistance and Essential Hypertension

As many as 25% to 47% of patients with essential hypertension may be insulin resistant. The metabolic syndrome is characterized by the concomitant presence of obesity, dyslipidemia, impaired glucose tolerance, and hypertension. Independent of body mass index or body fat distribution, patients with essential hypertension have higher fasting and postprandial insulin levels and greater reductions in insulin sensitivity compared with healthy normotensive patients. These findings suggest a direct correlation between blood pressure and plasma insulin levels, which indicates that insulin may be involved in the pathogenesis of essential hypertension.

The rise in plasma insulin levels is associated with increased sympathetic nervous system activity. This activity stimulates renal sodium reabsorption, which causes volume expansion and blood pressure elevation. Insulin resistance/hyperinsulinemia and visceral obesity also are associated with impaired endothelial function, which contributes to the development of atherosclerosis and cardiovascular disease.

Strategies to improve insulin resistance, such as aerobic exercise and treatment with thiazolidinediones and metformin, have been shown to lower blood pressure (8). These findings all indicate that insulin resistance and hypertension are causally related and that the treatment of either improves the other.

Although insulin resistance most likely helps to mediate obesity-related hypertension, additional mechanisms may be involved. These mechanisms include increased aldosterone levels and increased sympathetic activity, both of which cause increased renal sodium reabsorption and impaired pressure natriuresis. The hormone leptin also is increased in obese patients and may mediate increased sympathetic activity contributing to elevated blood pressure.

Obesity is related to obstructive sleep apnea, which may induce hypertension. The primary underlying mechanism is sympathetic activation triggered by apneic episodes. The cardiovascular effects of sleep apnea present early in the disease course, and young patients are particularly susceptible to its deleterious effect. Blood pressure profiles in these patients show higher diastolic pressures and a failure of blood pressure to decrease during sleep (nocturnal dipping). The renin–angiotensin axis, in conjunction with other vasoactive hormones, adds to the sympathetic activation in elevating blood pressure in sleep apnea. Treatment of sleep apnea using positive airway pressure, palatonasal surgery, and weight reduction corrects the associated hypertension, which may be resistant to conventional antihypertensive therapy.

KEY POINTS

- Impaired renal sodium excretion characterizes essential hypertension.
- Strategies to improve insulin resistance, such as aerobic exercise and treatment with thiazolidinediones and metformin, have been shown to lower blood pressure.
- Patients with sleep apnea have higher diastolic blood pressures and a failure of blood pressure to decrease with sleep.

Evaluation of Hypertension

Evaluation is indicated to identify known causes of hypertension, assess cardiovascular risk factors, and determine whether target organ damage or existing cardiovascular disease is present.

Measurement

Office blood pressure measurement remains the primary method of blood pressure evaluation in clinical practice. Several alternatives to the conventional Riva-Rocci/Korotkoff technique of blood pressure measurement exist. Various blood pressure measurement tools are available, including aneroid, electronic, and mercury devices, and guidelines provide protocols to evaluate the accuracy of these devices (9).

Ambulatory or home blood pressure monitoring, which measures blood pressure multiple times during a 24-hour period, also may be useful. Ambulatory blood pressure measurement (ABPM) shows blood pressure during the patient's usual daily activities and provides a profile of blood pressure away from the medical environment. This method may identify isolated clinic or white coat hypertension (office blood pressure >140/90 mm Hg; normal ambulatory pressure <135/85 mm Hg) and prevent unnecessary treatment.

White coat hypertension, present in 10% to 15% of patients with elevated office blood pressures, is associated with lower cardiovascular risk than sustained hypertension but may be a precursor to sustained hypertension and warrants monitoring. Although hypertension guidelines agree on the definition of white coat hypertension and recommend that "suspected" white coat hypertension is an indication for ABPM, there is no clear consensus regarding the specific criteria that should prompt evaluation for this condition. Therefore, the clinician must decide when evaluation for this condition is appropriate. The following factors may increase the probability of white coat hypertension: 1) office systolic pressure of 140 to 159 mm Hg or diastolic pressure of 90 to 99 mm Hg; 2) female sex; 3) not smoking cigarettes; 4) hypertension of recent onset; 5) a limited number of blood pressure measurements in the office; and 6) normal left ventricular mass.

ABPM also identifies abnormalities in the normal circadian rhythm, particularly failure of the blood pressure to decrease appropriately (10%–20%) during sleep, which has been associated with greater target organ damage and long-term cardiovascular risk. Recent studies suggest that ABPM correlates better with cardiovascular morbidity compared with office blood pressure measurement (10). However, until very recently, clinic blood pressure measurements have determined the benefits of antihypertensive treatment in most clinical trials.

In addition to identifying white coat hypertension, ABPM helps to evaluate patients with resistant hypertension (persistent hypertension despite full-dose therapy with three or more drugs, including a diuretic), in whom there may be a white coat effect (11). ABPM also may identify masked hypertension, characterized by a normal clinic blood pressure and a high ambulatory blood pressure (12). The clinic blood pressure measurement in these patients may underestimate the risk for cardiovascular events. This condition is the reverse of white coat hypertension and should be suspected when home blood pressure is higher than clinic blood pressure.

In elderly patients, ABPM also helps to document hypotensive episodes and avoid overtreatment. Home blood pressure monitoring provides additional blood pressure readings but has not been evaluated as comprehensively as ABPM.

Physical Examination and Laboratory Evaluation

A careful history and physical examination are indicated for all patients with hypertension and should include 1) measurement of all vital signs; 2) examination of optic fundi; 3) body mass index calculation; 4) auscultation of major blood vessels to identify bruits; 5) careful heart and lung examination; 6) examination of the abdomen for masses; 7) evaluation of extremities for edema and circulatory abnormalities; and 8) neurologic examination. Laboratory testing to screen for secondary causes and exclude comorbidity should include urinalysis, complete blood count, serum chemistry studies, and a 12-lead electrocardiogram. Essential or primary hypertension is the diagnosis in >90% of patients with hypertension.

KEY POINT

- **Ambulatory blood pressure monitoring may identify white coat hypertension and prevent unnecessary treatment.**

Identifiable Causes of Hypertension (Secondary Hypertension)

Patients with severe or resistant hypertension or who develop hypertension at young (<30 years) or older (>55 years) ages are more likely to have secondary hypertension. This condition is particularly likely if screening laboratory studies are abnormal (**Table 25**).

Renal Disease

Renal disease is the most common cause of secondary hypertension. Chronic and end-stage kidney disease are associated with hypertension in the majority of patients. Routine chemistry studies and urinalysis identify most cases of parenchymal renal disease. Renal ultrasonography may be indicated to diagnose patients with polycystic kidney disease. This study also should be considered in patients with a history of kidney failure in first-degree relatives or who have palpable abdominal masses.

Adrenal Hypertension: Primary Aldosteronism

Hypertension due to excess aldosterone should be considered in the setting of unprovoked hypokalemia and metabolic alkalosis or resistant hypertension. Primary hyperaldosteronism may be caused by a solitary autonomously functioning adrenal adenoma (aldosterone-producing adenoma) or idiopathic hyperaldosteronism caused by bilateral adrenal hyperplasia.

Hypertensive syndromes associated with hyperaldosteronism that occur less frequently include unilateral adrenal hyperplasia and glucocorticoid-remediable hyperaldosteronism. Hypokalemia is variably present, more often in the setting of adrenal adenoma.

An increased aldosterone–renin ratio (ARR) (ratio of plasma aldosterone concentration to plasma renin activity) accompanied by a plasma aldosterone level >15 ng/dL in

TABLE 25	Identifiable Causes of Hypertension
Chronic kidney disease
Coarctation of the aorta
Genetic mutations
Cushing's syndrome and corticosteroid excess
Obstructive uropathy
Pheochromocytoma
Primary aldosteronism and other mineralocorticoid excess states
Renovascular hypertension
Sleep apnea
Thyroid or parathyroid disease
Drug induced*
Alcohol

* Oral contraceptives, sympathomimetics, nonsteroidal anti-inflammatory drugs, erythropoietin, calcineurin inhibitors (cyclosporine, tacrolimus).

Modified with permission from Chobanian AV, Bakris GL, Black HR, Cushman WC, Green LA, Izzo JL Jr., et al. Seventh report of the Joint National Committee on Prevention, Detection, Evaluation, and Treatment of High Blood Pressure. Hypertension. 2003;42:1206-52. PMID: 14656957

patients who previously have been volume expanded with intravenous or oral salt loading is the best screen for primary aldosteronism. A 24-hour urine collection for aldosterone may be performed for confirmation; findings >12 µg/24 h establish the diagnosis. In healthy patients, the ARR ranges from 2 to 17 with a mean of 5.5. A recent study concluded that patients with an ARR <23.6 have an extremely low likelihood of primary hyperaldosteronism and that patients later diagnosed with aldosterone-producing adenoma or idiopathic hyperaldosteronism usually have an ARR >25 to 34 (13).

Recent reports of patients with hypertension screened using the ARR have suggested that primary aldosteronism is much more prevalent than previously recognized. In some studies, patients with hypertension reportedly had a prevalence of primary aldosteronism of 20% (14). However, this screening test may have a high rate of false-positive results, particularly in patients with very low plasma renin activity and only modestly elevated or even normal aldosterone levels (15). Therefore, these findings should be confirmed by demonstration of nonsuppressible aldosterone secretion.

Even in the absence of adrenal gland pathology, an elevated ARR in the setting of low plasma renin activity identifies patients who may benefit from therapy with aldosterone blockade. In patients with hyperaldosteronism and a strongly positive family history, glucocorticoid-remediable hyperaldosteronism should be considered.

CT scanning with thin cuts through the adrenal glands is indicated for patients with evidence of hyperaldosteronism. Removal of solitary adrenal adenomas may cure hypertension in carefully selected patients. Surgical removal of the adrenal gland is reasonable in patients <40 years of age, if there is biochemical evidence of hyperaldosteronism and radiographic demonstration of unilateral adrenal pathology.

Older patients are more likely to have bilateral adrenal hyperplasia that may not be apparent on CT. Therefore, adrenal vein sampling to document the presence of unilateral aldosterone secretion when a nodule is identified radiographically may be helpful. If unilateral aldosterone secretion with contralateral suppression is documented, then laparoscopic removal of the adrenal gland is recommended; cure rates for this procedure range from 60% to 70%.

Adrenal vein sampling also is useful when biochemical findings are consistent with primary aldosteronism but results of CT scanning are negative. Adenomas associated with Conn's syndrome are often <1 cm in diameter; therefore, false-negative CT scan findings are not unusual. If adrenal vein sampling shows unilateral hypersecretion, surgery should be considered.

In the presence of bilateral adrenal hyperplasia, aldosterone blockade is indicated. Dihydropyridine calcium antagonists also may effectively lower blood pressure in patients with primary aldosteronism, but additional therapy is needed to correct hypokalemia.

Pheochromocytomas

Pathology and Pathogenesis

Pheochromocytomas are chromaffin cell tumors of the adrenal medulla or extra-adrenal paraganglia that cause symptoms attributable to excess adrenaline production, including hypertension, autonomic disturbances, and feelings of heightened anxiety. Pheochromocytomas occur in only approximately 0.5% of patients evaluated because of hypertension and suggestive symptoms. Hypertension in patients with pheochromocytomas may be sustained or paroxysmal and may be accompanied by headache, sweating, and palpitations. Some affected patients may have normal blood pressure, and those with predominantly epinephrine-secreting tumors may have low blood pressure.

Pheochromocytomas may lead to serious complications, including myocardial infarction, stroke, and cardiovascular collapse. Surgical removal is curative in up to 90% of patients with this condition; therefore, diagnosis is important. Familial pheochromocytoma occurs in multiple endocrine neoplasia type II, von Hippel–Lindau disease, neurofibromatosis, and familial carotid body tumors and may be more common than previously thought. Genetic testing may detect these forms of pheochromocytoma even in asymptomatic individuals.

Diagnosis

Most pheochromocytomas occur sporadically; therefore, biochemical testing that detects excessive catecholamine production is indicated to establish a diagnosis. However, this approach is not definitive, because other conditions may be associated with excess catecholamine production and

sometimes pheochromocytomas do not secrete sufficient catecholamines to produce positive test results.

Recent evidence suggests that measurement of plasma free metanephrines has a higher sensitivity and specificity than measurement of plasma or urinary catecholamines, and urinary metanephrine and vanillymandelic acid. In most cases of pheochromocytoma, the plasma free metanephrine levels are elevated two- to fourfold. If these levels are only minimally elevated, additional biochemical testing, including repeat measurements of plasma metanephrines and measurement of plasma catecholamines, is indicated.

Clonidine suppression and glucagon stimulation testing may have increased specificity for pheochromocytoma but should be performed only by experienced clinicians. Imaging studies are indicated for patients with diagnostic or suggestive biochemical testing findings. CT is highly sensitive and specific for detecting adrenal pheochromocytoma. MRI has a lower sensitivity for adrenal tumors but is superior at detecting extra-adrenal pheochromocytomas.

Metaiodobenzylguanidine scanning has high specificity, is helpful in diagnosing extra-adrenal tumors, and often is performed to confirm positive CT or MRI findings. However, this test is not recommended as an initial imaging study.

Treatment

Surgical excision with appropriate preoperative blockade of catecholamine synthesis to prevent massive outpouring of catecholamines during surgery is indicated to treat pheochromocytoma. Administration of phenoxybenzamine, an α-adrenoreceptor blocker, is indicated; the subsequent addition of a β-blocker may oppose the reflex tachycardia associated with α-blockade. β-Blockade alone may exacerbate the effects of catecholamines and is contraindicated.

α-Methyl tyrosine inhibits catecholamine synthesis, reduces tumor stores of catecholamines, and is associated with better blood pressure control during surgery.

Pharmacologic treatment including α- and β-blockade, α-methyl tyrosine inhibition, and volume expansion should be initiated 10 to 14 days before surgery. A total of 27% to 40% of patients may have residual hypertension after tumor removal.

Renovascular Hypertension

Renovascular hypertension occurs in the setting of hemodynamically significant unilateral or bilateral renal artery stenosis. Hypertension is a consequence of stimulation of the renin–angiotensin system and, in patients with bilateral disease, excess plasma volume due to sodium retention.

Renovascular hypertension due to fibromuscular disease of the renal arteries usually presents in patients <35 years of age. Azotemia is rarely present. Atherosclerotic renovascular disease is more common in older patients and is frequently associated with vascular disease in other vessels (carotid or coronary arteries and peripheral vessels). Azotemia is often observed in patients with atherosclerotic renovascular hypertension. Patients with renovascular disease and azotemia may have ischemic nephropathy, which is attributed to the combined effects of nephrosclerosis, prolonged ischemia, and atheroembolic disease.

The gold standard for the diagnosis of renal artery stenosis is angiography, which may be performed using small amounts of contrast using digital subtraction techniques. Magnetic resonance angiography and computed tomographic angiography are less invasive. However, a recent multicenter study of >350 subjects who underwent digital subtraction, magnetic resonance, and computed tomographic angiography demonstrated that magnetic resonance angiography and computed tomographic angiography are not reproducible or sensitive enough to exclude renal artery stenosis in patients with hypertension (16).

Establishing a causal relationship between an anatomic lesion and hypertension or renal insufficiency may be difficult. Renal artery revascularization by either angioplasty with or without stenting or renal artery bypass will ameliorate true renovascular hypertension. However, these procedures are associated with technical difficulties and risks, including bleeding, vessel dissection, branch occlusion, atheroembolic renal failure, myocardial infarction, and stroke. In young patients with fibromuscular dysplasia, attributing hypertension to the presence of characteristic renal artery lesions usually is reasonable. In this setting, revascularization is almost always indicated to ameliorate or cure hypertension.

Patients with atherosclerotic renal artery stenosis may have coexistent essential hypertension, confounding diagnosis as well as treatment. In patients with atherosclerotic renal artery stenosis, certain clinical and laboratory features have been associated with improvement of blood pressure and/or renal function after revascularization (**Table 26**).

No single study has been demonstrated to be uniformly sensitive or specific for identifying reversible renovascular hypertension. The difficulty in determining the reversibility of hypertension before intervention may explain why, in observational as well as clinical trials, angioplasty rarely cures hypertension associated with atherosclerotic renal artery stenosis and improves blood pressure control in only 30% to 50% of affected patients (17–19).

Currently available antihypertensive therapy effectively controls blood pressure in many patients with atherosclerotic renovascular hypertension. Despite limited clinical trial data addressing the optimum treatment of atherosclerotic renovascular hypertension, renal revascularization should be considered when blood pressure cannot be adequately controlled.

Additional potential indications for renal artery revascularization include prevention of renal function deterioration and of renal artery occlusion. Ischemic nephropathy (renal function impairment beyond occlusive disease of the main renal arteries) has been reported to improve after renal revas-

TABLE 26 Features Associated with Improved Blood Pressure and/or Renal Function after Vascularization in Patients with Atherosclerotic Renal Artery Stenosis
Sudden acceleration of hypertension or renal insufficiency
Size discrepancy of kidneys
Renal resistive index <0.8 on ultrasonography*
Decrease in GFR determined by radionuclide scanning
Decrease in creatinine after oral captopril administration
Lateralization of renin secretion determined by renal vein renin sampling
Increased gradient across a stenosis demonstrated at the time of renal angiography

GFR = glomerular filtration rate

*The renal resistive index is determined by Doppler studies of the renal parenchymal vessels and is based on the following formula:

Peak Systolic Velocity – End Diastolic Velocity/Peak Systolic Velocity

cularization in 25% to 39% of affected patients. However, 19% to 25% of these patients experience a significant loss of kidney function, which may be associated with atheroemboli (20–22).

Renal artery stenosis also may progress to total occlusion. Prospective data suggest that progression is slow and that risk for total occlusion is related to the severity of the initial lesion and the patient's systolic blood pressure level.

Additional Causes of Secondary Hypertension

Additional causes of secondary hypertension include endocrine disorders and exogenous substances (Table 24). Suspicion for additional causes should be raised in the setting of atypical features and resistance to therapy.

KEY POINTS

- Patients with severe or resistant hypertension or who develop hypertension at <30 or >55 years of age are more likely to have secondary hypertension.

- Renal disease is the most common cause of secondary hypertension.

- Hyperaldosteronism may cause unprovoked hypokalemia and metabolic alkalosis or resistant hypertension.

- Hypertension associated with pheochromocytomas may be accompanied by headache, sweating, and palpitations.

- Surgical removal of pheochromocytomas is curative in up to 90% of affected patients.

- Measurement of plasma free metanephrines has a high specificity and sensitivity for pheochromocytoma.

- Angiography is the gold standard for diagnosing renal artery stenosis.

Treatment of Hypertension

The goal of hypertension treatment is to prevent cardiovascular morbidity and mortality by lowering blood pressure and modifying coexisting cardiovascular risk factors.

Lifestyle Modifications

Lifestyle modifications are recommended for all patients with hypertension, including prehypertension (**Table 27**). The Dietary Approaches to Stop Hypertension (DASH) study showed that 8 weeks of a diet of fruits, vegetables, low-fat dairy products, whole grains, poultry, fish, and nuts, along with a reduction in fats, red meat, and sweets, caused an 11.4-mm Hg decrease in systolic pressure and a 5.5-mm Hg decrease in diastolic pressure. In addition, patients using the DASH diet who consumed <100 mmol/d of sodium had a systolic pressure 3 mm Hg and a diastolic pressure 1.6 mm Hg less than those who consumed high amounts of sodium (23).

In patients with hypertension, sodium restriction to 2 g/d lowers systolic pressure by 3.7 mm Hg to 4.8 mm Hg and diastolic pressure by 0.9 mm Hg to 2.5 mm Hg. However, these values are population means and variability in individual responsiveness exists. Salt sensitivity is common in elderly patients with hypertension, and moderate sodium restriction is safe and effective in this population. The consensus of hypertension guidelines states that a modestly low-sodium diet (2–2.4 g/d) confers significant public health benefits without harm to the individual.

Weight reduction in a patient whose weight is 10% above ideal body weight lowers blood pressure by an average of 5 mm Hg to 7 mm Hg. Alcohol consumption should be limited to two drinks daily for men and one for women, because excess amounts of alcohol may contribute to hypertension and resistance to antihypertensive medications. Regular aerobic exercise also modestly decreases blood pressure.

Sustaining lifestyle modifications can be problematic. Long-term follow-up of patients treated with lifestyle modification alone suggests that these strategies are difficult to maintain. Most clinical trials assessing lifestyle modifications have been underpowered or of insufficient duration to evaluate their impact on major cardiovascular outcomes. However, these interventions are safe and inexpensive and therefore should be encouraged. When combined with drug therapy, lifestyle modifications may result in better blood pressure control and improved quality of life.

Pharmacologic Therapy

The benefits of lowering blood pressure have been demonstrated in all stages of hypertension. Dramatic reductions in mortality were first demonstrated after short-term treatment of malignant hypertension. Subsequent trials studying stages 1 and 2 hypertension showed that lowering systolic pressure by 10 mm Hg to 12 mm Hg and diastolic pressure by 5 mm Hg to 6 mm Hg reduces the relative risk of stroke by 40%,

TABLE 27 Lifestyle Modifications for Hypertension Prevention and Management

Maintain ideal body weight (1.6/1.1 mm Hg blood pressure reduction for 1 kg weight loss)
Increase aerobic physical activity (30–45 minutes most days of the week; may reduce BP by as much as 13/8 mm Hg)
Eat a diet including abundant fruits and vegetables, low-fat dairy products, and reduced saturated and total fat (may lower BP by as much as 11.4/5.5 mm Hg after 8 weeks)
Reduce sodium intake to <100 mmol/d (2.4 g sodium or 6 g sodium chloride; may lower BP by 3.7–4.8/0.9–2.5 mm Hg)
Limit alcohol intake to two drinks daily for men and one for women
Stop smoking

BP = blood pressure

coronary disease by 16%, and overall cardiovascular mortality by 20% (24).

Absolute cardiovascular risk, determined by the synergistic effect of all cardiovascular risk factors present, varies greatly depending on age, previous symptomatic cardiovascular disease, the presence of left ventricular hypertrophy and diabetes mellitus, renal function, cigarette smoking, gender, and lipid levels. A 50-year-old man with a blood pressure of 160/95 mm Hg has a 5-year risk for a major cardiovascular event of 2.5% to 5%; the risk doubles if this same patient has high cholesterol levels and triples if he also smokes cigarettes (25). The reductions in absolute risk are greater and the number needed to treat is smaller for individuals with higher blood pressure and multiple cardiovascular risk factors.

Initiation of drug therapy is based on a combined assessment of blood pressure level and absolute risk for cardiovascular disease (defined as the rate of stroke, heart attack, or cardiovascular death for a particular individual). The JNC guidelines previously recommended that patients with stage 1 hypertension with no other risk factors could be treated with lifestyle modifications alone for up to 1 year before instituting pharmacologic therapy to reach blood pressure targets. However, the most recent JNC 7 guidelines stress achieving appropriate blood pressure targets for all patients in a timely fashion. The British Hypertension Society Guidelines recommend institution of drug treatment for all patients with a sustained blood pressure ≥160/100 mm Hg and those with a systolic pressure of 140 mm Hg to 159 mm Hg or a diastolic pressure of 90 to 99 mm Hg who have complications of hypertension, target organ damage, or diabetes or if there is an estimated 10-year risk for cardiovascular disease of ≥20% despite lifestyle modifications. Similar to the JNC guidelines, the World Health Organization/International Society of Hypertension guidelines emphasize achieving blood pressure targets in all patients, even those with low overall cardiovascular risk.

TABLE 28 Compelling Indications, Contraindications, and Side Effects for Antihypertensive Drugs

Class of Drug	Compelling Indications	Contraindications	Side Effects
Diuretics	Heart failure; advanced age; systolic hypertension	Gout	Hypokalemia; hyperuricemia; glucose intolerance; hypercalcemia; hyperlipidemia; hyponatremia; impotence
β-Blockers	Angina; heart failure; postmyocardial infarction; tachyarrhythmias; migraine	Asthma and COPD; heart block	Bronchospasm; bradycardia; heart failure; impaired peripheral circulation; insomnia; fatigue, decreased exercise tolerance; hypertriglyceridemia
ACE inhibitors	Heart failure; left ventricular dysfunction; postmyocardial infarction; diabetic nephropathy; proteinuria	Pregnancy; hyperkalemia	Cough; angioedema; hyperkalemia; rash; loss of taste; leukopenia
Calcium antagonists	Advanced age; systolic hypertension; cyclosporine-induced hypertension; angina, coronary heart disease	Heart block (verapamil, diltiazem)	Headache; flushing; gingival hyperplasia; edema; constipation
α-Blockers	Prostatic hypertrophy	Orthostatic hypotension	Headache; drowsiness; fatigue; weakness; postural hypotension
Angiotensin II antagonists	ACE inhibitor cough; diabetic nephropathy; heart failure	Pregnancy; bilateral renal artery stenosis; hyperkalemia	Angioedema (rare); hyperkalemia

ACE = angiotensin-converting enzyme; COPD = chronic obstructive pulmonary disease

The goal of therapy is to reduce blood pressure to <140/90 mm Hg in all patients and to <130/80 mm Hg in those with diabetes or renal disease. Many experts believe that these treatment targets have not been low enough, because cardiovascular risk remains higher in treated patients with hypertension compared with normotensive patients. Recent studies suggest that more intensive blood pressure reduction is safe and beneficial, but few data are available to support lower targets.

In the Hypertension Optimal Treatment (HOT) trial, a blood pressure of 138.5/82.6 mm Hg was associated with the lowest risk for major cardiovascular events in subjects without diabetes; a blood pressure of 138.5/86.5 mm Hg was associated with the lowest risk for cardiovascular mortality (26). Additional decreases in blood pressure did not reduce events in patients without diabetes but were not harmful. In patients with diabetes, the lowest rates of major cardiovascular events and cardiovascular deaths were achieved with the lowest blood pressure, thus providing the rationale for current U.S. guidelines recommending a target blood pressure of ≤130/80 mm Hg in this group.

Lowering blood pressure slows renal disease progression. Based on the results of clinical trials, national guidelines such as JNC 7 recommend that the target blood pressure for patients with renal disease and proteinuria be ≤130/80 mm Hg for renal as well as cardiovascular protection, because the risk for cardiovascular events is increased in patients with chronic kidney disease compared with patients with essential hypertension.

Blood pressure in patients during or after an acute stroke should be lowered cautiously. Excessive lowering of blood pressure traditionally has been avoided to prevent a reduction in cerebral perfusion. Although there are no large clinical trials that address this issue, the American Stroke Association recommends lowering blood pressure by about 10% to 15%, if systolic pressure is >220 mm Hg or diastolic pressure is >120 mm Hg.

In elderly patients, a systolic pressure <160 mm Hg is associated with a decrease in cardiovascular morbidity and mortality. Whether a systolic pressure <140 mm Hg provides additional protection is uncertain.

Most antihypertensive agents reduce blood pressure by 10% to 15%. Monotherapy is effective in about 40% of unselected patients. More than one drug often is needed to treat patients with stage 2 or higher hypertension. Clinical trials have shown that diuretics, β-blockers, ACE inhibitors, angiotensin receptor blockers (ARBs), and calcium channel blockers reduce the complications of hypertension.

Patient characteristics, including comorbid conditions, age, race, and history of efficacy and adverse reactions to previously used drugs, determine the most appropriate initial therapy (**Table 28**). For example, in patients with a history of diabetic nephropathy or other proteinuric renal diseases, the treatment regimen should include an ACE inhibitor or an ARB. However, the primary goal of antihypertensive therapy is lowering blood pressure to the appropriate target. Many large trials have attempted to demonstrate the superiority of one antihypertensive agent over another in preventing adverse cardiovascular outcomes. However, most analyses conclude that differences in blood pressure may cause the differences in cardiovascular outcomes attributed to treatment with different drugs.

Diuretics

JNC 7 emphasizes the use of diuretics as first-line agents in the general population based on the results of numerous clinical trials conducted over a span of decades. Most recently, the Antihypertensive and Lipid-Lowering Treatment To Prevent Heart Attack Trial (ALLHAT) demonstrated in 40,000 individuals >55 years of age (35% black, 19% Hispanic) that diuretic-based therapy was equivalent to treatment regimens based on either a dihydropyridine calcium antagonist or an ACE inhibitor in preventing coronary heart disease (27).

Thiazide diuretics such as hydrochlorothiazide and chlorthalidone are often effective in doses as low as 12.5 mg/d to 25 mg/d. These low doses of these agents are well tolerated, and the associated metabolic side effects (insulin resistance, hyperglycemia, hyperuricemia, hypokalemia, hyponatremia, hyperlipidemia) are minimized. Diuretics are particularly effective in individuals with salt-sensitive hypertension, such as elderly and black patients.

The Perindopril Protection against Recurrent Stroke Study (PROGRESS) demonstrated that the addition of a diuretic to ACE inhibitor therapy, but not ACE inhibitor therapy alone, reduced recurrent stroke by 43%. However, several large clinical trials and a meta-analysis of >60,000 patients have demonstrated that, compared with other agents (particularly angiotensin receptor antagonists), long-term use of diuretics is associated with an increased risk for type 2 diabetes. Therefore, these agents should be used carefully in younger patients who are likely to need many years of therapy, particularly if these patients have risk factors for diabetes (28).

Higher doses of diuretics are associated with an increased risk for sexual dysfunction and hypokalemia-associated cardiac arrhythmias. Aldosterone antagonists also are effective antihypertensive agents, and the addition of low doses of these agents to standard therapy improves blood pressure control in resistant hypertension. Combination therapy with these agents and thiazides may increase antihypertensive efficacy and minimize hypokalemia. Loop diuretics such as furosemide have a shorter duration of action than thiazides, should be given twice daily, and are primarily used in patients with renal insufficiency in whom thiazides may not be effective.

β-Blockers

β-Blockers reduce blood pressure by decreasing cardiac output, heart rate, and renal renin secretion. All β-blockers antagonize β_1 receptors competitively but vary in their degree of β_2-receptor blockade in extracardiac tissue. β-Blockers with β_1 selectivity (selective β-blockers), such as atenolol or metoprolol, do not have increased efficacy in lowering blood pressure, but because of the lesser degrees of β_2 blockade may be associated with less bronchoconstriction and less severe disturbances in lipid and carbohydrate metabolism. β-Blockers with α-blocking properties such as carvedilol or labetalol have additional vasodilatory effects caused by selective α_1-receptor blockade.

β-Blockers may be more effective in younger patients. These agents are contraindicated in patients with asthma, heart block, or depression and should be used with caution in patients with diabetes who use insulin. β-Blockers may be associated with insulin resistance, lipid abnormalities, decreased exercise capacity, and sexual dysfunction.

Angiotensin-Converting Enzyme Inhibitors

ACE inhibitors block the conversion of angiotensin I to angiotensin II, causing lower angiotensin II and aldosterone levels. These agents increase bradykinin levels and decrease sympathetic nervous system activity, which may help to lower blood pressure. ACE inhibitors also have been shown to reduce fibrosis and inflammation, but whether these properties contribute to better clinical outcomes is uncertain.

ACE inhibitors are effective in a wide variety of clinical situations and are well tolerated. They are especially indicated to treat hypertension in patients with diabetes mellitus, renal disease, and congestive heart failure and other cardiovascular diseases. Compared with diuretics, β-blockers, and placebo, ACE inhibitors may help to improve insulin sensitivity.

The most common adverse effect associated with ACE inhibitors is cough, occurring in as many as 12% of treated individuals. These agents also may induce angioedema, hyperkalemia, and azotemia. ACE inhibitors are contraindicated in pregnancy because of adverse effects on fetal renal function and fetal death.

Angiotensin Receptor Blockers

ARBs block the effects of angiotensin II at the angiotensin receptor subtype 1, causing a decrease in peripheral resistance. These agents are indicated in similar clinical settings as ACE inhibitors, including heart failure and renal disease. Generally, their effects are comparable to ACE inhibitors.

ARBs have been shown to slow progression of renal disease in patients with type 2 diabetes. These agents are extremely well tolerated and are considerably less commonly associated with cough compared with ACE inhibitors. ARBs also have been associated with reduced incidence of new-onset diabetes, which may be related to their ability to stimulate peroxisome proliferator–activated receptor-γ and thus improve insulin sensitivity. ARBs also are contraindicated in pregnancy.

Calcium Antagonists

Calcium antagonists relax vascular smooth muscle and cause vasodilation. Unlike vasodilators such as hydralazine and minoxidil, these agents do not cause sodium retention and may be used effectively without concomitant diuretic therapy.

Dihydropyridine calcium antagonists, particularly those that have a relatively short onset of action and half life, may increase sympathetic tone. Nondihydropyridine calcium antagonists, such as verapamil and diltiazem, depress cardiac contractility and inhibit atrioventricular conduction.

Compared with placebo, calcium antagonists have been shown to reduce stroke, major cardiovascular events, and cardiovascular death, particularly in the elderly. Large clinical trials show that these agents are effective and safe and reduce cardiovascular morbidity and mortality at least as well as ARBs, ACE inhibitors, β-blockers, and diuretics (ALLHAT).

Calcium antagonists alone most likely are not as renoprotective as ACE inhibitors. However, when used in conjunction with ACE inhibitors or angiotensin receptor antagonists, calcium antagonists effectively help to decrease blood pressure and achieve blood pressure targets without jeopardizing renal protection in patients with renal disease and/or proteinuria.

The findings of larger clinical trials such as ALLHAT and Valsartan Antihypertensive Long-term Use Evaluation (VALUE) have not substantiated earlier concerns regarding an association between adverse cardiovascular outcomes and dihydropyridine calcium antagonists. Adverse effects associated with dihydropyridine calcium antagonists include headache, constipation, and dependent edema, which is caused by localized vasodilation, not fluid retention.

Additional Agents

Centrally acting α-agonists are used less frequently in patients with essential hypertension because of troublesome side effects, including dry mouth and postural hypotension. Methyldopa continues to be widely used in pregnancy because of its proven safety.

Direct-acting vasodilators such as minoxidil are reserved for patients with refractory hypertension, whereas hydralazine is effective in patients with heart failure. These agents are associated with fluid retention and tachycardia, and concomitant diuretic and β-blocker therapy usually is indicated.

Combination Therapy

Combining drugs with complementary mechanisms may lower blood pressure with fewer adverse effects, if low doses of two agents rather than higher doses of a single agent are used. Combination therapy usually includes small doses of a diuretic, which potentiates the effects of other drugs, such as ACE inhibitors, ARBs, and β-blockers. Combination therapy may improve compliance and more rapidly achieve target blood pressure. In most clinical trials that have demonstrated improved cardiovascular outcomes, two or more drugs were required to achieve target blood pressures. Therefore, hypertension guidelines support combination therapy as initial treatment.

KEY POINTS

- The target blood pressure for the general population is <140/90 mm Hg and is <130/80 mm Hg for patients with diabetes or renal disease.
- Blood pressure during and after an acute stroke should be lowered cautiously by about 10% to 15% if systolic pressure is >220 mm Hg or diastolic pressure is >120 mm Hg.
- More than one drug often is indicated for patients with stage 2 or higher hypertension.
- Diuretics are typically recommended for first-line treatment of hypertension.
- Low-dose therapy with two antihypertensive agents is associated with fewer adverse effects than higher doses of single-agent therapy.

Follow-up

Follow-up and medication adjustment are indicated at monthly intervals or more frequently until blood pressure targets are achieved. More frequent follow-up may be indicated for stage 2 hypertension or complicated comorbid conditions. If blood pressure control is inadequate after 1 to 3 months of monotherapy, an increase in the dose of the first drug, the addition of another drug from a different class, or the substitution of a drug from another class may be useful.

Serum chemistry studies, such as blood urea nitrogen, creatinine, and electrolyte measurements, should be performed once or twice yearly. When blood pressure goals are achieved, follow-up every 3 to 6 months is sufficient.

KEY POINT

- Follow-up at least every month is indicated for patients with hypertension until blood pressure targets are achieved.

Resistant Hypertension

A small percentage of patients with hypertension have truly resistant hypertension. Many patients who appear to be resistant to therapy are, in fact, inadequately treated because of nonadherence to therapy or inadequate dosing of medication. In addition, some patients may have white coat hypertension. ABPM is indicated for patients with clinical suspicion for this condition.

Drug interactions, most commonly associated with the volume-retaining effects of nonsteroidal anti-inflammatory drugs, may cause resistant hypertension. Other exogenous substances that may interfere with successful antihypertensive therapy include excessive alcohol, oral contraceptives, licorice, cyclosporine, erythropoietin, and antidepressants. Features contributing to resistant hypertension include obesity, sleep apnea, cigarette smoking, and panic attacks. Patients with secondary hypertension are more likely to have resistant hypertension, which should be considered when patients are unresponsive to adequate antihypertensive therapy (Table 25).

The most common factor contributing to resistant hypertension is excess sodium/volume and failure to address this condition adequately with appropriate dietary modifications and inadequate or inappropriate diuretic usage. In this setting, longer-acting diuretics (hydrochlorothiazide, chlorthalidone, spironolactone) are always more appropriate than shorter-acting agents (furosemide), which must be administered two to three times daily.

KEY POINTS

- Nonadherence to therapy or inadequate dosing may cause some patients to appear resistant to therapy.
- The most common factor contributing to resistant hypertension in compliant patients is excess sodium/volume.
- Longer-acting diuretics such as hydrochlorothiazide are more appropriate for resistant hypertension than shorter-acting agents such as furosemide.

References

1. Fields LE, Burt VL, Cutler JA, Hughes J, Roccella EJ, Sorlie P. The burden of adult hypertension in the United States 1999 to 2000: a rising tide. Hypertension. 2004;44:398-404. [PMID: 15326093]

2. Lloyd-Jones DM, Evans JC, Levy D. Hypertension in adults across the age spectrum: current outcomes and control in the community. JAMA. 2005;294:466-72. [PMID: 16046653]

3. Chobanian AV, Bakris GL, Black HR, Cushman WC, Green LA, Izzo JL Jr, et al. Seventh report of the Joint National Committee on Prevention, Detection, Evaluation, and Treatment of High Blood Pressure. Hypertension. 2003;42:1206-52. [PMID: 14656957]

4. Vasan RS, Larson MG, Leip EP, Evans JC, O'Donnell CJ, Kannel WB, et al. Impact of high-normal blood pressure on the risk of cardiovascular disease. N Engl J Med. 2001;345:1291-7. [PMID: 11794147]

5. Williams B, Poulter NR, Brown MJ, Davis M, McInnes GT, Potter JF, et al. Guidelines for management of hypertension: report of the fourth working party of the British Hypertension Society, 2004-BHS IV. J Hum Hypertens. 2004;18:139-85. [PMID: 14973512]

6. Whitworth JA. 2003 World Health Organization (WHO)/ International Society of Hypertension (ISH) statement on management of hypertension. J Hypertens. 2003;21:1983-92. [PMID: 14597836]

7. Lenders JW, Eisenhofer G, Mannelli M, Pacak K. Phaeochromocytoma. Lancet. 2005;366:665-75. [PMID: 16112304]

8. Dominguez LJ, Sowers JR. Metabolic syndrome therapy: prevention of vascular injury by antidiabetic agents. Curr Hypertens Rep. 2005;7:110-6. [PMID: 15748534]

9. O'Brien E, Asmar R, Beilin L, Imai Y, Mallion JM, Mancia G, et al. European Society of Hypertension recommendations for conventional, ambulatory and home blood pressure measurement. J Hypertens. 2003;21:821-48. [PMID: 12714851]

10. Clement DL, De Buyzere ML, De Bacquer DA, de Leeuw PW, Duprez DA, Fagard RH, et al. Prognostic value of ambulatory blood-pressure recordings in patients with treated hypertension. N Engl J Med. 2003;348:2407-15. [PMID: 12802026]

11. Kaplan NM. Resistant hypertension. J Hypertens. 2005;23:1441-4. [PMID: 16003165]

12. Pickering TG, Shimbo D, Haas D. Ambulatory blood-pressure monitoring. N Engl J Med. 2006;354:2368-74. [PMID: 16738273]

13. Tiu SC, Choi CH, Shek CC, Ng YW, Chan FK, Ng CM, et al. The use of aldosterone-renin ratio as a diagnostic test for primary hyperaldosteronism and its test characteristics under different conditions of blood sampling. J Clin Endocrinol Metab. 2005;90:72-8. [PMID: 15483077]

14. Mulatero P, Stowasser M, Loh KC, Fardella CE, Gordon RD, Mosso L, et al. Increased diagnosis of primary aldosteronism, including surgically correctable forms, in centers from five continents. J Clin Endocrinol Metab. 2004;89:1045-50. [PMID: 15001583]

15. Kaplan NM. The current epidemic of primary aldosteronism: causes and consequences. J Hypertens. 2004;22:863-9. [PMID: 15097219]

16. Vasbinder GB, Nelemans PJ, Kessels AG, Kroon AA, Maki JH, Leiner T, et al. Accuracy of computed tomographic angiography and magnetic resonance angiography for diagnosing renal artery stenosis. Ann Intern Med. 2004;141:674-82; discussion 682. [PMID: 15520423]

17. van Jaarsveld BC, Krijnen P, Pieterman H, Derkx FH, Deinum J, Postma CT, et al. The effect of balloon angioplasty on hypertension in atherosclerotic renal-artery stenosis. Dutch Renal Artery Stenosis Intervention Cooperative Study Group. N Engl J Med. 2000;342:1007-14. [PMID: 10749962]

18. Plouin PF, Chatellier G, Darné B, Raynaud A. Blood pressure outcome of angioplasty in atherosclerotic renal artery stenosis: a randomized trial. Essai Multicentrique Medicaments vs Angioplastie (EMMA) Study Group. Hypertension. 1998;31:823-9. [PMID: 9495267]

19. Webster J, Marshall F, Abdalla M, Dominiczak A, Edwards R, Isles CG, et al. Randomised comparison of percutaneous angioplasty vs continued medical therapy for hypertensive patients with atheromatous renal artery stenosis. Scottish and Newcastle Renal Artery Stenosis Collaborative Group. J Hum Hypertens. 1998;12:329-35. [PMID: 9655655]

20. Hallett JW Jr, Textor SC, Kos PB, Nicpon G, Bower TC, Cherry KJ Jr, et al. Advanced renovascular hypertension and renal insufficiency: trends in medical comorbidity and surgical approach from 1970 to 1993. J Vasc Surg. 1995;21:750-9; discussion 759-60. [PMID: 7769734]

21. Topol EJ, Yadav JS. Recognition of the importance of embolization in atherosclerotic vascular disease. Circulation. 2000;101:570-80. [PMID: 10662756]

22. Uzzo RG, Novick AC, Goormastic M, Mascha E, Pohl M. Medical versus surgical management of atherosclerotic renal artery stenosis. Transplant Proc. 2002;34:723-5. [PMID: 12009679]

23. Sacks FM, Svetkey LP, Vollmer WM, Appel LJ, Bray GA, Harsha D, et al. Effects on blood pressure of reduced dietary sodium and the Dietary Approaches to Stop Hypertension (DASH) diet. DASH-Sodium Collaborative Research Group. N Engl J Med. 2001;344:3-10. [PMID: 11136953]

24. Turnbull F. Effects of different blood-pressure-lowering regimens on major cardiovascular events: results of prospectively-designed overviews of randomised trials. Lancet. 2003;362:1527-35. [PMID: 14615107]

25. Anderson KM, Odell PM, Wilson PW, Kannel WB. Cardiovascular disease risk profiles. Am Heart J. 1991;121:293-8. [PMID: 1985385]

26. Hansson L, Zanchetti A, Carruthers SG, Dahlof B, Elmfeldt D, Julius S, et al. Effects of intensive blood-pressure lowering and low-dose aspirin in patients with hypertension: principal results of the Hypertension Optimal Treatment (HOT) randomised trial. HOT Study Group. Lancet. 1998;351:1755-62. [PMID: 9635947]

27. **ALLHAT Officers and Coordinators for the ALLHAT Collaborative Research Group.** The Antihypertensive and Lipid-Lowering Treatment to Prevent Heart Attack Trial. Major outcomes in high-risk hypertensive patients randomized to angiotensin-converting enzyme inhibitor or calcium channel blocker vs diuretic: The Antihypertensive and Lipid-Lowering Treatment to Prevent Heart Attack Trial (ALLHAT). JAMA. 2002;288:2981-97. [PMID: 12479763]

28. **Opie LH, Schall R.** Old antihypertensives and new diabetes. J Hypertens. 2004;22:1453-8. [PMID: 15257162]

ACUTE RENAL FAILURE

RECENT ADVANCES

- Less nephrotoxic radiocontrast agent
- Improving renal function in hepatorenal syndrome

Epidemiology

Acute renal failure is defined as an abrupt decrease in renal function sufficient to cause retention of metabolic waste products, such as urea and creatinine. Metabolic acidosis, hyperkalemia, disturbances in body fluid homeostasis, and secondary effects on other organ systems frequently develop in acute renal failure.

The incidence and prognosis of acute renal failure depends on the population under consideration. Prerenal acute renal failure, for example, accounts for 70% of community-acquired acute renal failure, with an observed mortality rate of 7%. In contrast, approximately 60% of hospital-acquired acute renal failure is due to ischemic or nephrotoxic tubular epithelial injury, with an attendant mortality rate of 50% to 70%.

Risk factors for acute renal failure include advanced age, preexisting renal parenchymal disease, diabetes mellitus, and underlying cardiac or liver disease. An increase in the serum creatinine level has been associated with increased mortality not only in the short term but persisting >5 years from the initial insult (1). Factors accounting for this association have yet to be determined but may include initiation of an ongoing inflammatory process (2).

The presence of oliguria, defined as a daily urine output <400 mL, portends a less favorable prognosis. Renal failure accompanied by oliguria is associated with a mortality rate of 75%, compared with 25% in nonoliguric patients. The correlation of oliguria with the severity of illness most likely accounts for this variance. The underlying disease process and infectious complications account for the majority of deaths associated with acute renal failure.

Hemodialysis has clearly reduced the incidence of certain complications related to acute renal failure, such as gastrointestinal hemorrhage and electrolyte disturbances. However, refinements in dialysis techniques over the past 30 years have had little impact on mortality. This finding likely reflects a greater tendency to intervene in patients with a higher index of illness severity.

KEY POINTS

- Advanced age, preexisting renal parenchymal disease, diabetes mellitus, and underlying cardiac or liver disease are risk factors for acute renal failure.
- Oliguria portends a less favorable prognosis in patients with acute renal failure.
- The underlying disease process and infectious complications account for the majority of deaths associated with acute renal failure.
- Prerenal acute renal failure accounts for 70% of community-acquired acute renal failure, with an observed mortality rate of 7%.
- Approximately 60% of hospital-acquired acute renal failure is due to ischemic or nephrotoxic tubular epithelial injury, with an attendant mortality rate of 50% to 70%.

Differential Diagnosis

Acute renal failure may develop in response to decreased renal perfusion (prerenal acute renal failure), obstruction (postrenal acute renal failure), or intrinsic renal parenchymal injury (intrarenal acute renal failure). Diagnosis of this condition first involves a clinical assessment, beginning with a thorough review of the history and medical record with a particular focus on nephrotoxic and hemodynamic insults (**Figure 6**).

The clinical setting often suggests the cause of acute renal failure. Recent exposure to a new medication or associated extrarenal manifestations may suggest the diagnosis. The history, physical examination, and other laboratory and hemodynamic parameters are then used to accurately define the status of the extracellular fluid volume. Analysis of the fractional excretion of sodium (FE_{Na}), defined as the percent of the filtered load of sodium excreted in the urine, is the most commonly used parameter in assessing oliguric renal failure. The FE_{Na} is calculated using the following equation based on simultaneously collected specimens of urine and plasma sodium and creatinine:

$$FE_{Na} = (Urine_{Na+} \times Plasma_{Creatinine})/(Plasma_{Na+} \times Urine_{Creatinine}) \times 100\%$$

A $FE_{Na} < 1\%$ suggests a prerenal cause of acute renal failure, whereas a value >2% is consistent with epithelial tubular injury. The FE_{Na} must be interpreted carefully in the context of the history; physical examination; and other laboratory findings, such as analysis of the urine sediment, because more than one process commonly occurs simultaneously. The FE_{Na}, for example, may be low early in the course of ischemic tubular injury and urinary tract obstruction, as well as in

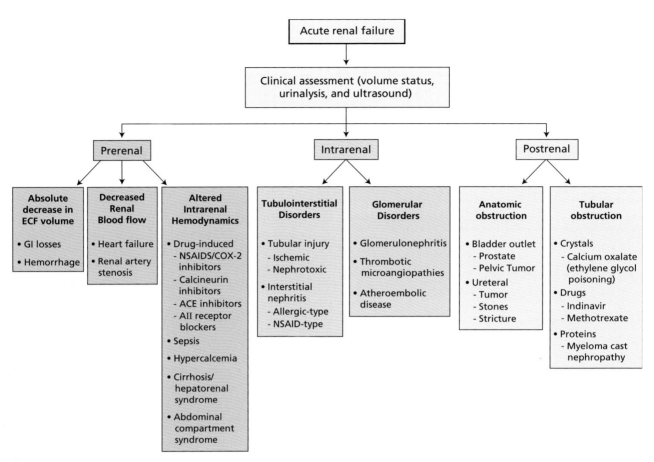

FIGURE 6.
Diagnosis of acute renal failure.

ECF = extracellular fluid; GI = gastrointestinal; NSAIDS = nonsteroidal anti-inflammatory drugs; COX-2 = cyclooxygenase-2; ACE = angiotensin-converting enzyme; AII = angiotensin II

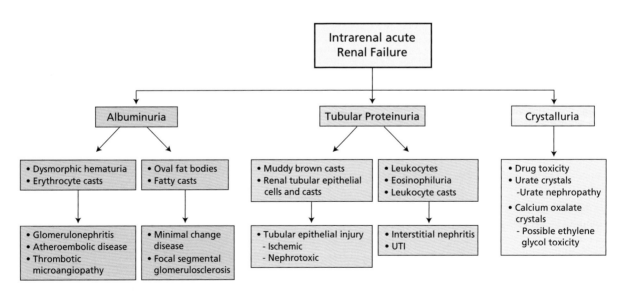

FIGURE 7.
Urinary sediment findings in intrarenal acute renal failure.

UTI = urinary tract infection

radiocontrast-induced tubular injury. Conversely, diuretics can increase the FE_{Na} in patients with prerenal azotemia. The FE_{Na} usually is low in patients presenting with the nephrotic syndrome or glomerulonephritis.

Because obstruction is a reversible cause of renal failure, ultrasonography is indicated early in the evaluation. Microscopic analysis of the urine sediment is essential in acute renal failure, particularly if pre- and postrenal causes have been excluded (**Figure 7**). If the diagnosis of intrarenal acute renal failure remains unclear after reviewing the aforementioned data, renal biopsy should be considered. Vascular insults such as renal artery thrombosis of a solitary kidney or renal vein thrombosis also should be considered because timely intervention is critical to preserve renal function.

KEY POINTS

- Careful attention to possible nephrotoxic or hemodynamic insults, new medications, and associated extrarenal manifestations is helpful in diagnosing acute renal failure.

- A fractional excretion of sodium <1% suggests a prerenal cause of acute renal failure, whereas a value >2% suggests an epithelial tubular injury.

- Because more than one process may occur simultaneously, the fractional excretion of sodium alone should not be used to diagnose the cause of acute renal failure.

- Because obstruction is a reversible cause of renal failure, ultrasonography is indicated early in the evaluation.

Acute Prerenal Failure

Prerenal azotemia is the most common cause of community-acquired acute renal failure. Normally, autoregulation of renal blood flow maintains the glomerular filtration rate at a fixed level until the mean arterial pressure decreases to less than approximately 60 mm Hg. Once renal perfusion decreases below this critical threshold, prerenal acute renal failure develops.

Patients with true volume depletion have decreased skin turgor and postural hypotension. Those with a >5% reduction in the extracellular volume have decreased capillary refill. The history and urinary indices are more useful in establishing a diagnosis in patients with milder degrees of volume depletion.

Patients with "functional" prerenal azotemia also may present with a normal or increased extracellular fluid volume. Patients with heart failure, sepsis, liver disease, or the nephrotic syndrome can develop prerenal acute renal failure because of decreased effective circulating volume with concomitant increased extracellular fluid volume.

A decrease in the glomerular capillary pressure, often in association with altered glomerular hemodynamics, also may

TABLE 29 Factors Altering Intraglomerular Hemodynamics Resulting in Decreased Glomerular Capillary Pressure

Factors Primarily Affecting Afferent Arteriolar Vasoconstriction
NSAIDs
COX-2 inhibitors
Cyclosporine A
Tacrolimus
Iodinated contrast
Hypercalcemia
Hepatorenal syndrome
Factors Primarily Affecting Efferent Arteriolar Vasodilation
ACE inhibitors*
ARBs*

NSAIDs = nonsteroidal anti-inflammatory drugs; COX-2 = cyclooxygenase-2; ACE = angiotensin-converting enzyme; ARBs = angiotensin receptor blockers

*Most apparent in patients with renovascular disease

cause functional prerenal acute renal failure. In these patients, the renal response and, therefore, the FE_{Na} mirror those of patients with true volume depletion (FE_{Na} <1%). Numerous medications, iodinated contrast agents, and hypercalcemia may reduce glomerular capillary pressure through afferent arteriolar vasoconstriction (**Table 29**). Patients with bilateral renal artery stenosis and intrarenal small-vessel disease are at increased risk for prerenal azotemia after administration of angiotensin-converting enzyme inhibitors and angiotensin receptor blockers.

Abdominal compartment syndrome is a form of prerenal acute renal failure that develops in patients with an expanded extracellular fluid volume. This syndrome can develop in patients who have received massive volume resuscitation resulting in accumulation of intra-abdominal fluid to the extent that renal perfusion is compromised. The diagnosis is established when the intra-abdominal bladder pressure increases to >25 mm Hg. Surgical or percutaneous decompression of the abdomen usually causes a prompt return of renal function.

Treatment of prerenal azotemia in patients with true volume depletion consists of restoring the extracellular fluid volume to normal with judicious administration of isotonic saline. Management of patients with functional prerenal failure should focus on reversing the underlying cause, which may include use of inotropic agents in patients with congestive heart failure or treatment of the underlying infection and use of vasopressors in patients with septic shock. Medications suspected of decreasing the glomerular capillary pressure should be discontinued.

Acute Postrenal Failure

Anatomic Obstruction

Renal ultrasonography to evaluate for obstruction is indicated for all patients presenting with acute renal failure. The presence of hydronephrosis is 90% sensitive and specific for obstruction but may not be evident in patients with concurrent volume depletion or retroperitoneal fibrosis. Urinary tract obstruction accounts for only 5% of all cases of acute renal failure and is often treatable, but a delay in the diagnosis can adversely affect outcomes. When urinary tract obstruction is diagnosed and corrected within 1 week of onset, the prognosis for complete renal recovery is excellent. Irreversible renal injury, characterized by interstitial fibrosis and tubular atrophy, may result from obstruction that persists for >12 weeks.

Urinary tract obstruction most commonly presents in men with prostatic hypertrophy or cancer, causing bladder outlet obstruction. A high index of clinical suspicion should be raised in patients with intra-abdominal and pelvic malignancies. The clinical presentation of urinary tract obstruction may vary from anuria (<50 mL/d of urine output) with complete obstruction to polyuria alternating with oliguria in partial obstruction. Hyperkalemic renal tubular acidosis is a common finding. Once ultrasonography confirms the diagnosis, MRI of the abdomen and pelvis is helpful in defining the etiology of the obstruction.

Functional recovery generally occurs over the course of 1 to 2 weeks after relief of obstruction. Tubular injury and excess retained solute may cause postobstructive diuresis, which usually is an appropriate response to the expanded extracellular fluid volume. Occasionally, frank volume depletion develops. However, routinely replacing urine output with intravenous fluids generally is not indicated because this intervention may potentially perpetuate the diuresis. Therefore, clinical assessment of the extracellular fluid volume should guide intravenous fluid administration.

Tubular Obstruction

Obstruction also may occur at the level of the renal tubule. Several drugs, including methotrexate, intravenous acyclovir, and sulfadiazine, as well as the protease inhibitor indinavir, are known to form crystals in the lumen of the tubule and cause obstruction on a microscopic level. Calcium oxalate crystal–induced acute renal failure may complicate ethylene glycol poisoning.

Urate nephropathy may develop after induction of cancer chemotherapy or may occur spontaneously in patients with tumors that have high proliferation rates, such as promyelocytic leukemia. The use of allopurinol prophylaxis has significantly decreased the incidence of this condition. The clinical presentation usually mimics acute oliguric renal failure, which is associated with high levels of plasma uric acid and a urine uric acid–creatinine ratio >1 mg/mg.

Early intervention with hemodialysis is indicated in this setting to clear the toxic metabolites. Often, renal function dramatically improves after a single hemodialysis treatment. Continuous renal replacement therapy may be helpful in patients with higher levels of serum uric acid and phosphate. Urinary alkalinization has been advocated but may worsen tubular obstruction by promoting formation of calcium phosphate crystals within the renal tubules. Therefore, volume expansion with normal saline is preferred.

Recently, a recombinant urate oxidase, rasburicase, has become available for the treatment of hyperuricemia in the setting of acute urate nephropathy, as well as for the prevention of tumor lysis syndrome in high-risk patients (3). This agent should be administered carefully because of the associated risks for hemolysis, hemoglobinuria, methemoglobinemia, and anaphylaxis.

Light chains produced in patients with multiple myeloma can induce tubular obstruction and acute renal failure known as myeloma cast nephropathy. The pathogenesis of this syndrome is not directly related to light chain burden but rather to the affinity of a particular light chain for Tamm–Horsfall protein. Therefore, low levels of highly avid light chains can result in acute renal failure. One controlled trial demonstrated a possible benefit of therapeutic apheresis in this setting, but this intervention appears to be most useful in patients with nonoliguric acute renal failure (4). A subsequent multicenter randomized trial, however, did not show improved outcomes with plasmapheresis (5). Unfortunately, these studies were underpowered to demonstrate benefit in certain subgroups of patients, such as those with the highest risk for renal failure, and the relative merits of plasmapheresis in addition to routine management with chemotherapy remains uncertain.

KEY POINTS

- The presence of hydronephrosis is 90% sensitive and specific for obstruction but may not be evident in patients with concurrent volume depletion or retroperitoneal fibrosis.
- Urinary tract obstruction is most common in men with prostatic hypertrophy or cancer and in patients with intra-abdominal and pelvic malignancies.
- The clinical presentation of urinary tract obstruction may vary from anuria to polyuria alternating with oliguria.
- Methotrexate, intravenous acyclovir, sulfadiazine, and indinavir may cause obstruction of the renal tubule.
- Allopurinol prophylaxis has significantly decreased the incidence of urate nephropathy after induction of cancer chemotherapy.
- Early intervention with hemodialysis is indicated for acute renal failure associated with tumor lysis syndrome.
- Urinary alkalinization has been advocated for the treatment of urate nephropathy but may worsen tubular obstruction by promoting formation of calcium phosphate crystals within the renal tubules.
- Rasburicase can be used to treat hyperuricemia associated with acute urate nephropathy.
- Rasburicase may be indicated as a prophylactic measure in patients with malignancies with a high proliferation rate.

Acute Intrarenal Failure

Tubulointerstitial Disorders

Ischemic

Ischemic tubular injury remains the most common form of intrinsic renal injury in critically ill patients. Traditionally, the term "acute tubular necrosis" has been used to define this syndrome. However, necrosis is not a constant morphologic finding, and the terms "ischemic tubular injury" or "nephrotoxic tubular injury" are more appropriate.

Conceptually, ischemic tubular injury has been divided into several phases: initiation, extension, maintenance, and recovery. The initiation phase occurs after a prerenal state of impaired renal perfusion, which causes decreased oxygen delivery and ischemic injury that is most prominent in the metabolically active corticomedullary junction. Sublethal tubular injury characterizes this phase, despite marked morphologic and functional changes.

Subsequently, the normal polarity of transport proteins and adhesion molecules is disrupted, leading to altered solute transport and sloughing of cells into the tubular lumen. Tubular obstruction results, which causes the glomerular filtrate to leak back into the interstitium. Activated endothelial cells upregulate adhesion molecules, thereby promoting endothelial–leukocyte interactions. Leukocytes trapped in the peritubular capillary cause mechanical obstruction that further potentiates ischemic injury.

The extension phase is marked by increased release of multiple inflammatory mediators, such as interleukin-1 and tumor necrosis factor, by renal tubular epithelial and endothelial cells. Ongoing cellular injury and apoptosis of the tubular epithelium characterize the maintenance phase. An imbalance between vasodilatory and vasoconstrictive mediators, such as nitric oxide and endothelin, mitigates further injury.

The recovery phase ensues with the return of renal perfusion. Viable tubular epithelial cells redifferentiate and reestablish normal polarity and solute transport. Diuresis often precedes full functional recovery, and repletion of fluid and electrolyte losses may be necessary. Even when renal function returns to baseline, the peritubular capillaries sustain permanent injury that is associated with tubulointerstitial fibrosis.

Treatment of established ischemic tubular injury is supportive and includes prevention of further renal parenchymal injury and, when possible, correction of the inciting event. Maintenance of fluid and electrolyte balance, tight glycemic control, and proper nutrition also are indicated. Despite appropriate supportive measures, many patients eventually require hemodialysis.

Nephrotoxic

Therapeutic agents are a common cause of acute renal failure and account for up to 30% of cases of intrarenal acute renal failure in hospitalized patients (**Table 30**). Aminoglycoside antibiotics are the most common cause of medication-induced renal failure. Aminoglycoside nephrotoxicity typically presents with nonoliguric acute renal failure occurring after 1 week of therapy. Cumulative uptake of the causative agent by the proximal tubular cells appears to be more important than trough levels in the development of nephrotoxicity. Aminoglycosides have been shown to exhibit less nephrotoxicity and equivalent efficacy when administered in higher doses on a once-daily basis.

Radiocontrast nephropathy is another common cause of acute renal failure, accounting for 10% of all cases in hospitalized patients. The incidence of radiocontrast nephropathy varies from approximately 2% in patients without diabetes who have normal renal function to up to 30% in patients with diabetes who have serum creatinine levels >3 mg/dL (6).

Radiocontrast nephropathy is most effectively prevented by avoiding use of radiocontrast in high-risk patients, unless no suitable alternatives exist. MRI with gadolinium enhancement is preferred compared with contrast CT. Simultaneous renal arteriography on a routine basis in patients undergoing cardiac catheterization is discouraged, particularly in patients with established renal parenchymal disease.

TABLE 30 Nephrotoxic Therapeutic Agents
Tubular Toxicity
Aminoglycosides
Nonoliguric ARF
Usually after 1 week of exposure
Renal Mg, K loss
Amphotericin B
Both direct membrane injury and vasoconstriction mediate toxicity
Deoxycholate detergent component of preparation may play a role in nephrotoxicity
Usually develops after 500 mg of exposure
Associated findings may include renal magnesium and potassium wasting, and distal RTA
Pretreatment isotonic saline or use of liposomal or lipid complex formulations decrease toxicity
Cisplatin
Intracellular formation of reactive hydroxyl radicals mediate toxicity
Hypomagnesemia common
Amifostine and theophylline may ameliorate toxicity
Foscarnet
Direct tubular toxicity and crystal formation involved in pathogenesis of tubular injury
Presents as nonoliguric ARF typically after about 1 week of exposure
Associated findings may include nephrogenic diabetes insipidus, hypocalcemia, as well as renal magnesium and potassium wasting
Tenofovir
Metabolic acidosis may be a prominent feature
Fanconi's syndrome
Adefovir
Mitochondrial DNA depletion important in pathogenesis
Fanconi's syndrome
Probenecid may limit nephrotoxicity
Cidofovir
Fanconi's syndrome
Probenecid may limit nephrotoxicity
Crystal Formation
Acyclovir
Most commonly follows IV administration, especially if volume depleted
Pretreatment volume expansion recommended
Indinavir
May cause crystal formation in both the tubules and collecting system
Often presents with flank pain, hematuria, pyuria
Can cause interstitial nephritis
Methotrexate
Crystals more likely to form in acidic urine
Pretreat with IV bicarbonate and volume expansion
Table continues

TABLE 30 Nephrotoxic Therapeutic Agents *(Continued)*
Leucovorin rescue for patients with high serum methotrexate levels
Carboxypeptidase G2 to rapidly decrease serum methotrexate levels that remain high in ARF
Sulfadiazine
Crystals more likely to form when urine pH is <5.5
May present with renal colic and collecting system stones
Urinary alkalinization and hydration with >3 L/d for prevention
Thrombotic Microangiopathy
Cancer chemotherapy*
Direct vascular toxicity implicated in pathogenesis
Role of therapeutic apheresis not well established
Calcineurin inhibitors[†]
Direct vascular toxicity and increased platelet aggregation may mediate pathogenesis
Quinine
Antiplatelet antibodies important in pathogenesis
OKT3
TNF release and direct vascular toxicity implicated in pathogenesis
Antiplatelet agents[‡]
Decreased ADAMTS13 activity has been documented
Osmotic Tubular Injury
Dextran 40
Variable presentation with both oliguric and nonoliguric acute renal failure
IVIG
Sucrose component in some preparations felt to mediate toxicity
Mixed Nephrotoxicity
Iodinated contrast
Vasoconstriction, increased osmotic stress, and generation of reactive oxygen species may mediate nephrotoxicity
Pretreatment NS or $NaHCO_3$ for prevention

ARF = acute renal failure; RTA = renal tubular acidosis; IV = intravenous; IVIG = intravenous immune globulin; TNF = tumor necrosis factor; NS = normal saline.

* Cisplatinum in conjunction with bleomycin, mitomycin C, and gemcitabine.

† Cyclosporine A, tacrolimus.

‡ Ticlopidine, clopidogrel.

The pathogenesis of radiocontrast nephrotoxicity is multifactorial. Alterations in intrarenal levels of adenosine, nitric oxide, and endothelin may mediate renal vasoconstriction. Increased osmotic and oxidative stress may cause direct cellular toxicity. First-generation ionic iodinated contrast agents pose the greatest risk and have an osmolarity of 1500 mosm/kg H_2O to 1800 mosm/kg H_2O. Second-generation, or low-osmolar nonionic, agents have an osmolarity

TABLE 31 Prevention of Radiocontrast Nephropathy

Intervention	Strength of Evidence	Clarity of Risk–Benefit	Grade of Recommendation*
Volume expansion with normal saline	Good	Clear	A
Volume expansion with sodium bicarbonate	Fair	Clear	B
Iso-osmolar contrast	Fair	Clear	B
Theophylline	Fair	Unclear	C
N-acetylcysteine	Good	Unclear	C
Hemofiltration	Fair	Unclear	I
Fenoldopam	Good	Unclear	D
Hemodialysis	Good	Unclear	D

* A = Intervention is always indicated and acceptable. B = Intervention may be effective and is acceptable. C = Intervention may be considered; minimal or no relative impact. I = Insufficient evidence to recommend for or against intervention. D = Not useful.

of 600 mosm/kg H_2O to 850 mosm/kg H_2O and are slightly less nephrotoxic. The nephrotoxicity of iodixanol, a third-generation iso-osmolar (osmolarity of 290 mosm/kg H_2O) nonionic dimeric contrast agent, recently was shown to exhibit less nephrotoxicity when compared with a second-generation agent (7).

Volume expansion with either isotonic saline or sodium bicarbonate is the most effective measure to decrease the incidence and severity of nephrotoxicity (8). The optimal timing and rate of administration have yet to be defined. However, most studies have followed a protocol requiring administration of 1 mL/kg/min of saline or sodium bicarbonate for several hours before the procedure and continuing for at least 6 hours postprocedure.

Measures that improve renal perfusion, such as optimization of cardiac output, as well as discontinuation of medications that may adversely affect renal perfusion (such as nonsteroidal anti-inflammatory drugs [NSAIDs] and high-dose aspirin) are indicated. N-acetylcysteine may help to decrease the oxidative stress and consequent tubular injury of radiocontrast agents. Multiple studies and meta-analyses have shown varying results, and use of this agent is not strongly recommended in this setting (9).

Potential benefit also has been shown for pretreating patients with theophylline, 200 mg. A small pilot study initially showed that fenoldopam may be beneficial (10). However, two well-designed randomized controlled trials have since demonstrated no benefit with this agent (11, 12). Therefore, use of fenoldopam is not recommended to prevent contrast nephropathy.

Conventional hemodialysis has been shown to be ineffective for removal of radiocontrast and does not decrease the incidence of contrast nephropathy. Hemofiltration is somewhat more effective in clearing radiocontrast and removes approximately 40% of the contrast load. A decreased incidence of contrast nephrotoxicity was demonstrated using this technique, but whether this effect was related to the bicarbonate contained in replacement fluids or to removal of contrast media is uncertain. Because of the costs and associated risks of hemofiltration, use of this therapy is not routinely recommended to prevent radiocontrast nephropathy. **Table 31** summarizes the relative merits of interventions to prevent contrast nephropathy.

Rhabdomyolysis accounts for 2% to 5% of all cases of acute renal failure in the intensive care unit. An elevated serum creatine kinase level, which closely parallels release of the nephrotoxin myoglobin, should raise suspicion for rhabdomyolysis. An important clue to the diagnosis is heme positivity on dipstick urinalysis in the absence of erythrocytes on microscopic analysis of the urine. Rhabdomyolysis most commonly develops after exposure to myotoxic drugs, infections, excessive exertion, or prolonged immobilization.

The risk for renal failure increases when the serum creatine kinase level exceeds 5000 U/L. The serum creatinine level may increase not only because of decreased renal function but also because of increased release of creatinine from injured muscle. Complications in this setting include hypocalcemia, hyperphosphatemia, hyperuricemia, metabolic acidosis, acute muscle compartment syndrome, and limb ischemia. Recent studies have shown no benefit from prophylactic fasciotomy, which is associated with a higher incidence of infectious complications.

Compartment syndrome presents with painful swelling in a limb after trauma. An intracompartmental pressure >30 mm Hg to 40 mm Hg with water or mercury manometry confirms the diagnosis. Compartment syndrome also should be suspected in patients who demonstrate a secondary increase in the serum creatine kinase level (called the "second-wave" phenomenon) after an initial decrease.

Expansion of the extracellular fluid volume with isotonic saline is the most effective measure to limit nephrotoxicity in patients with rhabdomyolysis. A serum creatinine level

>1.7 mg/dL on presentation to the emergency department was recently shown to be the most predictive factor for the subsequent development of renal failure (13). Patients who remain oliguric after initial resuscitation efforts and correction of volume depletion are at high risk for requiring dialysis, and fluids subsequently should be administered at a rate that matches losses once the effective circulating volume is optimized.

No salutary effect on renal outcomes has been demonstrated for the use of mannitol or urinary alkalinization. However, mannitol, which effects a decrease in intracompartmental pressure and muscle edema, may be beneficial in the treatment of acute muscle compartment syndrome (14). Calcium repletion is indicated only for patients with cardiac or neuromuscular irritability.

Interstitial Nephritis

Acute interstitial nephritis is a heterogeneous group of disorders that most commonly develop after exposure to drugs but also may result from various infectious and inflammatory conditions. Interstitial nephritis associated with infection may result from direct infection of the renal parenchyma, as occurs in pyelonephritis, or in reaction to systemic infection. Acute interstitial nephritis also may develop in patients with systemic immunologic disorders, such as Sjögren's syndrome, systemic lupus erythematosus, and sarcoidosis. Acute interstitial nephritis in association with uveitis predominantly affects adolescent girls.

Drug-induced allergic interstitial nephritis typically develops several days after exposure to agents such as penicillins, cephalosporins, fluoroquinolones, allopurinol, and phenytoin. Affected patients typically present with rash, pruritus, eosinophilia, and fever. Analysis of the urine sediment may reveal pyuria, leukocyte casts, microscopic hematuria, and tubular-range proteinuria.

Hansel's stain for eosinophils may be positive, but interpretation of the results of this study depends on the pretest probability of interstitial nephritis. A positive urine Hansel's stain is associated with an 80% likelihood of disease with a high pretest probability but only a 50% likelihood of disease with an intermediate pretest probability. Eosinophiluria also may develop in acute glomerulonephritis, atheroembolic disease, and acute prostatitis.

Treatment consists of discontinuation of the offending agent. Concomitant corticosteroid therapy may benefit patients with persistent severe renal failure, particularly when the renal biopsy reveals a high degree of acute interstitial inflammation. However, there are no published prospective randomized trials evaluating the efficacy of corticosteroids in this disorder.

Interstitial nephritis associated with NSAID and cyclooxygenase-2 (COX-2) inhibitors varies slightly from the classic allergic type. Renal failure due to these agents typically develops after several weeks to months rather than days and usually is not accompanied by rash, fever, and eosinophilia;

this presentation is characterized by nephrotic-range proteinuria. Renal biopsy may be needed to help distinguish this condition from NSAID-induced glomerular diseases such as minimal change disease, membranous nephropathy, or focal segmental glomerulosclerosis. NSAID-induced interstitial nephritis does not respond as well to corticosteroids compared with allergic-type disease, and progression to chronic kidney disease is more common than in allergic interstitial nephritis.

KEY POINTS

- Ischemic tubular injury is the most common form of intrinsic renal injury in critically ill patients.
- Initial treatment of established ischemic tubular injury includes prevention of further renal parenchymal injury; correction of the inciting event, when possible; maintenance of fluid and electrolyte balance; and tight glycemic control.
- Aminoglycoside antibiotics are the most common cause of medication-induced renal failure.
- In aminoglycoside-induced acute tubular injury, cumulative uptake of the causative agent by the proximal tubular cells appears to be more important than trough levels in the development of nephrotoxicity.
- Aminoglycosides have been shown to exhibit less nephrotoxicity and equivalent efficacy when administered in higher doses on a once-daily basis.
- To prevent radiocontrast nephropathy, routine simultaneous renal arteriography in patients undergoing cardiac catheterization is discouraged.
- Volume expansion with isotonic saline or sodium bicarbonate is the most effective means of preventing radiocontrast nephropathy.
- An elevated serum creatine kinase level and heme positivity on urine dipstick in the absence of erythrocytes on microscopic analysis of the urine suggest rhabdomyolysis.
- The risk for renal failure increases when the serum creatine kinase level exceeds 5000 U/L.
- Expansion of the extracellular fluid volume with isotonic saline is the most effective measure to limit nephrotoxicity in rhabdomyolysis.
- Interstitial nephritis associated with NSAIDs and cyclooxygenase-2 inhibitors responds only minimally to corticosteroids.

Atheroembolic Disease

Atheroembolic disease presents with acute renal failure in patients with erosive atherosclerosis. This condition may occur spontaneously but more commonly develops after manipulation of the aorta during surgery or after angiography. Anticoagulation with heparin, warfarin, and thrombolytic agents also may precipitate atheroembolic disease. Embolization of cholesterol clefts into the arterioles and glomerular capillaries leads to infiltration of inflammatory cells and intimal expansion, further limiting renal blood flow and resulting in ischemic tubular injury. The onset of renal failure is usually insidious, with a stuttering pace over several weeks.

Cutaneous manifestations of atheroembolic disease include livedo reticularis, as well as digital infarcts. Involvement of other organs, such as bowel ischemia and neurologic sequelae, can occur depending on the origin of the emboli. Fundoscopic examination may show evidence of cholesterol emboli known as Hollenhorst plaques.

Atheroembolic disease is often mistaken for systemic vasculitis, and dysmorphic hematuria and proteinuria may be prominent features. Eosinophilia is common in this condition, whereas only 15% of affected patients have low levels of serum C3.

Therapy in atheroembolic disease is supportive and should include management of risk factors such as dyslipidemia and hypertension. The prognosis for patients with atheroembolic disease is generally poor, because most affected patients have extensive cardiovascular disease. However, one recent series demonstrated a 1-year survival rate of 87% with judicious supportive care that included discontinuation of anticoagulants, as well as treatment of hypertension and congestive heart failure (15).

KEY POINTS

- Atheroembolic disease associated with acute renal failure may develop due to manipulation of the aorta during surgery; after angiography; or after treatment with heparin, warfarin, and thrombolytic agents.
- Atheroembolic disease often is mistaken for systemic vasculitis, and dysmorphic hematuria and proteinuria may be prominent features.
- Supportive care, including discontinuation of anticoagulants and treatment of hypertension and congestive heart failure, is indicated for atheroembolic disease.

The Thrombotic Microangiopathies

The thrombotic microangiopathies are a heterogeneous group of disorders that can cause acute renal failure in association with albuminuria and dysmorphic hematuria. The clinical presentation of these conditions may range from a renal-limited form without hematologic abnormalities to full-blown thrombotic thrombocytopenic purpura, characterized by microangiopathic hemolytic anemia, renal failure, fever, thrombocytopenia, and neurologic manifestations.

Multiple causes of thrombotic thrombocytopenic purpura have been identified, including drugs, diarrheal syndromes associated with Shiga toxin, antiphospholipid

TABLE 32 Diagnostic Criteria for the Hepatorenal Syndrome

Major Criteria

Chronic or acute liver disease with advanced hepatic failure and portal hypertension

Low GFR, as indicated by a serum creatinine >1.5 mg/dL or a creatinine clearance <40 mL/min

Absence of shock, ongoing bacterial infection, fluid loss, and current or recurrent treatment with nephrotoxic drugs

No sustained improvement in renal function (decrease in serum creatinine to 1.5 mg/dL or less or increase in creatinine clearance to ≥40 mL/min) after withdrawal of diuretics and expansion of plasma volume with 1.5 L of isotonic saline

Urine protein <500 mg/24 h and a lack of ultrasonographic evidence of obstructive uropathy or parenchymal renal disease

Minor Criteria

Urine volume <500 mL/24 h

Urine sodium <10 meq/L

Urine osmolality > plasma osmolality

Urine erythrocytes <50/hpf

Serum sodium concentration <130 meq/L

GFR = glomerular filtration rate; GI = gastrointestinal

antibodies, systemic lupus erythematosus, HIV infection, and hematopoietic stem cell transplantation (Table 30).

Thrombotic microangiopathy, as well as hypertension and acute renal failure, are predominant features of scleroderma renal crisis and malignant hypertension.

Acute Renal Failure in Patients with Liver Disease

Acute renal failure frequently complicates chronic liver disease and acute hepatic failure. Prerenal azotemia, ischemic or nephrotoxic tubular injury, and the hepatorenal syndrome most commonly cause acute renal failure in patients with liver disease. Distinguishing among these conditions often is difficult, because their clinical presentations overlap considerably. Therefore, major and minor criteria have been developed to aid in the diagnosis (**Table 32**) (16). Notably, a urinary sodium level <10 meq/L is not required to establish a diagnosis of hepatorenal syndrome, although this finding traditionally has been emphasized.

Two patterns of clinical presentation in the hepatorenal syndrome have been identified. Type I hepatorenal syndrome is defined as a doubling of the serum creatinine level to at least 2.5 mg/dL or a >50% decrease in the creatinine clearance over 2 weeks. An acute event such as a variceal bleed, infection, overly aggressive diuresis, or large-volume paracentesis often precipitates this condition. Type II hepatorenal syndrome develops more slowly in the setting of refractory ascites and edema.

Treatment of the hepatorenal syndrome is supportive until liver transplant can be performed in eligible patients. Recently, improvement in renal function has been observed with regimens of midodrine in conjunction with octreotide, as well as with terlipressin. Transjugular intrahepatic portosystemic shunts (TIPS) can improve renal perfusion and ameliorate ascites in patients with hepatorenal syndrome, but these benefits must be weighed against the risk for encephalopathy. In the absence of congestive heart failure, uncontrolled infection, and pulmonary hypertension, TIPS can be considered as a last-resort intervention in patients who are not candidates for liver transplantation. Use of TIPS is not recommended in hepatorenal syndrome because of the lack of controlled trials involving this particular indication.

KEY POINTS

- Acute renal failure frequently complicates chronic liver disease and acute hepatic failure.
- A urinary sodium level <10 meq/L is not required to establish a diagnosis of hepatorenal syndrome.
- Midodrine in conjunction with octreotide, as well as terlipressin, may help improve renal function in patients with the hepatorenal syndrome.

Management of Established Acute Renal Failure

Therapy for acute renal failure remains primarily supportive. Judicious fluid resuscitation and avoidance of further ischemic or nephrotoxic insults remain the mainstay of therapy. Careful titration of fluids to maximize renal perfusion and optimization of filling pressures and cardiac output are indicated. Excess fluid removal with diuretics, paracentesis, or dialysis should be avoided, and nephrotoxins such as iodinated contrast and aminoglycosides should be strictly avoided whenever possible.

Drug dosing should be modified according to the degree of renal impairment, and frequent monitoring of drug levels is indicated. Clinical trials examining use of "renal-dose" dopamine, loop diuretics, atrial natriuretic peptide, and growth factors such as insulin-like growth factor or thyroid hormone have shown no benefit in ameliorating the progression or improving the prognosis of acute renal failure.

Indications for dialysis include diuretic-resistant fluid overload, hyperkalemia, and acidosis, as well as uremic complications such as pericarditis or encephalopathy. Dialysis also increasingly is initiated earlier, particularly in oliguric, critically ill patients. This approach facilitates management of high levels of obligate fluid intake and permits ongoing aggressive nutritional support. However, a more conservative approach is reasonable in stable patients expected to recover renal function over the course of several days. In these patients, restriction of fluids, sodium, potassium, phosphorus, and protein may be appropriate to avoid the need for dialysis.

KEY POINTS

- Judicious fluid resuscitation and avoidance of further ischemic or nephrotoxic insults remain the mainstay of acute renal failure therapy.
- Modifying drug dosing according to the degree of renal impairment and frequent monitoring of drug levels are indicated for patients with acute renal failure.
- Indications for dialysis in patients with acute renal failure include diuretic-resistant fluid overload, hyperkalemia, acidosis, and uremic complications.
- Dialysis for acute renal failure increasingly is initiated earlier, particularly in oliguric, critically ill patients.
- Stable patients with acute renal failure expected to recover renal function within several days may benefit from restriction of fluids, sodium, potassium, phosphorus, and protein to avoid the need for dialysis.

References

1. **Loef BG, Epema AH, Smilde TD, Henning RH, Ebels T, Navis G, et al.** Immediate postoperative renal function deterioration in cardiac surgical patients predicts in-hospital mortality and long-term survival. J Am Soc Nephrol. 2005;16:195-200. [PMID: 15563558]

2. **Mehta RL.** Acute renal failure and cardiac surgery: marching in place or moving ahead? [Editorial]. J Am Soc Nephrol. 2005;16:12-4. [PMID: 15590755]

3. **Jeha S, Pui CH.** Recombinant urate oxidase (rasburicase) in the prophylaxis and treatment of tumor lysis syndrome. Contrib Nephrol. 2005;147:69-79. [PMID: 15604607]

4. **Zucchelli P, Pasquali S, Cagnoli L, Ferrari G.** Controlled plasma exchange trial in acute renal failure due to multiple myeloma. Kidney Int. 1988;33:1175-80. [PMID: 3043077]

5. **Clark WF, Stewart AK, Rock GA, Sternbach M, Sutton DM, Barrett BJ, et al.** Plasma exchange when myeloma presents as acute renal failure: a randomized, controlled trial. Ann Intern Med. 2005;143:777-84. [PMID: 16330788]

6. **Bartholomew BA, Harjai KJ, Dukkipati S, Boura JA, Yerkey MW, Glazier S, et al.** Impact of nephropathy after percutaneous coronary intervention and a method for risk stratification. Am J Cardiol. 2004;93:1515-9. [PMID: 15194023]

7. **Aspelin P, Aubry P, Fransson SG, Strasser R, Willenbrock R and Berg KJ.** Nephrotoxic effects in high-risk patients undergoing angiography. N Engl J Med. 2003; 348: 491-499. [PMID: 12571256]

8. **Mueller C, Buerkle G, Buettner HJ, Petersen J, Perruchoud AP, Eriksson U, et al.** Prevention of contrast media-associated nephropathy: randomized comparison of 2 hydration regimens in 1620 patients undergoing coronary angioplasty. Arch Intern Med. 2002;162:329-36. [PMID: 11822926]

9. **Kshirsagar AV, Poole C, Mottl A, Shoham D, Franceschini N, Tudor G, et al.** N-acetylcysteine for the prevention of radiocontrast induced nephropathy: a meta-analysis of prospective controlled trials. J Am Soc Nephrol. 2004;15:761-9. [PMID: 14978179]

10. **Tumlin JA, Wang A, Murray PT, Mathur VS.** Fenoldopam mesylate blocks reductions in renal plasma flow after radiocontrast dye infusion: a pilot trial in the prevention of contrast nephropathy. Am Heart J. 2002;143:894-903. [PMID: 12040355]

11. **Allaqaband S, Tumuluri R, Malik AM, Gupta A, Volkert P, Shalev Y, et al.** Prospective randomized study of N-acetylcysteine, fenoldopam, and saline for prevention of radiocontrast-induced nephropathy. Catheter Cardiovasc Interv. 2002;57:279-83. [PMID: 12410497]

12. **Stone GW, McCullough PA, Tumlin JA, Lepor NE, Madyoon H, Murray P, et al.** Fenoldopam mesylate for the prevention of contrast-induced nephropathy: a randomized controlled trial. JAMA. 2003;290:2284-91. [PMID: 14600187]

13. **Fernandez WG, Hung O, Bruno GR, Galea S, Chiang WK.** Factors predictive of acute renal failure and need for hemodialysis among ED patients with rhabdomyolysis. Am J Emerg Med. 2005;23:1-7. [PMID: 15672329]

14. **Better OS, Rubinstein I, Reis DN.** Muscle crush compartment syndrome: fulminant local edema with threatening systemic effects. Kidney Int. 2003;63:1155-7. [PMID: 12631101]

15. **Theriault J, Agharazzi M, Dumont M, Pichette V, Ouimet D, Leblanc M.** Atheroembolic renal failure requiring dialysis: potential for renal recovery? A review of 43 cases. Nephron Clin Pract. 2003;94:c11-8. [PMID: 12806187]

16. **Arroyo V, Gines P, Gerbes AL, Dudley FJ, Gentilini P, Laffi G, et al.** Definition and diagnostic criteria of refractory ascites and hepatorenal syndrome in cirrhosis. International Ascites Club. Hepatology. 1996;23:164-76. [PMID: 8550036]

CHRONIC KIDNEY DISEASE

RECENT ADVANCES

• Cinacalcet decreases the need for parathyroidectomy
• Corticosteroid-free regimen for maintaining renal allograft function

Chronic kidney disease (CKD) is characterized by an alteration in kidney function or structure of ≥3 months' duration. A progressive loss of renal function and/or complications due to decreased renal function accompany these alterations.

CKD is divided into five stages (**Table 33**). Abnormal findings on serum chemistry studies, renal imaging studies, or renal biopsy, as well as persistent urinary abnormalities, are diagnostic of this condition. An irreversible decline in glomerular filtration rate (GFR) (<60 mL/min for >3 months) also indicates the presence of CKD, but a decrease in the GFR is not needed to establish a diagnosis.

The most common cause of CKD is type 2 diabetes mellitus. CKD also is present in a significant number of patients with the metabolic syndrome, even in the absence of diabetes. In

patients with CKD who have a decreased GFR, reversible causes for the decrease in GFR should be excluded before diagnosing the declining GFR as chronic and irreversible. Reversible causes also may coexist with CKD in patients with impaired GFRs.

KEY POINT

• An alteration in kidney function or structure of ≥3 months' duration and a progressive loss of renal function and/or complications due to decreased renal function characterize chronic kidney disease.

Epidemiology

CKD affects an estimated 20 million patients in the United States. The current prevalence of stage 5 CKD or end-stage renal disease (ESRD) is >400,000, and this number is projected to increase by at least 50% by 2010.

The absolute rates of death and cardiovascular events are much higher in patients with stages 4 and 5 CKD. Therefore, measures to reduce cardiovascular risk in patients with early-stage CKD and to prevent ESRD are indicated. Management of ESRD is extremely costly, and patients with this condition have high morbidity and mortality and a reduced quality of life.

Pathophysiology

Progressive loss of renal function usually characterizes CKD. This progression may be due to the continuous presence and/or recurrence of the insult that incited the renal damage (for example, lupus nephritis or recurrent malignant hypertension). Therefore, treatment of the inciting condition is essential to prevent the onset of irreversible damage and development and progression of CKD. However, irrespective of the activity of the original disease, once the GFR declines to <50% of normal values (which signifies a >50% loss of renal mass), renal function continues to deteriorate.

The progressive decline in GFR usually is associated with proteinuria and systemic hypertension. In response to the reduction in renal mass and GFR, the remaining nephrons, glomeruli, and tubules undergo structural (hypertrophy) and

TABLE 33 Stages of Chronic Renal Disease

Stage	Description	GFR (mL/min)	Action
0	At increased risk	>90 (with CKD risk factors)	Screening, CKD risk reduction
1	Kidney damage with normal or increased GFR	≥90	Diagnose and treat, treat comorbid conditions, slow progression
2	Kidney damage with mildly decreased GFR	60–90	Estimate progression
3	Moderately decreased GFR	30–59	Evaluate and treat complications
4	Severely decreased GFR	15–29	Prepare for renal replacement therapy (dialysis or transplantation)
5	Kidney failure	<15 (or dialysis)	Replacement

GFR = glomerular filtration rate; CKD = chronic kidney disease functional (an increase in glomerular capillary pressure and single-nephron GFR) changes.

Angiotensin II elevates systemic blood pressure and vasoconstricts the efferent arterioles, which maintains the increase in glomerular capillary pressure. Angiotensin II also exerts trophic effects on glomerular and tubular cells that enhance matrix accumulation and attract inflammatory cells to the kidney; this mechanism contributes to the renal structural damage by further compromising the GFR. Therefore, therapeutic regimens to retard CKD progression heavily rely on blockade of the renin–angiotensin–aldosterone system and treatment of other risk factors, as well as specific treatment of the original disease.

The rate of progression of renal disease depends on the individual and the disease type. CKD progression can be monitored clinically using the reciprocal of serum creatinine over time and/or the GFR calculated from validated formulae.

KEY POINTS

- Treatment of the inciting condition in chronic kidney disease is essential.
- Once the glomerular filtration rate declines to <50% of normal values, renal function continues to deteriorate.
- The progressive decline in glomerular filtration rate in chronic kidney disease usually is associated with proteinuria and systemic hypertension.
- Therapy to retard chronic kidney disease progression relies heavily on blockade of the renin–angiotensin–aldosterone system.

Management of Chronic Kidney Disease

Diagnosis and Evaluation

Patients with CKD should be evaluated to establish the cause and determine the severity of renal disease. Certain types of renal disease require specific treatment, such as immunosuppressive agents. Systemic diseases or comorbid conditions such as hypertension and diabetes mellitus cause or contribute to CKD progression and should be treated. Prevention and treatment of cardiovascular disease and its risk factors, such as hyperlipidemia and cigarette smoking, also should be initiated during the early stages of CKD. However, multiple risk factor intervention may be ineffective in patients with stages 4 and 5 CKD.

Late referral of patients with CKD is associated with increased morbidity and poor outcome. A U.S. Renal Data System report indicates that approximately 40% of patients with CKD are not referred to a nephrologist until 3 months

TABLE 34 Strategies to Slow Progression of Renal Disease

Intervention	Goal
ACE inhibitor or ARB treatment (may consider combination therapy if goals not achieved with full-dose monotherapy)	Proteinuria <0.5 g/d GFR decline <2 mL/min per year
Additional antihypertensive therapy (as needed)	BP <130/80 mm Hg if proteinuria <1 g/d BP <125/75 mm Hg if proteinuria >1 g/d
Tight glycemic control in diabetic patients	HbA_{1c} <6.5%
Dietary protein restriction	0.8–1 g/kg per day
Cholesterol-lowering therapy	LDL <100 mg/dL
Erythropoietin therapy	Hb ≥12 g/dL
Dietary salt restriction	3–5 g/d
Smoking cessation	
Weight control	
Antiplatelet therapy	
Reduce elevated calcium–phosphate product	
Avoid nephrotoxic drugs, including some herbal remedies and dietary supplements	

ACE = angiotensin-converting enzyme; ARB = angiotensin receptor blocker; GFR = glomerular filtration rate; BP = blood pressure; HbA_{1c} = hemoglobin A_{1c}; HB = hemoglobin; LDL = low-density lipoprotein

before initiation of dialysis (1). Referral for initial nephrology consultation should occur as soon as a diagnosis of CKD is established.

A primary care physician may establish a partnership with a nephrologist who can recommend care and strategies to slow renal disease progression and to reduce cardiovascular risk (**Table 34**). Nephrologists should assume more responsibility as patients develop systemic complications secondary to CKD, which usually manifest in stage 4 disease when the GFR decreases to <30 mL/min.

Treatment

Intervention strategies aim to treat the underlying disease that resulted in CKD, reduce cardiovascular risk, and prevent loss of renal function. Strict blood pressure control; blockade of the renin–angiotensin system; and avoidance of nephrotoxic agents, including nonsteroidal anti-inflammatory drugs and, when possible, radiocontrast agents, are indicated to preserve GFR. The GFR should be estimated periodically to assess the degree of renal function and progression of CKD.

Hypertension

Early detection and effective treatment of hypertension are essential to retard the progression of renal disease in patients with CKD. Strict blood pressure control is the most important intervention to slow CKD progression. The target blood pressure for all patients with kidney disease is <130/80 mm Hg, whereas the goal for patients with proteinuria >1 g/24 h is <125/75 mm Hg.

Lifestyle modification, including weight loss and exercise, is indicated for patients with CKD. Angiotensin-converting enzyme (ACE) inhibitors and/or angiotensin receptor blockers are the preferred agents to treat hypertension, reduce proteinuria, and slow the progression of renal disease. In patients without diabetes, a diuretic also is appropriate for first-line pharmacologic therapy.

Most patients with CKD, particularly stages 3 and higher, require at least two to three medications for blood pressure control. Diuretics and nondihydropyridine calcium channel blockers such as verapamil or diltiazem or β-adrenergic receptor blockers can be added to the ACE inhibitor or angiotensin receptor blocker regimen as needed.

Recent evidence suggests that combination therapy with ACE inhibitors and angiotensin receptor blockers further reduces surrogate markers of CKD progression, including hypertension, albuminuria, and proteinuria. However, combination therapy with these agents is recommended only in patients who do not achieve goals with a maximum monotherapy dose. Close follow-up for side effects such as hyperkalemia and/or a significant elevation in serum creatinine levels is indicated.

Dietary Protein Restriction

Dietary protein restriction may be recommended for patients with CKD who are regularly monitored for dietary compliance and prevention of malnutrition. Patients with CKD and an impaired GFR should not consume >0.8 g/kg per day to 1 g/kg per day of protein; supervision by a renal dietitian is indicated in this setting to avoid the risk for protein malnutrition.

Anemia

A normochromic, normocytic anemia may accompany progressive CKD. The interstitial cells in the kidney cortex are the primary sites of erythropoietin synthesis in response to decreased renal tissue oxygenation. The anemia of CKD is attributable to reduced erythropoietin production due to a reduction in renal mass. However, other causes of anemia, such as gastrointestinal bleeding, iron or folate deficiency, and hemolysis, should be considered. Recombinant erythropoietin is very effective in treating anemia associated with ESRD or pre-ESRD.

The optimal target for hemoglobin levels has not been established in patients with pre-ESRD. However, a hemoglobin level of 12 g/dL may improve energy and physical function and reduce left ventricular mass.

Administration of erythropoietin before dialysis is initiated provides a survival benefit during the first 19 months of dialysis therapy. However, large, randomized, controlled clinical trials have not yet shown reductions in mortality with this therapy.

Patients with CKD who have hemoglobin levels <10 g/dL are candidates for recombinant erythropoietin therapy once iron deficiency has been excluded. Subcutaneous recombinant erythropoietin therapy, 75 U/kg to 125 U/kg weekly in divided doses, is indicated for adults with severe anemia or anemia-dependent angina. Low iron stores, inflammation or chronic infection, hemoglobinopathies, bone marrow fibrosis, aluminum toxicity, and vitamin B_{12} or folate deficiency are associated with erythropoietin resistance. In patients with ESRD, nonfunctioning vascular access and nonfunctioning transplanted kidneys contribute to erythropoietin resistance.

Erythropoietin therapy may worsen hypertension in approximately 30% of patients. Headaches and flu-like symptoms occur less frequently. Erythropoietin therapy and correction of anemia may slow progression of kidney disease as long as blood pressure is adequately controlled.

KEY POINTS

- Strict blood pressure control, blockade of the renin–angiotensin system, and avoidance of nephrotoxic agents are indicated to preserve the glomerular filtration rate in chronic kidney disease.
- Angiotensin-converting enzyme inhibitors and/or angiotensin receptor blockers are the preferred agents to treat hypertension, reduce proteinuria, and slow the progression of renal disease.
- In patients with chronic kidney disease, diuretics and nondihydropyridine calcium channel blockers can be added to the angiotensin-converting enzyme inhibitor or angiotensin receptor blocker regimen as needed.
- Protein restriction may reduce the rate of decline of the glomerular filtration rate and delays the need for dialysis.
- A normochromic, normocytic anemia usually accompanies progressive chronic kidney disease.
- Recombinant erythropoietin is very effective in treating anemia associated with end-stage renal disease or pre–end-stage renal disease.
- Administration of erythropoietin before dialysis is initiated provides a survival benefit during the first 19 months of dialysis therapy.
- Subcutaneous recombinant erythropoietin therapy, 75 U/kg to 125 U/kg weekly in divided doses, is indicated for adults with severe anemia or anemia-dependent angina.
- In patients with end-stage renal disease, nonfunctioning vascular access and nonfunctioning transplanted kidneys contribute to erythropoietin resistance.

Hyperparathyroidism and Renal Osteodystrophy

Hyperparathyroidism

Pathophysiology

Secondary hyperparathyroidism and bone disease affect almost all patients with CKD. Hyperphosphatemia, hypocalcemia, and deficiency of 1,25-dihydroxyvitamin D stimulate parathyroid hormone secretion.

Phosphate retention occurs when the GFR decreases to <60 mL/min to 80 mL/min. Hyperphosphatemia causes ionized calcium levels to decrease. The calcium-sensing receptor in the parathyroid gland detects hypocalcemia, which increases parathyroid hormone secretion. In this secondary hyperparathyroid response, serum calcium and phosphorus levels normalize, causing a persistently elevated parathyroid hormone level. Since 1,25-dihydroxyvitamin D (calcitriol) regulates calcium absorption in the gut and calcium release from bone, as well as has a direct inhibitory effect on the parathyroid gland, the reduction in renal calcitriol synthesis that occurs with a progressive decrease in the GFR results in hypocalcemia and increased parathyroid hormone secretion.

Management

Dietary phosphorus restriction is indicated if the GFR decreases to <60 mL/min. Oral calcium-containing phosphate binders (calcium acetate or calcium carbonate, taken with meals) or calcium-free phosphate binders prevent the increase of parathyroid hormone secretion in CKD. These agents should be administered as needed to prevent the increase in serum phosphorus levels (2).

Supplementation with oral calcitriol or other vitamin D analogs may be useful for prevention of secondary hyperparathyroidism in CKD as long as hypercalcemia and elevation of the serum–phosphorus product are avoided. Calcimimetics are a very promising new class of agents that suppress parathyroid hormone secretion by acting primarily on the calcium-sensing receptor in the parathyroid glands. Cinacalcet (not yet approved by the U.S. Food and Drug Administration for CKD) may suppress parathyroid hormone secretion and retard the development of renal bone disease while resulting in significantly less elevation in serum calcium and phosphorus levels.

The goal of therapy in hyperparathyroidism is to maintain serum parathyroid hormone levels at approximately two times the normal values. Intact parathyroid hormone (or *N*-terminal parathyroid hormone molecule) levels should be measured to assess parathyroid hormone activity, because inactive *C*-terminal parathyroid hormone molecules accumulate in CKD.

Osteodystrophy

Pathophysiology

Phosphate and calcium homeostasis abnormalities and the associated hyperparathyroidism that occurs in patients with CKD, as well as impaired GFR, result in osteodystrophy. This renal bone disease is classified as osteitis fibrosa, in which bone turnover is increased because of secondary hyperparathyroidism; osteomalacia, which is characterized by low bone turnover and increased noncalcified osteoid secondary to aluminum deposition in bone; and adynamic bone disease, which may be more prevalent in elderly individuals, diabetic patients, and patients treated with aluminum hydroxide. The pathophysiology of adynamic bone disease may relate to excessive parathyroid hormone suppression via calcitriol therapy.

Diagnosis and Evaluation

Patients with renal osteodystrophy may present with bone pain or fractures. Radiographic signs of osteitis fibrosa include subperiosteal bone resorption of phalanges, distal clavicles, and skull. Osteopenia and pseudofractures are more suggestive of osteomalacia. CKD secondary to chronic interstitial nephritis or other causes of CKD characterized by slow and protracted decline in renal function are associated with more severe forms of secondary hyperparathyroidism and renal osteodystrophy even before ESRD develops.

KEY POINTS

- Secondary hyperparathyroidism and bone disease affect almost all patients with chronic kidney disease.
- Dietary phosphorus restriction is indicated if the glomerular filtration rate decreases to <60 mL/min.
- Oral calcium-containing phosphate binders or calcium-free phosphate binders lessen the increase of parathyroid hormone secretion in chronic kidney disease.
- Calcimimetics suppress parathyroid hormone secretion.
- The goal of therapy in hyperparathyroidism is to maintain serum parathyroid hormone levels at approximately two times the normal values.
- Intact parathyroid hormone (or *N*-terminal parathyroid hormone molecule) levels should be used to assess parathyroid hormone activity.
- Patients with renal osteodystrophy may present with bone pain or fractures.

Medical Management of the Uremic State

Kidney function continues to decline with time in most patients with CKD. Inadequate sodium excretion leads to salt and water retention, hypertension, and edema, necessitating dietary sodium restriction and diuretic therapy. Use of ACE inhibitors and salt substitutes may induce hyperkalemia, which becomes more likely as the GFR decreases to <20 mL/min. Dietary potassium should be restricted, and other sources of potassium should be discontinued.

TABLE 35 Indications and Contraindications for Renal Replacement Therapy in End-Stage Renal Disease

Absolute Indications
Refractory hyperkalemia
CHF that is recurrent and/or resistant to diuretics and after load reduction
Progressive uremic neuropathy or encephalopathy
Pericarditis
Relative Indications
GFR <10 mL/min (or <15 mL/min in patients with diabetes mellitus)
Serum creatinine >8 mg/dL (or >6 mg/dL in patients with diabetes mellitus)
Uremic syndrome
Relative Contraindications
Severe irreversible dementia
Debilitating chronic disease

CHF = congestive heart failure; GFR = glomerular filtration rate

Correction of metabolic acidosis may improve muscle strength and lessen the effects of secondary hyperparathyroidism on bone. Medications should be reviewed, and doses should be adjusted as necessary to compensate for reduced renal metabolism and removal. Hypermagnesemia may potentially develop in patients who use magnesium-containing antacids and cathartics.

Uremia is the clinical state in which patients with advanced renal failure develop signs and symptoms related to azotemia. Poorly identified uremic toxins that accumulate as a result of the decreased GFR are believed to cause uremic symptoms, which include the following: anorexia, nausea, vomiting, pruritus, impaired cognitive functions, fatigue, sleep disturbances, sensory and motor neuropathy, asterixis, pericarditis, impaired myocardial contractility, and seizures. The improvement in symptoms with effective dialysis supports the hypothesis that retained toxins cause this condition.

Associated Endocrine Disorders
Several endocrine disorders accompany uremia in this setting. Levels of total thyroxine, triiodothyronine, and free triiodothyronine decrease, whereas levels of thyroid-stimulating hormone and free thyroxine usually are normal. Plasma prolactin and growth hormone levels are elevated. Peripheral resistance to insulin occurs, yet renal insulin clearance is impaired. Therefore, many patients with diabetes may reduce or discontinue insulin therapy.

Gonadal dysfunction occurs in men and women. This condition results in testicular atrophy, amenorrhea, sexual dysfunction, and infertility. Luteinizing hormone levels are elevated in men and women, and growth retardation frequently occurs in children with ESRD.

Renal Replacement Therapy
Renal replacement therapy may be appropriate in some settings, but preparation for this therapy is time consuming (Table 35). When the GFR is <30 mL/min, the patient and family should be counseled regarding the future need for replacement therapy and the most appropriate modality for the patient's condition and lifestyle. In addition to the GFR, the level of residual renal function, symptoms, biochemical abnormalities, nutritional status, and degree of disability determine when renal replacement therapy should be initiated.

KEY POINTS
- Kidney function continues to decline with time in most patients with chronic kidney disease.
- Inadequate sodium excretion leads to salt and water retention, hypertension, and edema, necessitating dietary sodium restriction and diuretic therapy.
- Use of angiotensin-converting enzyme inhibitors and salt substitutes may induce hyperkalemia in patients with chronic kidney disease.
- Hypermagnesemia may potentially develop in patients who use magnesium-containing antacids and cathartics.
- Poorly identified uremic toxins that accumulate as a result of the decreased glomerular filtration rate are believed to cause uremic symptoms.
- When the glomerular filtration rate is <30 mL/min, counseling regarding the future need for replacement therapy is indicated.
- The level of residual renal function, symptoms, biochemical abnormalities, nutritional status, and degree of disability help determine when renal replacement therapy should be initiated.

Tubulointerstitial Disorders
Epidemiology
Tubulointerstitial disorders are characterized by diseases that affect the vascular and interstitial compartments of the kidney with relative sparing of the glomeruli. An estimated 10% to 15% of end-stage renal disease results from tubulointerstitial disorders. These disorders develop because of various toxic, genetic, autoimmune, and chronic medical conditions (Table 36). Tubulointerstitial disorders also may develop secondary to other chronic kidney diseases, such as

TABLE 36 Causes of Chronic Tubulointerstitial Disorders

Toxic
Analgesics
Aristolochic acid
Calcineurin inhibitors
Cisplatin
Lithium
Medical
Hypertension-induced nephrosclerosis
Atheroemboli
Lymphoproliferative disorders
Heavy metals
Chronic urinary tract obstruction
Genetic
Alport's syndrome
Cystinosis
Polycystic kidney disease
Medullary cystic kidney disease
Autoimmune
SLE
Sarcoidosis
Sjögren's syndrome

SLE = systemic lupus erythematosus

diabetic nephropathy or glomerular disorders. The most common causes of tubulointerstitial disorders are hypertensive nephrosclerosis, myeloma kidney (discussed in Glomerular Disorders), and analgesic nephropathy.

Pathophysiology

Regardless of the cause of tubulointerstitial disease, the pathogenesis involves a nonspecific immunologic mechanism of renal injury with exposure of new antigens on tubular cells, causing an inflammatory reaction and destruction of the interstitium. Lymphocytic infiltration and fibrosis in the interstitium with tubular atrophy, arterial sclerosis, and global glomerulosclerosis are characteristic findings on renal histology in affected patients.

In multiple myeloma, glomerular filtration of light chains, or Bence–Jones proteins, is toxic to the renal tubular cells (3, 4). Light chains also may bind to Tamm–Horsfall protein, causing cast formation and renal tubular obstruction.

Hypertensive Nephrosclerosis

Epidemiology

The underlying causative disease primarily determines the risk factors for tubulointerstitial disorders. Hypertensive nephrosclerosis is more common in black patients compared with white or Asian individuals (5). Uncontrolled hypertension

and concomitant underlying chronic kidney disease increase the risk for and progression of nephrosclerosis.

Diagnosis

The diagnosis of tubulointerstitial disorders is largely clinical, because the majority of patients do not undergo kidney biopsy for histologic confirmation. Evaluation consists of a careful history and physical examination particularly focusing on chronic medical conditions, family history, medication and analgesic use, and environmental exposures.

Hypertensive nephrosclerosis is a diagnosis of exclusion in patients with a history of hypertension. This condition is characterized by modest elevations in the blood urea nitrogen (BUN) and creatinine levels that gradually worsen over time. The urine sediment is characterized as bland, or without formed elements, and the urinary protein level typically is <1 g/24 h. Renal ultrasonography is a helpful diagnostic study in this setting, because the kidneys in affected patients are characteristically small and echogenic; these findings are consistent with chronic kidney disease.

Treatment

For all individuals with chronic kidney disease, blood pressure control slows progressive loss of kidney function. In the African American Study of Kidney Disease and Hypertension (AASK) trial, patients with a clinical diagnosis of hypertensive nephrosclerosis were randomized to antihypertensive therapy with ramipril, amlodipine, or metoprolol. The ramipril group was significantly less likely to achieve the secondary outcomes of a reduction in the glomerular filtration rate, development of renal failure, or death compared with the other two medication groups (6). The seventh Joint National Committee on Prevention, Detection, Evaluation, and Treatment of High Blood Pressure (JNC 7) thus recommends angiotensin-converting enzyme inhibitors or angiotensin II receptor blockers as first-line therapy for chronic kidney disease, with a target blood pressure <130/80 mm Hg (7). For patients with CKD and proteinuria >1 g/24h, a target blood pressure <125/75 mm Hg is recommended (2).

Prognosis and Follow-up

Despite optimal blood pressure control, patients with hypertensive nephrosclerosis develop reduced kidney function over time; this finding suggests that the associated kidney injury involves other factors. Diagnosis and treatment of other causes of hypertension, such as renovascular disease, are indicated to prevent accelerated loss of kidney function. Concomitant use of nephrotoxins, such as nonsteroidal anti-inflammatory drugs and intravenous contrast agents, should be avoided.

Analgesic Nephropathy

Epidemiology

The prevalence of analgesic nephropathy is five times more common in women than men. This condition usually presents after the fifth decade of life. The incidence of analgesic nephropathy is declining, particularly in Europe, since the offending agent phenacetin was removed from the market (8).

Combination analgesics, such as acetaminophen and aspirin with caffeine or codeine, are believed to increase the risk for analgesic nephropathy. However, epidemiologic studies have not proven a direct causal relationship. A cumulative analgesic dose >3 kg over time is associated with analgesic nephropathy.

Diagnosis

A history of chronic analgesic use, elevations in the BUN and creatinine levels, and a bland urine sediment that may contain occasional granular casts or leukocytes establish a diagnosis of analgesic nephropathy. Renal ultrasonography in affected patients typically reveals small, echogenic kidneys.

Treatment

The treatment of analgesic nephropathy is largely supportive. Most affected patients have a good prognosis with stabilization of kidney function after discontinuation of the offending agents. However, patients with advanced kidney failure at the time of diagnosis are more likely to progress to end-stage renal disease.

Prognosis and Follow-up

Analgesic nephropathy has been associated with a 10% increased risk for transitional-cell carcinomas of the urinary collecting system (9). Therefore, urine cytology and cystoscopy are recommended to further evaluate patients with analgesic nephropathy who have persistent hematuria.

KEY POINTS

- **Lymphocytic infiltration and fibrosis in the interstitium with tubular atrophy, arterial sclerosis, and global glomerulosclerosis are characteristic renal histology findings in tubulointerstitial disorders.**
- **Renal ultrasonography in patients with hypertensive nephrosclerosis typically reveals small, echogenic kidneys.**
- **A history of chronic analgesic use, elevations in the blood urea nitrogen and creatinine levels, and a bland urine sediment that may contain occasional granular casts or leukocytes establish a diagnosis of analgesic nephropathy.**
- **Renal ultrasonography in patients with analgesic nephropathy typically reveals small, echogenic kidneys.**
- **Urine cytology and cystoscopy to evaluate for transitional-cell carcinomas of the urinary collecting system are recommended in patients with analgesic nephropathy and persistent hematuria.**

Treatment of End-Stage Renal Disease

End-stage renal disease (ESRD) is characterized by severe, irreversible kidney failure for which affected patients require dialysis or renal transplantation for survival. In the United States, ESRD is currently treated by hemodialysis (60%), peritoneal dialysis (10%), and renal transplantation (30%) (1). The primary care physician plays a key role in initiating the treatment process and in counseling patients who decline dialysis. Early referral to a nephrologist is essential for adequate patient education and preparation for treatment options.

Dialysis versus Renal Transplantation

Patients with ESRD should receive counseling about their options for dialysis or transplantation, as well as information comparing survival and quality of life with all modalities. Renal transplantation is associated with superior quality of life and is less expensive compared with long-term dialysis. All patients with ESRD are considered candidates for renal transplantation unless they have systemic malignancy, chronic infection, severe cardiovascular disease, or neuropsychiatric disorders.

Annual mortality rates for patients on dialysis in recent years range from 21% to 25%, whereas these rates are <8% for cadaveric transplant recipients and <4% for living related transplant recipients. Recognition that healthier patients generally receive transplantation is needed when comparing patient outcomes with transplantation versus dialysis. However, patients who have undergone a successful transplantation have lower mortality rates than those maintained on dialysis while awaiting a renal transplant, which suggests that transplantation is associated with a clear-cut survival advantage.

Transplantation is particularly beneficial in young patients and those with diabetes mellitus (**Figure 8**). For example, the projected years of life in a patient 20 to 39 years of age on dialysis without diabetes is 31 with a renal transplant and 20 without a transplant. The projected years of life for a patient in the same age group on dialysis who has diabetes is 25 with a transplant and only 8 without a transplant.

The current shortage of donor organs in the United States severely limits patient access to transplantation, despite its superior results and reduced long-term costs. Patients are encouraged to find their own donors to avoid prolonged waiting. Results of renal transplantation from living related or unrelated donors are excellent.

Principles of Dialysis Therapy

Dialysis refers to the diffusion of small molecules down their concentration gradient across a semipermeable membrane. In hemodialysis, blood is withdrawn from the patient's body and passed through a membrane that separates the blood from a dialysate solution on the other side, which contains electrolytes and glucose. Small molecules such as urea, potassium, and phosphorus diffuse down their concentration gradients from the blood into the dialysate solution. At the same time, small molecules such as calcium and bicarbonate move down their concentration gradients from the dialysate solution into the blood. The net effect is removal of low-molecular-weight toxins from the blood while increasing the plasma concentration of molecules that may be deficient in patients with renal failure. Dialysis also may achieve fluid removal.

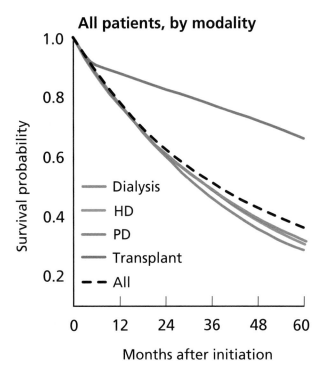

All patients, by modality

FIGURE 8.
Survival curves for different treatment modalities for ESRD. Adjusted survival: 1988–1992 incident patients.
Incident dialysis patients and patients receiving a first transplant in the calendar year. All probabilities are adjusted for age, gender, and race; overall probabilities are also adjusted for primary diagnosis. All ESRD patients, 1996, used as reference cohort. Modality determined on first ESRD service date; excludes patients transplanted or dying during the first 90 days.

ESRD = end-stage renal disease; HD = hemodialysis; PD = peritoneal dialysis

Adapted with permission from www.usrds.org.

Dialysis Techniques
In-center hemodialysis, home hemodialysis, and home peritoneal dialysis (chronic ambulatory or cycler peritoneal dialysis) are available to most U.S. patients with ESRD. Almost 85% of patients receive in-center hemodialysis, whereas only 1% of patients receive home hemodialysis, despite better survival statistics with this method.

High-efficiency hemodialysis uses a membrane with a large surface area that can remove large amounts of low-molecular-weight solute, whereas high-flux hemodialysis uses a membrane with a larger pore size that can remove larger molecules and allow for more rapid fluid removal. Use of these modalities is believed to decrease symptoms associated with dialysis. Long-term use of high-flux membranes is believed to reduce morbidity.

Approximately 10% of patients undergo peritoneal dialysis. Patient survival with this therapy is equivalent to in-center hemodialysis in patients without diabetes. Data from the U.S. Renal Data System show a slight increase in mortality in diabetic and elderly patients treated with chronic ambulatory

peritoneal dialysis (see also Reference 1). However, this finding is not universal, and patients in these population groups who have hemodynamic instability frequently undergo peritoneal dialysis.

Peritoneal dialysis catheters should be placed approximately 1 month before therapy is initiated. In patients with catheters, one episode of peritonitis occurs every 3 years on average; the majority of these episodes are successfully treated with outpatient intraperitoneal antibiotics.

Maintaining access for hemodialysis is a major challenge. A native arteriovenous fistula or a synthetic polytetrafluoroethylene vascular graft should be placed weeks to months before initiation of dialysis. Once mature, native fistulas have excellent long-term patency rates and, when compared with other forms of vascular access, consistently are associated with the lowest mortality risk (10). Referral for arteriovenous fistula creation is indicated once the serum creatinine level increases to approximately 4 mg/dL or the glomerular filtration rate decreases to <30 mL/min.

Use of cephalic veins for phlebotomy or intravenous cannulation can prevent successful fistula construction. Therefore, venipuncture and intravenous cannulation above the level of the hands, particularly in the nondominant extremity, are contraindicated in patients with chronic kidney disease. Synthetic polytetrafluoroethylene grafts are an alternative option for patients with inadequate anatomy to support a fistula.

As a last resort, dialysis can proceed via a cuffed double-lumen silastic or silicone catheter inserted through a subcutaneous tunnel into the internal jugular vein. However, this method is associated with a high rate of infection and an inability to achieve adequate solute clearance, both of which contribute to excess mortality. Therefore, this modality is the least desirable form of vascular access.

Medical Problems in Patients Undergoing Dialysis
Cardiovascular disease, infection, and discontinuation of dialysis primarily due to poor functional status are the most common causes of death in patients undergoing dialysis. Cardiovascular disease accounts for almost 50% of deaths of patients on dialysis. Cardiovascular risk factors in patients on dialysis include hypertension, hyperlipidemia, and hyperhomocystinemia; diabetes is frequently an underlying disorder in these patients, as well. Dialysis-induced hypertension, increased oxidant stress, and vascular calcification may contribute to atherosclerotic risk. Cardiomyopathy and left ventricular hypertrophy also may occur.

The 1-year mortality rate after an acute myocardial infarction is >50% in patients undergoing dialysis. Coronary angioplasty without stenting is less effective in patients on dialysis, because rates of restenosis are 70% to 80% at 6 months in this population. Therefore, coronary artery bypass grafting is often favored over angioplasty in these patients. However, long-term outcomes of percutaneous transluminal angioplasty with stent placement in patients with ESRD are uncertain pending further clinical trials.

Altered calcium–phosphorus metabolism has been identified as a significant risk factor in cardiovascular disease and mortality (11). Elevated serum calcium and phosphorus levels contribute to increased vascular calcification and have been associated with higher mortality rates in patients with ESRD. Traditional methods to control serum parathyroid hormone levels and to prevent high-turnover renal osteodystrophy, such as use of calcium-based phosphate binders and vitamin D sterols, may increase serum calcium and phosphorus levels.

The Kidney Disease Outcomes Quality Initiative's practice guidelines recommend maintaining serum calcium levels <9.5 mg/dL and serum phosphorus levels <5.5 mg/dL (6). Achieving this goal using vitamin sterols and calcium-based phosphate binders to reduce increased parathyroid hormone secretion traditionally has been difficult.

Recently, the oral calcimimetic agent cinacalcet has been approved by the U.S. Food and Drug Administration to treat secondary hyperparathyroidism in patients on dialysis. This agent facilitates control of serum parathyroid hormone levels while maintaining both serum calcium and phosphate within recommended levels. Non–calcium-based phosphate binders such as sevelamer and lanthanum carbonate also are frequently needed to achieve these goals. Whether this approach favorably impacts mortality awaits controlled prospective clinical trials.

Infection accounts for 15% to 20% of all deaths in patients on dialysis. Infection of the vascular access site, frequently with gram-positive organisms, may occur with few local findings, which underscores the need to maintain a high index of clinical suspicion (12). Ultrasonography and radionucleotide imaging studies such as indium-labeled leukocyte scanning can aid in the diagnosis.

Although 1-year survival rates in patients on dialysis have improved and are now approximately 80%, U.S. rates are lower than those in other countries. One possible explanation for this finding is insufficient dosing of dialysis. However, dialysis doses are now monitored frequently and adjusted accordingly. Short-term daily daytime or nocturnal dialysis dosing appears to improve patients' well-being and decrease frequency of hospitalization.

Renal Transplantation

Renal transplantation is considered successful if the glomerular filtration rate after transplantation is >50 mL/min. Advantages of successful transplantation include improved quality of life and survival, correction of anemia, and restoration of endocrine function, which allow a return to an unrestricted lifestyle. Renal transplantation stabilizes or improves autonomic neuropathy, retinopathy, and gastroenteropathy, which have an accelerated course in patients with diabetes who have ESRD. A lack of adequate numbers of donor organs, surgical risk, complications, and the cost of immunosuppression are the major barriers to wider use of transplantation.

Contraindications

Contraindications for renal transplantation include active substance abuse or noncompliance, metastatic cancer, severe arterial disease involving the iliac arteries, active infection, active ischemic cardiac and cerebrovascular disease, advanced dementia, and debility. Chronological age is no longer considered an absolute exclusion criterion in patients with few comorbid conditions.

Patient and Graft Survival

The source of the transplanted organ significantly influences patient survival after renal transplantation. Recipients of a living related kidney have survival rates of 97% at 1 year and 90% at 5 years, whereas recipients of a living unrelated kidney have survival rates of 96% at 1 year and 84% at 5 years. Recipients of a cadaveric kidney have survival rates of 93% at 1 year and 81% at 5 years.

Patients with diabetes who are >60 years of age have 1-year survival rates of approximately 90% but 5-year survival rates of 45% to 70%. Cardiovascular disease is the most frequent cause of death in adult renal transplant recipients; acute myocardial infarction accounts for one third of these cardiovascular-related deaths. Infection and cancer account for 18% and 10% of deaths in renal transplant recipients, respectively.

Patient and allograft survival advantages have recently been demonstrated for preemptive transplantation and for transplantation performed after shorter periods of dialysis (13). These findings highlight the importance of early referral for patients with progressive chronic kidney disease to facilitate timely identification of potential living donors.

One-year deceased-donor transplant allograft survival is 88% nationally. Short-term graft survival is influenced by factors such as source of the kidney, HLA mismatch, panel-reactive antibody status, and dialysis history. However, acute rejection is the primary cause of short-term renal allograft loss. Five-year renal allograft survival is approximately 65%.

Long-term graft survival is affected by HLA matching, episodes of acute rejection, hypertension, and recurrent or new glomerular disease. Use of newer immunosuppressive agents has significantly improved short-term graft survival, but long-term survival has only improved slightly. For transplants performed in the United States between 1988 and 1996, the half-life was 18.8 years for cadaveric allografts and 21.6 years for one-haplotype–mismatched living related grafts (14).

Immunosuppressive Treatment

Indefinite immunosuppressive therapy is indicated to maintain allograft function; discontinuation of immunosuppression leads to allograft rejection. Multiple drugs generally are required to inhibit T-cell function and prevent rejection. In the early post-transplant period, larger doses of immunosuppressants are used; over time, dosages are tapered. Induction therapy often entails use of either lymphocyte-depleting agents, such as alemtuzumab (a humanized monoclonal antibody to CD52); thymoglobulin; or anti–interleukin-2 agents, such as basiliximab and daclizumab. Use of these agents has permitted successful maintenance of renal allograft function without the use of corticosteroids.

The benefits of a successful renal transplant outweigh the risks of immunosuppression. The major risks of chronic immunosuppressive therapy are infection and malignancy. The cyclophilin inhibitors cyclosporine and tacrolimus (FK506) are the cornerstones of immunosuppressive therapy (**Table 37**). Both drugs may cause hypertension, hyperkalemia, and nephrotoxicity. Unlike cyclosporine, tacrolimus does not cause hirsutism or gum hypertrophy but can induce seizures, encephalopathy, diarrhea, and glucose intolerance.

Nephrotoxicity limits the use of single-agent therapy with calcineurin inhibitors. Therefore, most immunosuppressive regimens use steroids or purine metabolism inhibitors such as mycophenolate mofetil or azathioprine. Mycophenolate mofetil acts more selectively on lymphocytes compared with azathioprine but induces dose-related diarrhea and leukopenia. This agent also may be associated with a higher frequency of viral infections. Unlike azathioprine, mycophenolate mofetil does not prolong the half-life of allopurinol.

Special Problems in Renal Transplant Recipients

Cardiovascular disease, especially myocardial infarction, is the most common cause of morbidity and mortality in renal transplant recipients. Cutaneous and lymphoid neoplasms occur at a significantly higher rate in these patients compared with the general population. Aseptic necrosis of the hips and knees and cataracts related to use of high-dose corticosteroids was previously a significant problem in this setting. However, incidence of these conditions is decreasing after introduction of corticosteroid-sparing immunosuppressive regimens.

Infections within the first month of transplantation usually are associated with complications of surgery and include wound and urinary tract infections, postoperative pneumonia, and catheter-related sepsis. Opportunistic infections may particularly develop during the first post-transplant year. Reduction or discontinuation of immunosuppression during episodes of life-threatening infection should be considered.

Routine post-transplant management includes prophylaxis against *Pneumocystis* and cytomegalovirus (CMV). Symptomatic CMV is the most common opportunistic infection in renal transplant recipients. The likelihood of symptomatic infection is highest in recipients who are CMV negative who receive a kidney from a CMV-positive donor.

Presenting features of CMV may include fever, headache, diarrhea, or pulmonary symptoms. Elevated liver chemistry studies, leukopenia, and thrombocytopenia are common in affected patients. CMV infection also can precipitate acute rejection.

TABLE 37 Classes of Maintenance Immunosuppressive Drugs
Cyclophilin Inhibitors
Calcineurin inhibitors
Cyclosporine
Tacrolimus (FK506)
Calcineurin-independent agents
Sirolimus (rapamycin)
Corticosteroids
Antimetabolites
Nonselective purine inhibitors
Azathioprine
Lymphocyte selective purine inhibitors
Mycophenolate mofetil
Mycophenolate

Infection with *Listeria* is the most common cause of meningitis in renal transplant recipients. Therefore, empiric therapy should be considered if these patients have findings suggestive of meningitis until the specific microbiological diagnosis is confirmed.

Since the advent of more aggressive induction regimens and mycophenolate mofetil, BK (human polyomavirus) virus nephropathy has become an increasing problem in renal transplant recipients. This condition typically presents with an asymptomatic rise in the serum creatinine level. In affected patients, quantitative polymerase chain reaction assays reveal an elevated BK viral load in the blood and urine. Urine cytology in affected patients reveals the presence of decoy cells. Immunohistochemical staining for simian virus 40 viral antigen in renal biopsy specimens establishes the diagnosis of this condition.

The mainstay of therapy in BK nephropathy is a reduction in immunosuppression, often with discontinuation of mycophenolate mofetil. Both cidofovir and leflunomide have been used with varying success.

Most cases of post-transplant lymphoproliferative disorder (PTLD) are associated with Epstein–Barr virus infection. The clinical spectrum of disease varies widely. In mild disease, a mononucleosis-like condition develops and is associated with polyclonal B cell proliferation and normal cytogenetics. Intermediate disease has similar clinical features but is characterized by polyclonal B-cell proliferation associated with cytogenetic abnormalities and immunoglobulin gene rearrangements. Reduction of immunosuppression and antiviral therapy with agents such as ganciclovir or acyclovir, in combination with rituximab, have been used successfully in polyclonal PTLD, often without loss of allograft function.

Monoclonal B-cell proliferation associated with malignant cytogenetic abnormalities and immunoglobulin gene rearrangements characterize a more aggressive extranodal form of PTLD. Clinical features of this condition may include localized solid tumors; lymphadenopathy; and pulmonary, cutaneous, hepatic, central nervous system, gastrointestinal, and renal allograft involvement. Chemotherapy in conjunction with rituximab generally is indicated for affected patients. Discontinuation of immunosuppression often is indicated; consequently, allograft function may be lost.

KEY POINTS

- Renal transplantation is associated with a superior quality of life and a clear-cut survival advantage and is less expensive compared with long-term dialysis.

- Contraindications for renal transplantation include active substance abuse or noncompliance, metastatic cancer, severe iliac arterial disease, active infection, active ischemic cardiac or cerebrovascular disease, and advanced dementia or debility.

- Chronological age is no longer considered an absolute exclusion criterion for renal transplantation.

- In hemodialysis, a native arteriovenous fistula or a synthetic polytetrafluoroethylene vascular graft should be placed weeks to months before initiation of dialysis.

- In peritoneal dialysis, catheter placement should occur approximately 1 month before therapy is initiated.

- In hyperparathyroidism, cinacalcet helps to control serum parathyroid hormone levels and to maintain serum calcium and phosphate within recommended levels.

- Nephrotoxicity limits the use of single-agent immunosuppressive therapy with calcineurin inhibitors in renal transplant recipients.

- Most cases of post–renal transplantation lymphoproliferative disorder are associated with Epstein–Barr virus infection.

References

1. **USRDS 2004 Annual data report.** Am J Kid Dis. 2005;45:8-280.

2. K/DOQI clinical practice guidelines for bone metabolism and disease in chronic kidney disease. Am J Kidney Dis. 2003;42:S1-201. [PMID: 14520607]

3. **Solomon A, Weiss DT, Kattine AA.** Nephrotoxic potential of Bence Jones proteins. N Engl J Med. 1991;324:1845-51. [PMID: 1904132]

4. **Bladé J, Fernández-Llama P, Bosch F, Montolíu J, Lens XM, Montoto S, et al.** Renal failure in multiple myeloma: presenting features and predictors of outcome in 94 patients from a single institution. Arch Intern Med. 1998;158:1889-93. [PMID: 9759684]

5. **Perneger TV, Klag MJ, Feldman HI, Whelton PK.** Projections of hypertension-related renal disease in middle-aged residents of the United States. JAMA. 1993;269:1272-7. [PMID: 8437305]

6. **Agodoa LY, Appel L, Bakris GL, Beck G, Bourgoignie J, Briggs JP, et al.** Effect of ramipril vs amlodipine on renal outcomes in hypertensive nephrosclerosis: a randomized controlled trial. JAMA. 2001;285:2719-28. [PMID: 11386927]

7. **Chobanian AV, Bakris GL, Black HR, Cushman WC, Green LA, Izzo JL Jr, et al.** Seventh report of the Joint National Committee on Prevention, Detection, Evaluation, and Treatment of High Blood Pressure. Hypertension. 2003;42:1206-52. [PMID: 14656957]

8. **De Broe ME, Elseviers MM.** Analgesic nephropathy. N Engl J Med. 1998;338:446-52. [PMID: 9459649]

9. **Piper JM, Tonascia J, Matanoski GM.** Heavy phenacetin use and bladder cancer in women aged 20 to 49 years. N Engl J Med. 1985;313:292-5. [PMID: 4010740]

10. **Dhingra RK, Young EW, Hulbert-Shearon TE, Leavey SF, Port FK.** Type of vascular access and mortality in U.S. hemodialysis patients. Kidney Int. 2001;60:1443-51. [PMID: 11576358]

11. **Block GA, Hulbert-Shearon TE, Levin NW, Port FK.** Association of serum phosphorus and calcium x phosphate product with mortality risk in chronic hemodialysis patients: a national study. Am J Kidney Dis. 1998;31:607-17. [PMID: 9531176]

12. **Ayus JC, Sheikh-Hamad D.** Silent infection in clotted hemodialysis access grafts. J Am Soc Nephrol. 1998;9:1314-7. [PMID: 9644644]

13. **Mange KC, Joffe MM, Feldman HI.** Effect of the use or nonuse of long-term dialysis on the subsequent survival of renal transplants from living donors. N Engl J Med. 2001;344:726-31. [PMID: 11236776]

14. **Hariharan S, Johnson CP, Bresnahan BA, Taranto SE, McIntosh MJ, Stablein D.** Improved graft survival after renal transplantation in the United States, 1988 to 1996. N Engl J Med. 2000;342:605-12. [PMID: 10699159]

THE KIDNEY IN PREGNANCY

Renal Anatomy and Physiology in Pregnancy

Anatomic and Functional Changes in the Urinary Tract

Kidney length increases approximately 1 cm during normal gestation. However, the major anatomic alterations of the urinary tract during pregnancy occur in the collecting system, where calyces, renal pelvices, and ureters dilate. This dilation often resembles obstructive uropathy.

Hormonal mechanisms, as well as mechanical obstruction by the enlarging uterus, may cause ureteral dilatation in pregnancy. These morphologic changes result in stasis in the urinary tract and a propensity of pregnant women with asymptomatic bacteriuria to develop frank pyelonephritis.

Renal Hemodynamics

Pregnancy is characterized by marked vasodilatation, which is detectable in the first trimester. Recent studies of the menstrual cycle show that vasodilatation also is present in the late luteal phase, before conception (1). Throughout gestation, blood pressure and renal vascular resistance are decreased and the renal plasma flow (RPF) and glomerular filtration rate (GFR) are increased.

Because the RPF increases slightly more than the GFR, filtration fraction is constant or slightly lower in pregnancy. Increases in renal hemodynamics reach a maximum during the first trimester and are approximately 50% higher than nonpregnant levels. Creatinine production is unchanged during pregnancy. Therefore, increments in creatinine clearance result in decreased serum creatinine levels.

The increased GFR and RPF cause an increased excretion of glucose, amino acids, calcium, and urinary protein. In this setting, the upper limit of normal for urinary protein excretion (150–300 mg/24 h) is elevated.

Acid–Base Regulation in Pregnancy

Bicarbonate excretion in pregnant patients increases, most likely in response to chronic respiratory alkalosis. Plasma bicarbonate concentration decreases by approximately 4 μmol/L, averaging 22 μmol/L. The hypocapnia that occurs during pregnancy is probably a result of progesterone-mediated hyperventilation. P_{CO_2} averages only 30 mm Hg. Therefore, because both P_{CO_2} and HCO_3 levels are already diminished, pregnant women may be disadvantaged when threatened by acute metabolic acidosis.

Water Metabolism

Pregnant women typically have a plasma osmolality 5 mosm/kg H_2O to 10 mosm/kg H_2O lower than nongravid patients. Responses to water loading and dehydration in these patients are appropriate and suggest a resetting of the osmoreceptor system. Clinical studies demonstrating decreased osmotic thresholds for thirst and arginine vasopressin release in pregnant women support this hypothesis.

Pregnant women metabolize arginine vasopressin more rapidly because of increased production of placental vasopressinases. The increased metabolism of arginine vasopressin also may cause transient diabetes insipidus, which is infrequently observed and may be treated with desmopressin.

Volume Regulation

Total body water increases by 6 L to 8 L during pregnancy, 4 L to 6 L of which are extracellular. Plasma volume increases 50% during gestation, with the largest rate of increment occurring in midpregnancy. During pregnancy, there is a gradual cumulative retention of approximately 900 meq/L of sodium, which is distributed between the products of conception and the maternal extracellular space. Serum potassium levels may be slightly lower due to increased levels of aldosterone.

The marked vasodilatation observed early in the first trimester may be the stimulus for increased sodium retention and increased plasma volume. The significant decrease in blood pressure and stimulation of the renin–angiotensin system that occur during normal pregnancy are consistent with this hypothesis (2).

KEY POINTS

- **Pregnant patients have an elevated upper limit of normal for urinary protein excretion.**
- **Because P_{CO_2} and HCO_3 levels are diminished in pregnancy, pregnant women may be disadvantaged when threatened by acute metabolic acidosis.**
- **During normal pregnancy, blood pressure significantly decreases.**

Kidney Disease in Pregnancy

Fertility and the ability to sustain an uncomplicated pregnancy are related to a patient's degree of renal functional impairment, not the specific underlying disorder. The greater the functional impairment and the higher the blood pressure, the less likely the pregnancy is to be successful (3).

Women with moderate or severe renal dysfunction (serum creatinine ≥1.5 mg/dL) should be discouraged from conceiving, because up to 40% of pregnancies in this setting are complicated by hypertension or deterioration in renal function that may be irreversible (**Table 38**) (4). The level of blood pressure at the time of conception is an important variable in pregnancy outcome. In the absence of hypertension, irreversible deterioration in renal function during pregnancy is significantly less likely.

When hypertension is present, and especially when it is severe, pregnancy outcome is rarely uncomplicated. Premature delivery and deterioration in renal function in this setting are likely. Urinary protein excretion may increase markedly in pregnant women with underlying renal disease. The increments in urinary protein excretion during pregnancy

TABLE 38 Pregnancy and Renal Disease: Functional Renal Status and Prospects*

Outcome	Category Mild (Cr <1.5 mg/dL)	Moderate (Cr = 1.5–3.0 mg/dL)	Severe (Cr >3.0 mg/dL)
Pregnancy complications	25%	47%	86%
Successful obstetric outcome	96% (85%)	90% (59%)	47% (8%)
Long-term sequelae	<3% (9%)	25% (71%)	53% (92%)

Cr = creatinine clearance

* Estimates are based on 1862 women with 2799 pregnancies (1973–1992) and do not include collagen diseases. Numbers in parentheses refer to prospects when complications develop before 28 weeks' gestation. Modified with permission from Davison JM, Lindheimer MD. Renal disorders. In: Creasy RK, Resnik RK, eds. Maternal Fetal Medicine. 4th ed. Philadelphia: Saunders; 1999.

may not necessarily reflect worsening of the underlying kidney disease. However, increased proteinuria is associated with worse fetal prognosis.

Renal Diseases Associated with Systemic Illness
Diabetes

Diabetes mellitus is one of the most common medical disorders present during pregnancy, and the majority of cases are due to gestational diabetes. Preexisting diabetes poses significant risks to pregnancy. Many younger women with pregestational diabetes have type 1 diabetes. If these patients have a 10- to 15-year history of this condition, they may have early signs of diabetic nephropathy.

Women with microalbuminuria, well-preserved renal function, and normal blood pressure have a good prognosis for pregnancy and low risk for deterioration in renal function (5). However, these patients have increased risk for preeclampsia and urinary infection. Urinary protein excretion may increase significantly but transiently during pregnancy. Women with overt nephropathy before conception, particularly those with impaired renal function and hypertension (as in any other renal disease), have a high incidence of premature delivery and deterioration in maternal renal function.

Strict glucose control is crucial, because of the relationship between tight glucose control and improved fetal outcome. Blood pressure control also is important. Angiotensin-converting enzyme inhibitors and angiotensin receptor blockers are contraindicated during pregnancy (6). Therefore, a switch to other agents before conception is indicated.

Systemic Lupus Erythematosus

Because systemic lupus erythematosus tends to flare, this condition is unpredictable. Lupus may become more active during pregnancy and therefore may be associated with significant maternal and fetal risk (7). When lupus is active at conception, outcomes are worse. Therefore, conception is not recommended unless disease has been inactive for the preceding 6 months.

Women with lupus may have clinically significant titers of antiphospholipid antibodies and the lupus anticoagulant, which are associated with spontaneous fetal loss; hypertensive syndromes indistinguishable from preeclampsia; and thrombotic events, including deep vein thrombosis, pulmonary embolus, myocardial infarction, and stroke. Aspirin, 80 mg/d to 325 mg/d, is recommended when anticardiolipin antibody titers are elevated or the lupus anticoagulant is detected. If there is a history of thrombotic events, combination therapy with heparin and aspirin is recommended (8).

In the latter half of pregnancy, distinguishing between a renal lupus flare and preeclampsia may be difficult. Unfortunately, delivery may be necessary if immunosuppressive therapy and supportive care fail to stabilize the condition. Appropriate therapy for lupus nephritis during pregnancy includes steroids and azathioprine. Cyclophosphamide is not recommended during pregnancy, because of potential fetal toxicity. Results from animal studies and anecdotal reports of human use show that mycophenolate mofetil also may compromise fetal safety and is not indicated to treat lupus nephritis in pregnant patients. Patients who are already using this agent who are contemplating pregnancy should switch to another agent, such as a glucocorticoid or azathioprine.

Chronic Glomerulonephritis

Various forms of chronic glomerulonephritis are common in women of childbearing age, including IgA nephropathy, focal and segmental glomerulosclerosis, membranoproliferative glomerulonephritis, minimal change nephritis, and membranous nephropathy. Because pregnant patients undergo frequent blood pressure measurement and urinalyses, renal disease is sometimes first diagnosed during pregnancy. Renal diagnostic testing during pregnancy may include serum chemistry studies, urine testing, and ultrasonography.

Patients with chronic glomerulonephritis may have urinary abnormalities and/or abnormal renal function at their first antepartum visit. When these abnormalities are first detected in the latter half of pregnancy, preeclampsia should be considered in the differential diagnosis. Significant azotemia (serum creatinine ≥1.5 mg/dL) with or without proteinuria is more consistent with glomerulonephritis. Chronic glomerulonephritis also is more likely when azotemia and proteinuria are present in a normotensive woman.

Renal biopsy in pregnant patients usually is deferred until after delivery, unless there is acute deterioration in renal function or morbid nephrotic syndrome. There are insufficient data to suggest that histologic subtype confers a specific prognosis for pregnancy; in the setting of normal renal function with an absence of hypertension, prognosis is good.

Polycystic Kidney Disease

Young women with autosomal dominant polycystic kidney disease are frequently asymptomatic, have normal renal function and normal blood pressure, and may be undiagnosed. Older women with progressive disease, functional impairment, and hypertension who are pregnant are at risk for preeclampsia and premature delivery and have an increased incidence of urinary tract infection (9).

Chronic Pyelonephritis

Chronic pyelonephritis is characterized by recurrent urinary tract infections that are often associated with urinary tract abnormalities, such as vesicoureteral reflux. The dilation and stasis in the urinary tract associated with pregnancy may exacerbate this condition. High fluid intake and frequent screening for bacteriuria are indicated for affected patients.

Acute Renal Failure in Pregnancy

The incidence of acute renal failure from obstetric causes is less than 1 in 20,000 pregnancies. Acute renal failure early in pregnancy (12 to 18 weeks' gestation) usually is associated with septic abortion or prerenal azotemia due to hyperemesis gravidarum. Most cases of acute renal failure in pregnancy occur between gestational week 35 and the puerperium and are primarily caused by preeclampsia and bleeding complications.

Preeclampsia is rarely associated with renal failure. However, the HELLP syndrome (hemolysis, elevated liver enzymes, and low platelets), which is a variant of preeclampsia, may be associated with significant renal dysfunction, especially if not treated promptly.

Although rare, thrombotic microangiopathies (thrombotic thrombocytopenic purpura and hemolytic uremic syndrome) are associated with considerable morbidity. Therefore, these conditions are an important cause of pregnancy-related acute renal failure. These conditions also share several clinical and laboratory features of pregnancy-specific disorders, such as the HELLP variant of preeclampsia and acute fatty liver of pregnancy, including elevated blood pressure, thrombocytopenia, and renal insufficiency. Renal biopsy may be appropriate if there has been no improvement in renal function within 1 to 3 weeks after delivery. However, caution is indicated because of low platelet counts and an increased risk for bleeding in this setting.

Delivery and supportive care are indicated to treat preeclampsia and the HELLP syndrome, and renal function usually returns to normal within days or a few weeks of delivery. Treatment of thrombocytopenic purpura/hemolytic uremic syndrome includes plasma infusion/exchange and other modalities used in nonpregnant patients with these conditions. Hemolytic uremic syndrome often is associated with renal failure, which often develops in the postpartum period and may be resistant to treatment with plasma infusion/exchange.

Bilateral Renal Cortical Necrosis

Abruptio placentae associated with obstetric hemorrhage may induce bilateral renal cortical necrosis. Primary disseminated intravascular coagulation and severe renal ischemia may initiate bilateral renal cortical necrosis. Affected patients typically present with oliguria or anuria, hematuria, and flank pain. Ultrasonography or CT scanning may demonstrate hyperechoic or hypodense areas in the renal cortex. Most patients ultimately require dialysis, but 20% to 40% have partial recovery of renal function.

Management of acute renal failure occurring in pregnancy or immediately post partum is similar to that in nongravid patients. Because urea, creatinine, and other metabolites that accumulate in uremia traverse the placenta, dialysis should be performed early, with the goal of maintaining the blood urea nitrogen at approximately 50 mg/dL.

Therapy of End-Stage Renal Disease during Pregnancy

Pregnancy is rare and often unsuccessful in women on dialysis. Prematurity, very low birthweight, and intrauterine growth restriction are common fetal complications in this setting. Possible maternal complications include accelerated hypertension and mortality.

Women with end-stage renal disease may have a successful pregnancy after renal transplantation (10). These patients should wait 1 to 2 years post transplant before conceiving, and pregnancy should be discouraged if serum creatinine is >2 mg/dL. Complications in these patients include impaired glucose tolerance, hypertension, increased infection, ectopic pregnancy, and uterine rupture. Fetal complications include a higher incidence of premature delivery, intrauterine growth restriction, congenital anomalies, hypoadrenalism, thrombocytopenia, and infection.

KEY POINTS

- Fertility and the ability to sustain an uncomplicated pregnancy are related to a patient's degree of renal functional impairment, not the specific underlying disorder.

- The greater the functional renal impairment and the higher the blood pressure, the less likely the pregnancy is to be successful.

- Women with moderate or severe renal dysfunction (serum creatinine >1.5 mg/dL) should be discouraged from conceiving.

- Diabetes is one of the most common medical disorders present during pregnancy, with the majority of presentations due to gestational diabetes.

- Preexisting diabetes poses significant risks to pregnancy.

- Angiotensin-converting enzyme inhibitors and angiotensin receptor blockers are contraindicated during pregnancy.

- Patients with lupus whose disease has been active within the past 6 months should not conceive.

- Aspirin, 80 mg/d to 325 mg/d, is indicated for pregnant patients with lupus whose antiphospholipid antibody titers are elevated.

- Distinguishing between a renal lupus flare and preeclampsia may be difficult in the latter half of pregnancy.

- High fluid intake and frequent bacteriuria screening are indicated for pregnant patients with chronic pyelonephritis.

- Preeclampsia and bleeding complications primarily cause acute renal failure in pregnancy.

- Pregnancy is rare and often unsuccessful in women on dialysis.

- Women with end-stage kidney disease may have a successful pregnancy after renal transplantation but should wait 1 to 2 years post transplant before conceiving.

Hypertensive Disorders of Pregnancy

Hypertensive disorders are the most common medical conditions complicating pregnancy. In the United States, hypertension complicates approximately 8% to 10% of all pregnancies; 50% of these cases are attributable to the pregnancy-specific disorder preeclampsia. Additional hypertensive disorders in pregnancy are chronic hypertension, chronic hypertension with superimposed preeclampsia, and transient hypertension. Hypertension in pregnancy is a leading cause of maternal death and morbidity and may cause considerable fetal morbidity and mortality in association with preterm birth.

Preeclampsia

Preeclampsia is characterized by hypertension (blood pressure ≥140/90 mm Hg) and proteinuria (urinary protein ≥300 mg/24 h) that usually develops in the third trimester and occurs less frequently in the second trimester and extremely rarely as early as 20 weeks gestation. Edema, thrombocytopenia, and liver function abnormalities also may be present. The fetal manifestations are poor placentation, growth restriction, and possibly death. Eclampsia is the convulsive form of preeclampsia.

Preeclampsia is more common in nulliparous women and those with preexisting renal disease, hypertension, diabetes and obesity, multiple gestations, positive family history, extremes of reproductive age, and hydatiform mole. Thrombophilic disorders, particularly the factor V Leiden mutation, and the antiphospholipid antibody syndrome also are associated with an increased risk for preeclampsia.

The cause of preeclampsia is not known. Current research regarding the pathophysiology of the maternal manifestations of preeclampsia has focused on the associated alterations in maternal endothelial cell function, including reductions in nitric oxide and prostacyclin and increased endothelin. There is evidence that the placenta may be critically involved in the genesis of preeclampsia, and failure of trophoblastic invasion of the uterine spiral arteries is one of the earliest manifestations of this disorder. Failure of trophoblast cells to invade these vessels results in more constricted spiral arteries and decreased placental perfusion. Recent evidence suggests a role for dysregulated angiogenic factors in the pathogenesis of preeclampsia (11).

Glomerular capillary endotheliosis is the characteristic renal histologic lesion seen in preeclampsia, which is characterized by swollen glomerular capillary endothelial cells. Both GFR and RPF decrease in preeclampsia with average decrements of approximately 25% in most patients, but GFR remains above pregravid values in most cases (12). Changes occur in the renal handling of urate in preeclampsia. Uric acid clearance decreases, accompanied by an increase in blood levels, which may precede other clinical signs of preeclampsia.

TABLE 39 Antihypertensive Therapy in Preeclampsia
Imminent Delivery
Hydralazine (IV, IM)
Labetalol (IV)
Calcium channel blockers
Diazoxide (IV)
Delivery Postponed
Methyldopa
Labetalol, other β-blockers
Calcium channel blockers
Hydralazine
α-Blockers
Clonidine

IV = intravenous; IM = intramuscular

Management

Management of preeclampsia includes accurate early diagnosis, bed rest, judicious use of antihypertensive therapy, close monitoring of both maternal and fetal condition, prevention of convulsions with magnesium sulfate, and appropriately timed delivery. Rest is an important aspect of therapy, as it improves uteroplacental perfusion. Delivery should be considered in all patients at term and in patients remote from term if signs of impending eclampsia (hyperreflexia, headaches, epigastric pain) are present or if blood pressure cannot be controlled.

Lowering blood pressure does not cure preeclampsia, and aggressive lowering of blood pressure compromises uteroplacental perfusion, which may be hazardous to fetal well-being. There is no consensus regarding how high blood pressure should increase before treatment is initiated in women with preeclampsia. However, levels >150/100 mm Hg may be hazardous in women who previously had low-normal blood pressure.

Parenteral therapy is recommended when delivery is likely to occur in the next 24 hours (**Table 39**). If postponement of delivery appears safe, oral therapy is recommended. Magnesium sulfate effectively prevents eclamptic convulsions. Although this agent is not classified as an antihypertensive, it lowers blood pressure to a mild degree in some women.

Magnesium sulfate usually is administered immediately after delivery, because convulsions are most likely to occur in the immediate postpartum period. However, magnesium may slow the progress of labor and complicate anesthesia and intraoperative monitoring during cesarean section. Therefore, this agent is rarely administered antepartum.

Prevention

Prevention of preeclampsia has not yet been successful. Small studies have suggested that low-dose aspirin or calcium supplementation may be beneficial. However, subsequent large, placebo-controlled trials have all failed to demonstrate a significant benefit of these prophylactic strategies except in women with the antiphospholipid antibody syndrome or other thrombophilias who may be at risk for early, severe, recurrent preeclampsia. Anticoagulation with heparin and aspirin administered throughout pregnancy particularly has been shown to benefit women with the antiphospholipid antibody syndrome. Therefore, although there are no published data regarding the benefits of treatment, some experts recommend treating other thrombophilias with similar approaches.

Chronic Hypertension

Women with preexisting or chronic hypertension may have essential or secondary hypertension. Most women with stage 1 or 2 essential hypertension do well during pregnancy. However, the risk for developing superimposed preeclampsia may be as high as 25% in these patients. Preexisting maternal hypertension also is associated with an increased risk for placental abruption, intrauterine growth restriction, and midtrimester fetal death.

Management

The approach to treatment of chronic hypertension during pregnancy and in nonpregnant patients differs. The primary concern in nongravid patients is reducing long-term cardiovascular risk. Treatment of pregnant patients primarily concerns maintaining maternal health during the period of gestation and maintaining a favorable intrauterine environment to allow fetal maturity while minimizing fetal exposure to potentially harmful drugs (**Table 40**).

There are little data to support a target level of blood pressure that should be attained during pregnancy. Similarly, no data exist that suggest that maintaining blood pressure levels close to normal prevents the development of superimposed preeclampsia. The current standard of care is to treat maternal hypertension when systolic pressure is >145 to 150 mm Hg and diastolic pressure is >95 to 100 mm Hg (13).

Although secondary hypertension is considerably less common than essential hypertension, failure to recognize the presence of these conditions may result in adverse pregnancy outcomes. Pheochromocytoma and renovascular hypertension are associated with poor maternal and fetal prognosis, but accelerated hypertension, superimposed preeclampsia, and fetal demise are more common events.

Women with primary aldosteronism may have relatively uncomplicated pregnancies, particularly if hypertension is only stage 1. However, if more severe hypertension is present, pregnancy may be complicated and dangerous. It is preferable to diagnose secondary hypertension before conception,

TABLE 40 Antihypertensive Drugs and Pregnancy
α₂-Adrenergic Receptor Agonists
Methyldopa is the most extensively used drug in this group. Its safety and efficacy are supported by evidence from randomized trials and a 7.5-year follow-up study of children born to mothers treated with this agent.
β-Adrenergic Receptor Antagonists
These drugs appear to be safe and efficacious in late pregnancy, but fetal growth restriction has been reported when treatment is started in early or midgestation. Fetal bradycardia can occur, and animal studies suggest that the fetus' ability to tolerate hypoxic stress may be compromised.
α-Adrenergic Receptor and β-Adrenergic Receptor Antagonists
Labetalol is as effective as methyldopa, but there is limited information regarding follow-up of children born to mothers given labetalol. Rare cases of hepatotoxicity have been reported.
Arterial Vasodilators
Hydralazine is frequently used as adjunctive therapy with methyldopa and β-adrenergic antagonists. Rarely, neonatal thrombocytopenia has been reported. Trials with calcium channel blockers look promising. The experience with minoxidil is limited, and this drug is not recommended.
Calcium Channel Blockers
Small uncontrolled studies and a meta-analysis suggest that these agents are safe and effective in pregnancy. There is limited information regarding follow-up of children exposed to calcium channel blockers in utero.
Angiotensin-Converting Enzyme Inhibitors
Captopril causes fetal death in diverse animal species, and several angiotensin-converting enzyme inhibitors have been associated with oligohydramnios and neonatal renal failure when administered to humans. Contraindicated during pregnancy.
Angiotensin II Receptor Blockers
These drugs have not been used in pregnancy. In view of the deleterious effects of blocking angiotensin II generation, angiotensin II receptor antagonists also are considered to be contraindicated in pregnancy.
Diuretics
Many authorities discourage the use of diuretics, but others continue these medications if they were prescribed before conception or there is evidence of salt sensitivity.

because the physiologic changes associated with pregnancy make diagnosis more difficult.

Gestational Hypertension

High blood pressure that first develops after midpregnancy is characterized as gestational hypertension. This condition is distinguished from preeclampsia by an absence of proteinuria.

Manifestations of gestational hypertension vary. Some patients later develop diagnostic criteria for preeclampsia, whereas others may have chronic hypertension but develop a decrease in blood pressure in early pregnancy, masking the true diagnosis. Gestational hypertension that resolves post partum, excluding preeclampsia, is more likely to occur in women who develop essential hypertension later in life.

KEY POINTS

- Hypertensive disorders, particularly preeclampsia, are the most common medical conditions complicating pregnancy.
- Preeclampsia is characterized by hypertension and proteinuria and usually develops in the third trimester.
- Management of preeclampsia includes bed rest, anti-hypertensive therapy, and immediate postpartum therapy with magnesium sulfate.
- Delivery may be indicated for patients with signs of impending preeclampsia or uncontrollable blood pressure.
- Aggressive lowering of blood pressure in patients with preeclampsia may be harmful to the fetus.
- Treatment for pregnant patients is indicated when systolic pressure increases to >145 to 150 mm Hg and diastolic pressure increases to >95 to 100 mm Hg.
- Gestational hypertension first develops in midpregnancy and is not associated with proteinuria.

References

1. **Chapman AB, Abraham WT, Zamudio S, Coffin C, Merouani A, Young D, et al.** Temporal relationships between hormonal and hemodynamic changes in early human pregnancy. Kidney Int. 1998;54:2056-63. [PMID: 9853271]

2. **August P, Mueller FB, Sealey JE, Edersheim TG.** Role of renin-angiotensin system in blood pressure regulation in pregnancy. Lancet. 1995;345:896-7. [PMID: 7707813]

3. **Fischer MJ, Lehnerz SD, Hebert JR, Parikh CR.** Kidney disease is an independent risk factor for adverse fetal and maternal outcomes in pregnancy. Am J Kidney Dis. 2004;43:415-23. [PMID: 14981599]

4. **Jones DC, Hayslett JP.** Outcome of pregnancy in women with moderate or severe renal insufficiency. N Engl J Med. 1996;335:226-32. [PMID: 8657238]

5. **Rossing K, Jacobsen P, Hommel E, Mathiesen E, Svenningsen A, Rossing P, et al.** Pregnancy and progression of diabetic nephropathy. Diabetologia. 2002;45:36-41. [PMID: 11845221]

6. **Cooper WO, Hernandez-Diaz S, Arbogast PG, Dudley JA, Dyer S, Gideon PS, et al.** Major congenital malformations after first-trimester exposure to ACE inhibitors. N Engl J Med. 2006;354:2443-51. [PMID: 16760444]

7. **Moroni G, Quaglini S, Banfi G, Caloni M, Finazzi S, Ambroso G, et al.** Pregnancy in lupus nephritis. Am J Kidney Dis. 2002;40:713-20. [PMID: 12324905]

8. **Noble LS, Kutteh WH, Lashey N, Franklin RD, Herrada J.** Antiphospholipid antibodies associated with recurrent pregnancy loss: prospective, multicenter, controlled pilot study comparing treatment with low-molecular-weight heparin versus unfractionated heparin. Fertil Steril. 2005;83:684-90. [PMID: 15749498]

9. **Chapman AB, Johnson AM, Gabow PA.** Pregnancy outcome and its relationship to progression of renal failure in autosomal dominant polycystic kidney disease. J Am Soc Nephrol. 1994;5:1178-85. [PMID: 7873727]

10. **Armenti VT, Radomski JS, Moritz MJ, Gaughan WJ, McGrory CH, Coscia LA.** Report from the National Transplantation Pregnancy Registry (NTPR): outcomes of pregnancy after transplantation. Clin Transpl. 2003:131-41. [PMID: 15387104]

11. **Maynard SE, Min JY, Merchan J, Lim KH, Li J, Mondal S, et al.** Excess placental soluble fms-like tyrosine kinase 1 (sFlt1) may contribute to endothelial dysfunction, hypertension, and proteinuria in preeclampsia. J Clin Invest. 2003;111:649-58. [PMID: 12618519]

12. **Moran P, Baylis PH, Lindheimer MD, Davison JM.** Glomerular ultrafiltration in normal and preeclamptic pregnancy. J Am Soc Nephrol. 2003;14:648-52. [PMID: 12595500]

13. **Report of the National High Blood Pressure Education Program Working Group on High Blood Pressure in Pregnancy.** Am J Obstet Gynecol, 2000;183: S1-S22. [PMID: 10920346]

NEPHROLITHIASIS

Epidemiology

Nephrolithiasis, or kidney stones, affects 5% of women and 12% of men and often develops before the sixth decade of life (1). This condition is more common in white patients compared with black, hispanic, or Asian patients. The incidence of nephrolithiasis varies geographically and is more frequent in warm, arid climates compared with colder regions.

Pathophysiology

Kidney stones predominantly are composed of calcium, but other substrates, such as uric acid, struvite, and cystine, also may form kidney stones. The pathogenesis of nephrolithiasis is complex and depends on the saturation of crystalloid molecules and the concentration of promoters or inhibitors of stone formation in the urine. Typically, molecules such as calcium that normally are soluble in the urine become super-saturated. These molecules undergo nucleation to form microscopic particles on renal tubular surfaces or on cellular debris. Crystal aggregation and growth of the microscopic particles develop into a kidney stone.

It is unclear why microscopic crystalloid particles are not excreted with the urine, but this circumstance may result from preexisting renal epithelium damage, urinary stasis, or conditions associated with low urinary volume that predispose patients to stone formation.

Risk Factors

A constellation of dietary, metabolic, and genetic factors, as well as certain chronic medical conditions, most likely cause stone formation and recurrence (**Table 41**).

Diet

Fluid intake is one of the most important dietary factors influencing stone development. In several large cohort studies, patients in the highest quartile of fluid intake (>2500 mL/d)

TABLE 41 Risk Factors for the Development of Nephrolithiasis
Dietary
Low fluid intake
High sodium intake
High protein intake
Low calcium intake
Metabolic
Hypercalciuria
Hypocitraturia
Hyperuricosuria
Hyperoxaluria
Medical Conditions
Gout
Obesity
Renal tubular acidosis
Sarcoidosis
Primary hyperparathyroidism
Medullary sponge kidney
Horseshoe kidney
HIV/AIDS with protease inhibitors
Metabolic syndrome/type 2 diabetes mellitus
Genetic
Polycystic kidney disease
Dent's disease
Cystinuria
Primary hyperoxaluria

Metabolism

High levels of stone promoters, such as calcium, uric acid, and oxalate, and/or a decreased level of stone inhibitors, such as urinary citrate, are among the metabolic factors that increase the risk for nephrolithiasis. Hypercalciuria is the most common metabolic abnormality affecting individuals with nephrolithiasis; this condition is present in 60% of these patients. Typically, calcium levels >250 mg/d in women and >300 mg/d in men characterize hypercalciuria. However, some experts suggest that calcium levels >200 mg/d for both men and women are normal.

Sources of excess calcium usually are related to increased calcium absorption in the gastrointestinal tract. However, excess calcium from bone and renal tubular defects in calcium absorption also may contribute to hypercalciuria. Patients with a history of gout and levels of urinary uric acid >1000 mg/d, or hyperuricosuria, have a 40% to 50% increased risk for uric acid stones compared with the general population.

Elevated urinary oxalate levels, typically >45 mg/d, account for only 8% of the metabolic abnormalities in nephrolithiasis, although calcium oxalate is the most prevalent type of kidney stone. Hyperoxaluria is associated with a low-calcium diet and malabsorption syndromes that increase oxalate absorption in the gastrointestinal tract, as well as prolonged use of antibiotics that alter enteric flora, such as *Oxalobacter formigenes*, that degrade oxalate.

Approximately one third of patients with nephrolithiasis may have low urinary citrate levels. Citrate inhibits crystal formation and binds to urinary calcium, therefore preventing stone formation. Chronic metabolic acidosis associated with renal tubular defects or diarrhea increases the proximal reabsorption of citrate. This increase results in hypocitraturia, defined by urinary citrate levels <320 mg/d.

Genetics and Medical Conditions

Genetic and chronic medical conditions associated with nephrolithiasis are less common than dietary or metabolic factors. Genetic disorders such as polycystic kidney disease favor calcium stone formation with urinary stasis and Dent's disease with hypercalciuria, as well as cystinuria with a renal tubular defect in cystine metabolism that results in cystine stones and primary hyperoxaluria with an enzymatic defect in glyoxylate metabolism that causes calcium oxalate stones. Medical disorders, such as primary hyperparathyroidism with hypercalciuria, cause calcium oxalate stones. The metabolic syndrome and type 2 diabetes mellitus have an increased risk for calcium-containing and uric acid stones associated with hypocitraturia and acidic urine, respectively (4). Recurrent urinary tract infections with urease-splitting organisms such as *Klebsiella* and *Proteus* species are associated with struvite stones.

had a 30% reduction in stone formation compared with those in the lowest quartile (<1275 mL/d in men and <1400 mL/d in women) (2). The type of fluid consumed also may affect stone disease; for example, grapefruit juice is associated with an increased risk for this condition, whereas moderate alcohol or coffee intake is associated with a decreased risk.

Increased dietary sodium and protein intake also increase the risk for kidney stones. Conversely, higher amounts of dietary calcium correlate with a 45% reduction in the risk for nephrolithiasis, most likely because dietary calcium binds and prevents oxalate absorption (see also Reference 2). Supplemental calcium has not demonstrated this protective effect, because this agent often is taken between meals. Supplemental calcium may even slightly predispose patients to stone formation (3).

- Increased fluid and dietary calcium consumption decrease the risk for kidney stones.
- Consumption of grapefruit juice and increased dietary sodium and protein intake increase the risk for kidney stones.
- Calcium, uric acid, and oxalate promote kidney stones.
- Hypercalciuria usually related to increased calcium absorption in the gastrointestinal tract is the most common metabolic abnormality affecting individuals with nephrolithiasis.
- Hyperoxaluria is associated with a low-calcium diet, malabsorption syndromes that increase oxalate absorption in the gastrointestinal tract, and prolonged use of certain antibiotics.
- Chronic metabolic acidosis associated with renal tubular defects or diarrhea increases the proximal reabsorption of citrate.

Screening and Prevention

There is no standard approach for the primary prevention of kidney stones. The history and risk factors for stone recurrence determine whether evaluation after a first kidney stone should be limited or complete.

Routine kidney chemistry studies and bicarbonate, calcium, phosphorous, and uric acid measurements are recommended for patients without appreciable risk factors. In addition, parathyroid hormone measurement is indicated if hypercalcemia is present. A more complete evaluation is warranted in patients with a high risk for stone recurrence, such as white men and patients with chronic diarrheal and malabsorption syndromes, osteoporosis, gout, or a family history of nephrolithiasis.

In addition to the serum chemistry studies obtained for a limited stone evaluation, a 24-hour urine collection is recommended to measure urine volume, pH, creatinine, sodium, calcium, uric acid, oxalate, and citrate excretion. Because of dietary variations, the sensitivity and specificity of studies to identify a metabolic abnormality in the urine increase if three 24-hour collections are obtained compared with a single collection (5).

- White men and patients with chronic diarrheal and malabsorption syndromes, osteoporosis, gout, or a family history of nephrolithiasis have a high risk for stone recurrence.
- The sensitivity and specificity of studies to identify a metabolic abnormality in the urine increase if three 24-hour collections are obtained compared with a single collection.

Diagnosis

The clinical presentation, urinalysis, stone analysis, and imaging studies establish a diagnosis of acute nephrolithiasis. The classic symptoms of nephrolithiasis are acute flank pain and hematuria. Other conditions, such as ectopic pregnancy, pyelonephritis, aortic aneurysm, papillary necrosis, or bowel ischemia, should be considered in the differential diagnosis.

Urinalysis in patients with nephrolithiasis reveals blood, and the urine sediment has intact, nondysmorphic erythrocytes. Microscopic analysis of the urine for crystals may suggest the type of stone present in the urinary collecting system (**Table 42**). Straining and analyzing the urine for stone collection is necessary to definitively establish the stone type.

Imaging studies such as a kidney, ureter, and bladder (KUB) film; renal ultrasonography; intravenous pyelography;

TABLE 42 Types and Treatment of Nephrolithiasis

Metabolic Abnormality	Stone Type	Crystals	Treatment
Low urine volume	All stone types		Increase fluid intake
Hypercalciuria	Calcium oxalate Calcium phosphate	Envelope, dumbbell Irregular, elongated	Thiazide diuretic
Hyperuricosuria	Uric acid	Rhomboid, diamond	Potassium citrate Allopurinol
Hypocitraturia	Calcium oxalate Calcium phosphate	Envelope, dumbbell Irregular, elongated	Potassium citrate
Hyperoxaluria	Calcium oxalate	Envelope, dumbbell	Dietary restriction of oxalate Increase dietary calcium
Cystinuria	Cystine	Hexagon	Potassium citrate Penicillamine Tiopronin Captopril
Recurrent urinary infection	Struvite	Coffin lid	Surgical removal Antibiotic therapy

and noncontrast helical abdominal CT may be used to diagnose nephrolithiasis. The majority of kidney stones are radio opaque and visualized on KUB film. However, limiting factors of a KUB film include small and non–radio-opaque stones, such as those composed of uric acid or that result from protease inhibitors.

Renal ultrasonography detects kidney stones and urinary tract obstruction but is less sensitive for smaller stones. Intravenous pyelography has a high sensitivity and specificity for the diagnosis of kidney stones and anatomic abnormalities in the urinary collecting system. However, this study requires the use of radiocontrast, which is contraindicated in renal insufficiency. Noncontrast helical abdominal CT detects stones as small as 1 mm in diameter and is considered the gold standard for the diagnosis of nephrolithiasis.

KEY POINTS

- **The classic symptoms of nephrolithiasis are acute flank pain and hematuria.**
- **The differential diagnosis of nephrolithiasis includes ectopic pregnancy, pyelonephritis, aortic aneurysm, papillary necrosis, or bowel ischemia.**
- **Urinalysis in patients with nephrolithiasis reveals blood, and the urine sediment has intact, nondysmorphic erythrocytes.**
- **The majority of kidney stones are radio opaque and visualized on kidney, ureter, and bladder film.**
- **Renal ultrasonography detects kidney stones and urinary tract obstruction but is less sensitive for smaller stones.**
- **Intravenous pyelography is highly sensitive and specific for kidney stones but is contraindicated in patients with renal insufficiency.**
- **Noncontrast helical abdominal CT is the gold standard for diagnosing nephrolithiasis.**

Treatment

Hydration and pain control with nonsteroidal anti-inflammatory drugs or narcotics if renal insufficiency is present are indicated to treat nephrolithiasis in the acute setting. Kidney stones <5 mm in diameter typically pass spontaneously, whereas stones >10 mm often require invasive measures. The most common procedures for the treatment of kidney stones include percutaneous nephrostolithotomy, ureterorenoscopy, and shock-wave lithotripsy.

Percutaneous nephrostolithotomy is indicated for stones >2 cm in diameter; staghorn calculi; anatomic abnormalities, such as horseshoe kidney; and stones comprised of cystine that are resistant to shock-wave lithotripsy. Rigid or flexible ureterorenoscopy is recommended for stones in the ureteral tract; this study involves direct visualization of the kidney stone and/or stone fragments.

Shock-wave lithotripsy is the most common stone removal technique. This treatment generates high-energy shock waves that fragment the stone and allow smaller fragments to pass spontaneously or incorporates ureterorenoscopy for stone and fragment removal. Repeat interventions may be required if stone fragments remain, because these fragments may act as a nidus for further stone formation and growth. Open surgery for stone removal is indicated for procedural failures, large staghorn calculi, or renal anatomic abnormalities but is rarely used.

Prevention of recurrent nephrolithiasis includes pharmacologic and nonpharmacologic therapies. Identification and treatment of underlying chronic medical conditions that are associated with nephrolithiasis are indicated to avoid stone recurrence. Fluid consumption >2 L/d and restriction of sodium intake are recommended for all patients with a history of nephrolithiasis, regardless of stone composition. Targeted therapy is recommended for patients with an identifiable metabolic abnormality that favors stone formation (Table 42).

Increasing dietary calcium to 1 g/d to 4 g/d is recommended to decrease oxalate absorption in patients with hyperoxaluria. Restriction of foods high in oxalate, such as spinach, rhubarb, beets, and chocolate, also is indicated in these patients. Consumption of dietary sources of citrate, such as 4 oz of lemon juice or 60 meq/d to 80 meq/d of oral potassium citrate or bicarbonate, is recommended to increase urinary citrate levels and decrease urinary calcium levels in order to decrease the development of recurrent calcium oxalate stones. Potassium salts are preferred over sodium salts, because excess sodium causes volume expansion that may worsen hypercalciuria and increase stone formation.

Calcium phosphorous stones are associated with renal tubular acidosis and hypocitraturia. These stones form in alkaline urine, and citrate therapy may increase stone recurrence. In this setting, careful monitoring of citrate use is required. In patients with hypercalciuria, low-dose thiazide diuretics, such as chlorthalidone or hydrochlorothiazide, 12.5 mg/d to 25 mg/d, increases renal calcium absorption in the distal convoluted tubule and decreases urinary calcium excretion.

For uric acid stones, alkalization of the urine to a pH >6 using potassium citrate increases the solubility of uric acid and decreases the recurrence of kidney stones. Allopurinol, 100 mg/d to 300 mg/d, also is recommended to treat uric acid stones and is associated with an 80% reduction in stone recurrence. Identification and treatment of underlying infection are indicated for patients with struvite stones. Chronic suppressive antibiotic therapy may be beneficial in this setting, but stone removal is the standard treatment.

In cystinuria, the goal is to decrease the solubility of cystine in the urine via increased fluid intake; urine alkalization; sodium restriction; and medications, such as penicillamine, tiopronin, or captopril. In patients with cystinuria and end-stage renal disease, transplantation resolves the renal tubular defect associated with cystinuria.

KEY POINTS

- Hydration and pain control with nonsteroidal anti-inflammatory drugs or narcotics if renal insufficiency is present are indicated to treat acute nephrolithiasis.
- Kidney stones <5 mm in diameter typically pass spontaneously, whereas stones >10 mm often require invasive measures.
- Percutaneous nephrostolithotomy is indicated for stones >2 cm in diameter, staghorn calculi, anatomic abnormalities, and stones comprised of cystine that are resistant to shock-wave lithotripsy.
- Shock-wave lithotripsy is the most common stone removal technique, but repeat interventions may be indicated if fragments remain.
- Open surgery for stone removal is indicated for procedural failures, large staghorn calculi, or renal anatomic abnormalities.
- Fluid consumption >2 L/d and restriction of sodium intake are recommended for all patients with a history of nephrolithiasis.
- Increasing dietary calcium and restricting foods high in oxalate are recommended for hyperoxaluria.
- Consumption of dietary sources of citrate may decrease the development of recurrent calcium oxalate stones.
- Low-dose thiazide diuretics may benefit patients with hypercalciuria.
- Alkalization of the urine to a pH >6 using potassium citrate and allopurinol therapy may decrease uric acid stone recurrence.
- Identification and treatment of underlying infection and stone removal are indicated for patients with struvite stones.
- In patients with cystinuria and end-stage renal disease, transplantation resolves the renal tubular defect associated with cystinuria.

Prognosis and Follow-up

Nephrolithiasis is a chronic, recurring condition. Fifteen percent of affected patients have a stone recurrence at 1 year, 35% to 40% at 5 years, and 50% at 10 years. Kidney stones discovered incidentally are likely to cause acute symptoms that often develop within 3 to 5 years of diagnosis and typically require medical intervention.

Treatment of identifiable metabolic abnormalities and dietary modifications decrease the recurrence rate of kidney stones. However, only 15% to 40% of patients followed prospectively over 3 years in a kidney stone clinic complied with recommended therapy (6). Imaging studies such as a KUB film for radio-opaque stones or renal ultrasonography are recommended annually after the first stone, then every 2 to 4 years to evaluate for recurrence. Noncontrast helical CT or intravenous pyelography generally is not used for stone surveillance, because they are more costly and expose patients to radiation and contrast agents.

KEY POINT

- Imaging studies such as a kidney, ureter, and bladder film for radio-opaque stones or renal ultrasonography are recommended annually after the first stone, then every 2 to 4 years.

References

1. **Johnson CM, Wilson DM, O'Fallon WM, Malek RS, Kurland LT.** Renal stone epidemiology: a 25-year study in Rochester, Minnesota. Kidney Int. 1979;16:624-31. [PMID: 548606]
2. **Curhan GC, Willett WC, Rimm EB, Stampfer MJ.** A prospective study of dietary calcium and other nutrients and the risk of symptomatic kidney stones. N Engl J Med. 1993;328:833-8. [PMID: 8441427]
3. **Curhan GC, Willett WC, Speizer FE, Spiegelman D, Stampfer MJ.** Comparison of dietary calcium with supplemental calcium and other nutrients as factors affecting the risk for kidney stones in women. Ann Intern Med. 1997;126:497-504. [PMID: 9092314]
4. **Taylor EN, Stampfer MJ, Curhan GC.** Diabetes mellitus and the risk of nephrolithiasis. Kidney Int. 2005;68:1230-5. [PMID: 16105055]
5. **Parks JH, Goldfisher E, Asplin JR, Coe FL.** A single 24-hour urine collection is inadequate for the medical evaluation of nephrolithiasis. J Urol. 2002;167:1607-12. [PMID: 11912373]
6. **Parks JH, Asplin JR, Coe FL.** Patient adherence to long-term medical treatment of kidney stones. J Urol. 2001;166:2057-60. [PMID: 11696706]

GENETIC DISORDERS AND RENAL DISEASE

The most common inherited mendelian (monogenic) kidney diseases are polycystic kidney disease, medullary sponge kidney, Alport's syndrome, and cystinuria. These disorders have an autosomal dominant, autosomal recessive, or X-linked pattern of transmission (**Table 43**).

Pathophysiology

The genetics of even single-gene disorders are complex, because multiple distinct genotypes can cause several disorders that appear to have the same phenotype (clinical manifestations), such as autosomal dominant polycystic kidney disease (ADPKD) or Bartter's syndrome. Moreover, intrafamilial phenotypic variability indicates that even the same germ-line mutation does not entirely dictate the phenotype; environmental and genetic modifiers also are important determinants of clinical manifestations. A complete and continuously updated list of these single-gene disorders, most of which are rare, is located at www.ncbi.nlm.nih.gov/Omim (1).

Complex interactions between genetic predisposition and environmental factors also cause various common conditions that affect the kidney. Subtle variations in multiple genes that

TABLE 43 Monogenic Renal Disorders			
Disease	**Mode of Inheritance**	**Gene Locus**	**Frequency**
Polycystic kidney disease	Autosomal dominant (common) Autosomal recessive (rare) X linked (80%)	Chromosomes 16 and 4	1:400 to 1:1000 1:40,000
Alport's syndrome	Autosomal recessive (10%)	Xq22 2q35–37	
Benign familial hematuria	Autosomal recessive (carrier)	2q and 13q	
Nephrogenic diabetes insipidus	X linked		
Bartter's syndrome	Autosomal recessive	Not known	1:2,000,000
Gitelman's syndrome	Autosomal recessive	Chromosome 16	Not known
Cystinosis	Autosomal recessive	Chromosome 2p	1:7000
Fabry's disease	X linked	Xq21, 22	1:40,000
Hyperoxaluria, type I, II, and III	Autosomal recessive	2q36–37	

interact with multiple environmental factors cause these genetically complex traits, known as polygenic disorders. In these disorders, the clinical expression of disease varies according to the interaction between genetic predisposition and key environmental or host factors. Examples of these interactions include the correlation between hypertension and salt intake, or a predisposition to diabetes and obesity.

Genetic Disorders That Cause Direct Renal Effects

Polycystic Kidney Disease

Pathophysiology

Polycystic kidney disease is characterized by multiple epithelial-lined renal cysts scattered throughout the cortex and medulla of both kidneys. Autosomal recessive polycystic renal disease is caused by a mutation on chromosome 16. An abnormal gene on the short arm of chromosome 16 causes ADPKD in 85% to 90% of patients with ADPKD. An abnormal gene on chromosome 4 and a third gene, which have not been cloned, account for most of the remainder of cases of ADPKD.

Epidemiology

ADPKD typically is diagnosed in patients 30 to 50 years of age, whereas autosomal recessive disease usually is expressed at birth and causes death during the neonatal period (2). ADPKD is the most common heritable cystic disease and the fourth leading cause of renal failure. This condition occurs at a frequency of approximately 1 in 400 to 1 in 1000 individuals. Conversely, autosomal recessive polycystic renal disease is rare.

ADPKD usually manifests in patients >30 years of age, with the highest incidence of onset occurring between 45 and 65 years of age. Approximately 50% of affected patients develop renal insufficiency before 70 years of age, and renal function declines linearly over several years. ADPDK affects all racial and ethnic groups.

Diagnosis and Evaluation

Early clinical manifestations of ADPKD include back and flank pain, hematuria, renal stones, hypertension, urinary tract infections, and stroke. ADPKD is associated with cerebral aneurysms (especially if there is a family history of aneurysm), hepatic cysts (40% to 60% of patients), mitral and aortic valve prolapse, colonic diverticular disease, pancreatic cysts, and thoracic and abdominal aortic aneurysms.

Certain manifestations of ADPKD tend to cluster in families. However, family members of some affected patients may die of other causes; ADPKD in these patients is diagnosed at a later age, when symptoms and signs are first observed.

Medullary Sponge Kidney

Medullary sponge kidney is a benign disease characterized by small or large cysts in the medulla. Most patients are asymptomatic, but some patients present with hematuria, which does not cause renal failure. Medullary sponge kidney also is characterized by hypercalciuria, nephrocalcinosis, recurrent urinary tract infection, and hemihypertrophy. Familial occurrence accounts for some cases (3). Intravenous pyelography showing small cystic outpouchings of the renal papillary ducts establishes the diagnosis in this condition.

Alport's Syndrome

Alport's syndrome is an X-linked disorder in 80% of patients and an autosomal recessive disorder in 10% of patients. Mutations in the α5 chain of type IV collagen on Xq22 cause the classic or X-linked form of this disease, whereas mutations in the α3 and α4 chains of type IV collagen cause the autosomal recessive form (4).

Men with Alport's syndrome develop hematuria, proteinuria, and progressive chronic kidney disease in the second or third decade of life. X-linked Alport's syndrome in women has a much milder course. Microscopic hematuria is present in 90% of affected women.

Benign Familial Hematuria

Benign familial hematuria or thin glomerular basement membrane disease is an inherited disorder characterized by microscopic or gross hematuria. Mutations in the α3 and α4 chains of type IV collagen in affected patients suggest that this disorder represents a carrier state of autosomal recessive Alport's syndrome (4). However, unlike Alport's syndrome, this condition usually does not result in renal failure. Benign familial hematuria usually presents in childhood, and a family history of hematuria is suggestive of the condition.

Nephrogenic Diabetes Insipidus

Tubular unresponsiveness to antidiuretic hormone in nephrogenic diabetes insipidus (NDI) causes urinary concentrating defects, polyuria, and thirst. In most cases, NDI is X linked and caused by mutations in the type 2 vasopressin receptor. Mutations in the aquaporin-2 water channel gene cause autosomal recessive and rare dominant forms of NDI. NDI usually is diagnosed in infancy or early childhood.

Bartter's and Gittelman's Syndromes

Genetic mutations in the chloride transporters in the ascending loop of Henle characterize Bartter's syndrome, whereas genetic mutations in the distal tubule characterize Gittelman's syndrome (5). These conditions cause hypokalemia, hypochloremic metabolic alkalosis, renal potassium wasting, and low blood pressure.

Bartter's Syndrome

Antenatal Bartter's syndrome is the most severe variant of Bartter's syndrome. Bartter's syndrome classically occurs in young children with less severe renal functional abnormalities and, less often, nephrocalcinosis.

Bartter's syndrome results from defects in the genes that encode the basolateral chloride channel (classic Bartter's syndrome), Na-K-2Cl cotransporter, or adenosine triphosphate–sensitive renal outer medullary potassium channel (6, 7). Therefore, the defect occurs in solute transport in the thick ascending limb. Findings in patients with this condition are similar to those associated with loop diuretics that inhibit the Na-K-2Cl transporter.

Gittelman's Syndrome

The presence of hypocalciuria, as well as hypomagnesemia, distinguishes Gittelman's syndrome from Bartter's syndrome (7). Gittelman's syndrome results from mutations in the gene encoding the thiazide-sensitive sodium chloride transporter. This condition presents in patients who are older than those who present with Bartter's syndrome and predominantly manifests with musculoskeletal signs and symptoms.

Hereditary Tubulointerstitial Kidney Disease

Nephronophthisis and medullary cystic disease are related conditions characterized by multiple cysts located in the corticomedullary junction and medulla that arise from the distal and collecting tubules. This disease complex causes tubular atrophy, interstitial inflammation and scarring, and renal failure.

Familial nephronophthisis is a recessive disorder that causes renal failure before 20 years of age. Medullary cystic disease, an autosomal dominant condition, causes renal failure in early adulthood. Polyuria, polydipsia, nocturia (due to a renal concentrating disorder), and renal salt wasting characterize the initial clinical presentation of these disorders; the tubular injury produced by the cystic and scarring process causes these manifestations. Subsequently, azotemia and end-stage renal failure develop.

Cystinuria is described in the Nephrolithiasis section. Mutations also occur in many podocyte cytoskeletal and slit diaphragm proteins in proteinuric renal diseases, particularly congenital nephrotic syndromes.

KEY POINTS

- Polycystic kidney disease is characterized by multiple epithelial-lined renal cysts scattered throughout the cortex and medulla of both kidneys.
- Early clinical manifestations of autosomal dominant polycystic kidney disease include back and flank pain, hematuria, renal stones, hypertension, urinary tract infections, and stroke.
- Medullary sponge kidney is a benign disease characterized by small or large cysts in the medulla.
- Men with Alport's syndrome develop hematuria, proteinuria, and progressive chronic kidney disease in the second or third decade of life.
- Microscopic or gross hematuria characterizes benign familial hematuria.
- Nephrogenic diabetes insipidus causes urinary concentrating defects, polyuria, and thirst.
- Nephrogenic diabetes insipidus usually is diagnosed in infancy or early childhood.
- Bartter's and Gittelman's syndromes cause hypokalemia, hypochloremic metabolic alkalosis, renal potassium wasting, and low blood pressure.
- The presence of hypocalciuria, as well as hypomagnesemia, distinguishes Gittelman's syndrome from Bartter's syndrome.
- Gittelman's syndrome predominantly manifests with musculoskeletal signs and symptoms.
- Multiple cysts located in the corticomedullary junction and medulla characterize nephronophthisis and medullary cystic disease.
- The disease complex of nephronophthisis and medullary cystic disease causes tubular atrophy, interstitial inflammation and scarring, and renal failure.
- Familial nephronophthisis and medullary cystic disease initially manifest with polyuria, polydipsia, nocturia, and renal salt wasting.
- Azotemia and end-stage renal failure characterize the later stages of nephronophthisis and medullary cystic disease.

Genetic Metabolic Disorders That Affect the Kidney

Fabry's Disease

Pathophysiology

Fabry's disease is an X-linked disorder that results from deficiency of the α-galactosidase A enzyme. This condition causes ceramide trihexoside, also known as globotriaosylceramide, to accumulate in multiple tissues, including glomerular, tubular, endothelial, epithelial, and smooth muscle cells throughout the body.

Diagnosis and Evaluation

Clinical features of Fabry's disease include mild proteinuria, slow deterioration in kidney function, cutaneous angiokeratomas, painful paresthesias of the hands, and premature coronary artery disease. Progression to end-stage renal disease during the third or fourth decade of life is the most common complication in affected men and the primary cause of premature death in all patients with Fabry's disease. This condition affects men more frequently than women.

Electron microscopy of the kidney and of spun urine sediment in patients with Fabry's disease reveals characteristic inclusion bodies in the cytoplasm with concentric lamellation and zebra or onion-skin appearance (8).

Management

Treatment of Fabry's disease is symptomatic and supportive. Intravenous replacement with recombinant human α-galactosidase A appears to be a promising therapeutic modality (8). Affected family members of patients with Fabry's disease should be identified and undergo genetic counseling.

Hyperoxalurias

Pathophysiology

Primary hyperoxaluria results from an inborn metabolism defect in which glyoxalate cannot be converted to glycine because of a functional deficiency of the enzyme alanine glyoxalate aminotransferase or glyoxalate reductase in the liver. An abnormal gene on chromosome 2q36-37 causes type 1 hyperoxaluria, which is the most common hyperoxaluria.

Diagnosis and Evaluation

Type 1 and 2 hyperoxaluria have similar clinical presentations. Patients with these conditions typically develop nephrolithiasis and nephrocalcinosis before 20 years of age, and 50% of affected patients develop end-stage renal failure by 15 years of age. Renal biopsy in this setting demonstrates marked calcium oxalate deposition, but oxalate deposition is found in many other tissues, as well (2–8).

KEY POINTS

- Clinical features of Fabry's disease include mild proteinuria, slow deterioration in kidney function, cutaneous angiokeratomas, painful paresthesias of the hands, and premature coronary artery disease.

- Electron microscopy of the kidney and of spun urine sediment in Fabry's disease reveals inclusion bodies in the cytoplasm with concentric lamellation and zebra or onion-skin appearance.

- Intravenous replacement with recombinant human α-galactosidase A appears to be a promising therapeutic modality in Fabry's disease.

- Affected family members of patients with Fabry's disease should be identified and undergo genetic counseling.

- Patients with type 1 and 2 hyperoxaluria typically develop nephrolithiasis and nephrocalcinosis before 20 years of age.

- Fifty percent of patients with hyperoxaluria develop end-stage renal failure by 15 years of age.

- Renal biopsy in hyperoxaluria reveals marked calcium oxalate deposition.

References

1. **Sessa A, Conte F, Meroni M, Battini G.** Hereditary kidney diseases. Introduction. Contrib Nephrol. 1997;122:XI-XII. [PMID: 9399028]

2. **Igarashi P, Somlo S.** Genetics and pathogenesis of polycystic kidney disease. J Am Soc Nephrol. 2002;13:2384-98. [PMID: 12191984]

3. **Fick GM, Gabow PA.** Hereditary and acquired cystic disease of the kidney. Kidney Int. 1994;46:951-64. [PMID: 7861721]

4. **Moller CC, Pollak MR, Reiser J.** The genetic basis of human glomerular disease. Adv Chronic Kidney Dis. 2006;13:166-73. [PMID: 16580618]

5. **Simon DB, Lifton RP.** The molecular basis of inherited hypokalemic alkalosis: Bartter's and Gitelman's syndromes. Am J Physiol. 1996;271:F961-6. [PMID: 8945989]

6. **Ellison DH.** Divalent cation transport by the distal nephron: insights from Bartter's and Gitelman's syndromes. Am J Physiol Renal Physiol. 2000;279:F616-25. [PMID: 10997911]

7. **Peters M, Jeck N, Reinalter S, Leonhardt A, Tonshoff B, Klaus G G, et al.** Clinical presentation of genetically defined patients with hypokalemic salt-losing tubulopathies. Am J Med. 2002;112:183-90. [PMID: 11893344]

8. **Warnock DG, West ML.** Diagnosis and management of kidney involvement in Fabry disease. Adv Chronic Kidney Dis. 2006;13:138-47. [PMID: 16580615]

GLOMERULAR DISEASES

Glomerular Anatomic Regions and Clinicopathologic Syndromes

Glomeruli are bundles of capillaries that, when injured, cause proteinuria, hematuria, edema, hypertension, and renal insufficiency. Glomeruli are composed of several cell types, including mesangial cells that support the glomerular capillary wall and endothelial and epithelial cells located on opposite sides of the glomerular basement membrane (GBM).

Damage to the glomerular epithelial cells (podocytes) or the GBM alters the permeability of the capillary wall and results in proteinuria. Rupture of the capillary wall or proliferation of the resident mesangial cells of the glomerulus causes hematuria. Inflammatory infiltrations into the glomerulus may cause areas of necrosis and crescent formation that invades and sometimes replaces Bowman's space. Consequently, a rapidly progressive glomerulonephritis with acute renal failure develops.

Glomerular damage can produce several clinical patterns of kidney disease classified as the nephrotic syndrome or the nephritic syndrome (**Table 44**). The nephrotic syndrome is characterized by proteinuria, edema, hypoalbuminemia, hyperlipidemia, and lipiduria. This condition may occur because of a disease process limited to the kidney or as part of a systemic disease.

The main characteristics of the nephritic syndrome are hematuria, oliguria, hypertension, and renal insufficiency. Most nephritic diseases are immune mediated. Many of the patterns of glomerular injury are part of a systemic process, including the vasculitides (systemic lupus erythematosus and antineutrophil cytoplasmic autoantibody [ANCA]–associated small-vessel vasculitis).

The nephrotic and nephritic syndromes are not always distinct entities, and patients commonly have characteristics of both syndromes. Kidney biopsy provides a precise diagnosis.

KEY POINTS

- **Glomeruli are bundles of capillaries that, when injured, cause proteinuria, hematuria, edema, hypertension, and renal insufficiency.**
- **Most nephritic diseases are immune mediated.**
- **Many patterns of glomerular injury are part of a systemic process, including the vasculitides.**
- **Kidney biopsy is used to differentiate between the nephrotic and nephritic syndromes.**

Clinical Syndromes of Glomerular Disease

The Nephrotic Syndrome

In the nephrotic syndrome, proteinuria typically is asymptomatic until 24-hour urinary protein excretion is >2 g. Severe proteinuria >3000 mg/24 h results in the nephrotic syndrome, which is characterized by hypoalbuminemia, decreased plasma oncotic pressure, and the transudation of fluid into the interstitium (edema). The perceived decrease in effective arterial volume causes the kidney to avidly retain salt and water because of the activation of the

TABLE 44 Tendencies of Glomerular Diseases To Manifest Nephrotic and Nephritic Features*

Condition	Nephrotic Features	Nephritic Features
Minimal change glomerulopathy	++++	—
Membranous glomerulopathy	++++	+
Diabetic glomerulosclerosis	++++	+
Amyloidosis	++++	+
Focal segmental glomerulosclerosis	+++	++
Fibrillary glomerulonephritis	+++	++
Mesangioproliferative glomerulopathy†	++	++
Membranoproliferative glomerulonephritis‡	++	+++
Proliferative glomerulonephritis†	++	+++
Acute diffuse proliferative glomerulonephritis§	+	++++
Crescentic glomerulonephritis‖	+	++++

* Most diseases can manifest both nephrotic and nephritic features, but there usually is a tendency for one to predominate.

† Mesangioproliferative and proliferative glomerulonephritis (focal or diffuse) are structural manifestations of a number of glomerulonephritides, including IgA nephropathy and lupus nephritis.

‡ Both type I (mesangiocapillary) and type II (dense deposit disease)

§ Often a structural manifestation of acute poststreptococcal glomerulonephritis

‖ Can be immune complex or anti–glomerular basement membrane antibody mediated, or associated with antineutrophil cytoplasmic antibodies.

Modified with permission from Jennette JC, Mandal AK: The nephrotic syndrome. In: Mandal AK, Jennette JC, eds. Diagnosis and Management of Renal Disease and Hypertension. Durham, NC: Academic Press; 1994.

renin–angiotensin–aldosterone system and as yet unclear distal tubular mechanisms of sodium retention. Clinically evident edema usually prompts affected patients to come to the office.

The loss of plasma proteins into the urine has various consequences. Hypoalbuminemia and decreased oncotic pressure stimulate the liver to produce cholesterol. However, hypercholesterolemia is a consequence of more than just increased synthesis of cholesterol. Levels of cholesteryl ester transfer protein (the enzyme that converts cholesterol to low-density lipoprotein) are significantly increased in patients with the nephrotic syndrome.

Hypercholesterolemia in this setting is severe, with total cholesterol levels of 300 mg/dL to 400 mg/dL. This conversion process not only accelerates the development of atherosclerotic disease but also exacerbates the progression of chronic kidney disease.

Treatment of hypercholesterolemia in the nephrotic syndrome is difficult. Lifestyle modification is important but only marginally effective. A 3-hydroxy-3-methylglutaryl coenzyme A (HMG-CoA) reductase inhibitor and other lipid-lowering agents are indicated to try to decrease the low-density lipoprotein cholesterol levels to 100 mg/dL to 129 mg/dL. Patients with the nephrotic syndrome also have substantially elevated triglyceride levels that are equally difficult to decrease. Fibric acid derivatives have been used in this setting.

Additional consequences of urinary protein loss include coagulation abnormalities that increase the risk for deep venous and renal vein thrombosis. Numerous factors cause these abnormalities, including the urinary loss of fibrinolytic factors and antithrombin III with concomitant increased platelet aggregation and increased serum fibrinogen levels. Renal vein thrombosis may worsen proteinuria and renal insufficiency and result in pulmonary emboli. This process occurs in virtually all patients with the nephrotic syndrome, but monitoring is particularly indicated for those with membranous nephropathy.

Numerous endocrine abnormalities are associated with the nephrotic syndrome, particularly hypothyroidism due to urinary losses of thyroid-binding globulin and thyroxine. Nevertheless, the majority of affected patients remain euthyroid.

Calcium balance abnormalities also are more common in the nephrotic syndrome than previously recognized. Most affected patients are hypocalcemic due to low plasma albumin levels. However, the loss of vitamin D–binding protein into the urine causes low levels of 25 hydroxyvitamin D and 1, 25-dihydroxyvitamin D. Patients with the nephrotic syndrome tend to be anemic due to urinary losses of transferrin and erythropoietin. Recombinant erythropoietin therapy is beneficial if the hemoglobin level decreases to <10 g/dL.

The Nephritic Syndrome

The nephritic syndrome is characterized by the presence of hypertension, edema, oliguria, azotemia, and hematuria. The urine sediment may reveal hematuria with or without proteinuria and may contain erythrocytes, pigmented casts, and cellular debris. The nature and severity of glomerular inflammation usually correlate with the clinical pattern of disease.

The most common causes of asymptomatic glomerular hematuria without evidence of proteinuria or glomerular abnormality are thin basement membrane nephropathy and IgA nephropathy. These conditions exemplify the structural basis of hematuria. The thinning of the basement membrane most likely allows erythrocytes to enter the urine. The perturbation of the glomerular capillary wall as it faces the mesangium (perimesangial basement membrane) due to the proliferation of mesangial cells results in hematuria in IgA nephropathy.

Focal proliferation of mesangial cells, which involves <50% of the glomeruli, may result in asymptomatic hematuria.

Proliferation that involves >50% of the glomeruli may induce more hematuria and proteinuria and the development of erythrocyte casts in the urine sediment. With the influx of leukocytes, especially neutrophils and mononuclear phagocytes, destructive necrotizing and crescentic lesions develop.

Rapidly progressive glomerulonephritis is characterized by an increase in creatinine over days to weeks associated with a ≥50% loss of kidney function. The pathologic processes producing this clinical syndrome have either proliferative or necrotizing glomerular lesions that spill into Bowman's space and produce crescents. The diagnostic term "crescentic glomerulonephritis" is used when crescents affect >50% of the glomeruli. Related inflammatory changes cause scarring of the glomerulus (glomerulosclerosis) and scarring or fibrosis of the tubulointerstitial compartment. The scarring process occurs within days to weeks of the onset of a destructive glomerular lesion.

Lupus nephritis is characteristic of a proliferative glomerular disease. This condition ranges from a very mild proliferative process to rampant inflammation resulting in rapidly progressive glomerulonephritis due to a diffuse proliferative glomerulonephritis. The latter usually is accompanied by crescent formation and chronic glomerulonephritis that develops after the inflammatory disease resolves.

KEY POINTS

- **Urinary protein excretion >3 g/24 h characterizes severe proteinuria and results in the nephrotic syndrome.**
- **Severe hypercholesterolemia associated with the nephrotic syndrome accelerates the development of atherosclerotic disease and exacerbates chronic kidney disease progression.**
- **Lifestyle modification and a 3-hydroxy-3-methylglutaryl coenzyme A (HMG-CoA) reductase inhibitor and other lipid-lowering agents are indicated to decrease low-density lipoprotein cholesterol levels in the nephrotic syndrome.**
- **Urinary protein loss in patients with the nephrotic syndrome increases the risk for deep venous and renal vein thrombosis.**
- **Rapidly progressive glomerulonephritis is characterized by an increase in creatinine over days to weeks associated with a ≥50% loss of kidney function.**

Disorders That Cause the Nephrotic Syndrome

Diabetic nephropathy is the most common cause of the nephrotic syndrome. Other causes of this syndrome include minimal change disease; focal segmental glomerulosclerosis (FSGS); membranous nephropathy; membranoproliferative glomerulonephritis; and plasma cell dyscrasias, including amyloidosis and light-chain deposition disease (LCDD). These conditions affect the glomerular capillary wall, resulting in its permeability to plasma proteins. Kidney biopsy is indicated to diagnose minimal change disease, FSGS, membranous nephropathy, and membranoproliferative glomerulonephritis.

Epidemiology

Age is a major factor in the epidemiology of certain causes of the nephrotic syndrome. In children <10 years of age, minimal change glomerulopathy causes approximately 80% of cases of the nephrotic syndrome. Throughout adulthood, the frequency of minimal change disease decreases, whereas diabetic nephropathy, FSGS, and membranous nephropathy become much more common. Amyloidosis frequently causes the nephrotic syndrome in older adults. The incidence of FSGS in renal biopsies in adults has increased from approximately 4% in 1975 to ≥12% in 1995.

Race also may influence the predilection for glomerular diseases, excluding diabetic nephropathy. FSGS is the most common cause of the nephrotic syndrome in black adults, whereas membranous glomerulonephropathy is the most common cause in white adults.

Treatment

Careful control of blood pressure to 125/75 mm Hg with either angiotensin-converting enzyme (ACE) inhibitors or angiotensin receptor blockers has become the standard of care for all forms of the nephrotic syndrome. Single-agent or combination therapy with these medications helps to decrease proteinuria and ameliorate the nephrotic syndrome. Lipid-lowering agents, particularly HMG-CoA reductase inhibitors (statins), are needed to control the hyperlipidemia. Vitamin D analogues may be needed to prevent deficiency of this vitamin. Some patients require recombinant erythropoietin to ameliorate anemia.

Minimal Change Disease
Pathology

In minimal change disease, light microscopy reveals no discernible abnormalities and immunofluorescence microscopy shows no immunoreactants. Effacement or flattening of glomerular epithelial cells on electron microscopic evaluation establishes the diagnosis in this condition.

The cause of minimal change disease is unknown, but this condition may develop because of a product derived from circulating lymphocytes. In adults, this condition may be associated with drug use (especially nonsteroidal anti-inflammatory drugs) or occur as a consequence of a lymphoproliferative disease.

Clinical Presentation

In minimal change disease, proteinuria develops suddenly and can be massive; 24-hour urinary protein excretion in this setting may exceed 9 g. In both children and adults, minimal change disease is a relapsing and remitting disease. Approximately one third of affected patients have only one episode with a long-term remission, whereas the majority of patients have a relapsing course; the first relapse typically occurs within the first 6 months. Frequently relapsing disease (characterized by four or more episodes per year) is more common in children.

Approximately 10% of patients with minimal change disease become dependent on corticosteroid therapy or are resistant to it. Hypertension and end-stage renal disease are rare in this setting; however, acute renal failure occurs in adult patients with a baseline atherosclerosis and rapid development of proteinemia or edema. Controlling proteinuria resolves the acute renal failure.

Treatment

Prednisone, 60 mg on a daily or alternate-day basis for 4 weeks and then 40 mg/m² every other day for 4 weeks, is indicated to treat minimal change disease. Corticosteroid resistance is characterized by a lack of full response (such as urinary protein excretion <300 mg/24 h) after 8 weeks of therapy. Older adults require a longer corticosteroid treatment period to induce a response and may require daily therapy for 12 to 16 weeks. In frequently relapsing corticosteroid-dependent or corticosteroid-resistant adults, cyclosporine and cyclophosphamide may be useful.

Focal Segmental Glomerulosclerosis
Pathology

FSGS usually is idiopathic; genetic; or related to other associated conditions, such as secondary focal sclerosis (**Table 45**). There are several hereditary forms of FSGS that are a consequence of mutations that encode proteins that constitute the podocyte and the slit diaphragm between podocytes (1). A structural adaptation to nephron loss may cause FSGS, as in reflux nephropathy, chronic pyelonephritis, or interstitial diseases. Obesity-related FSGS is becoming increasingly common.

The primary lesion in FSGS is a focal scarring process that involves only a few glomeruli and segments of the glomerular tuft. Immunofluorescence microscopy in affected patients reveals coarse deposits of immunoglobulins, C3, and usually fibrin trapped in the segmentally involved glomeruli. Electron microscopy shows diffuse obliteration of the foot processes and foam cells that often occupy the lumina of collapsed capillaries.

Clinical Presentation

FSGS is a more indolent form of the nephrotic syndrome. Some affected patients present with non-nephrotic proteinuria (24-hour urinary protein excretion <3 g) and typically have secondary forms of FSGS. In secondary FSGS, there is little edema, and the full spectrum of the nephrotic syndrome is rare. Patients with primary FSGS have a wide range of proteinuria,

TABLE 45 Causes of Focal Segmental Glomerulosclerosis

Primary (Idiopathic) FSGS
FSGS with hyalinosis
Progression from minimal change disease
Progression from IgM nephropathy
Progression from mesangial proliferative glomerulonephritis
Superimposed on other primary glomerulonephritis conditions (membranous glomerulonephritis, IgA nephropathy)
Variants of primary FSGS
Collapsing form
Cellular variant (endocapillary and extracapillary hypercellularity)
FSGS with mesangial hypercellularity
FSGS with glomerular tip lesions
Secondary FSGS
Drugs
Intravenous heroin
Analgesics
Viruses
Hepatitis B
HIV
Parvovirus
Hemodynamic factors with reduced renal mass
Solitary kidney
Renal allograft
Renal dysplasia
Renal agenesis
Oligomeganephronia
Segmental hypoplasia
Vesicoureteric reflux
Hemodynamic causes without reduced renal mass
Massive obesity
Sickle cell nephropathy
Congenital cyanotic heart disease
Malignancies
Lymphomas
Other malignancies
Scarring*
Miscellaneous
Hypertensive nephrosclerosis
Alport's syndrome
Sarcoidosis
Radiation nephritis

FSGS = focal segmental glomerulosclerosis; IgM = immunoglobulin M; IgA = immunoglobulin A

* Postinflammatory in postinfectious glomerulonephritis.

and their prognosis is based largely on whether there is massive proteinuria (24-hour urinary protein excretion >10 g) or if therapy can induce remission. Patients who achieve complete or even partial remission have a better prognosis than those who have no treatment response (2).

Treatment

Spontaneous remission is rare in FSGS, and the majority of affected patients require some form of therapy. In non-nephrotic patients, ACE inhibitors, angiotensin receptor blockers, or both are indicated. In patients with FSGS and persistent nephrotic syndrome, 16 weeks of daily or alternate-day prednisone, cyclosporine, or mycophenolate mofetil is indicated. A randomized, controlled trial demonstrated that cyclosporine was useful in achieving remission in up to 70% of corticosteroid-resistant patients. However, relapses occurred in nearly 40% of these patients when cyclosporine therapy was discontinued.

Membranous Nephropathy

Pathology

Membranous nephropathy derives its name from the electron-dense deposits that are arranged within the GBM. These deposits are immune complexes presumably derived from an antigen deposited in the GBM with subsequent antibody–antigen interaction. This *in situ* immune complex formation activates the complement cascade that in animal studies has been shown to cause glomerular capillary wall permeability and proteinuria.

Clinical Presentation

In membranous nephropathy, one third of all patients have a spontaneous remission within 3 to 4 years; one third have persistent proteinuria that over decades may cause renal insufficiency; and one third have a more rapidly progressive course leading to end-stage kidney disease. Numerous predictors portend a poor prognosis, including male sex, the amount and persistence of proteinuria, and the degree of renal insufficiency at the time of presentation. A practical predictor of long-term outcome is the amount and duration of proteinuria. Patients with 24-hour urinary protein excretion >6 g that persists for 6 months have a worse prognosis than those with 24-hour urinary protein excretion <3 g. Kidney survival in patients who have never been nephrotic is excellent, as is the outcome for those who have a complete or partial remission of their nephrotic syndrome.

Certain pharmaceutical agents and several systemic diseases may cause membranous nephropathy. These systemic diseases include infections (such as hepatitis B and syphilis) and malignancies (such as breast, colon, lung, and ovarian cancers and other solid tumors). Patients >55 years of age with membranous nephropathy should be screened for solid tumors. Patients with membranous nephropathy also have a high risk for developing renal vein thrombosis with resultant pulmonary emboli, but prophylactic anticoagulation therapy in this setting is controversial.

Treatment

Corticosteroid therapy alone has been proved to be ineffective for membranous nephropathy. Pulse corticosteroid therapy combined with cytotoxic therapy has been effective in persistent nephrosis. Cyclosporine has been proved to be an appropriate alternative therapy. However, the process returns when cyclosporine is discontinued (3).

Membranoproliferative Glomerulonephritis
Pathology

Membranoproliferative glomerulonephritis can be idiopathic but most often is associated with autoimmune diseases such as lupus or Sjögren's syndrome or infections such as hepatitis C, bacterial endocarditis, or certain types of cancer. This condition results from deposits of immune complexes in the glomeruli, mesangial and endothelial cell proliferation, and expansion of the mesangial matrix; thickening of the peripheral capillary walls by subendothelial immune and/or intramembranous dense deposits; and mesangial interposition into the capillary wall, which causes the classic "tram-track" appearance on light microscopy.

Clinical Presentation

Membranoproliferative glomerulonephritis may affect any age group and usually results in the nephrotic syndrome. Patients with this condition frequently have glomerular hematuria, unlike those with membranous nephropathy. Activation of the alternative pathway of the complement system results in a low or depressed C3. Without activation of the classical complement cascade, a normal C4 results.

Hepatitis C may cause membranoproliferative glomerulonephritis with or without associated cryoglobulinemia. The presence of cryoglobulins accompanied by abnormal liver chemistry studies, a positive rheumatoid factor, and a circulating C4 level that is decreased more than the C3 level establishes a diagnosis of cryoglobulinemia.

Cryoglobulin measurement is difficult to perform. Results of cryoglobulin studies are frequently false-negative if the specimen is not drawn in warm conditions and analyzed by an experienced laboratory. A footprint for the diagnosis of cryoglobulinemia in the setting of glomerulopathy is suggested by the presence of low C4 and low normal C3 levels.

Treatment

Treatment of membranoproliferative glomerulonephritis varies depending on the signs and symptoms, but this condition usually improves with successful treatment of the associated disease. For example, treatment of hepatitis C–induced disease is aimed at eradicating hepatitis C with pegylated interferon-α2 plus ribavirin. In patients with cryoglobulinemia, therapy focuses on removing immune complexes with plasmapheresis or, more recently, B-cell antibodies.

KEY POINTS

- Diabetic nephropathy is the most common cause of the nephrotic syndrome.
- Diabetic nephropathy, minimal change disease, focal segmental glomerulosclerosis, membranous nephropathy, membranoproliferative glomerulonephritis, and plasma cell dyscrasias may cause the nephrotic syndrome.
- Effacement or flattening of glomerular epithelial cells on electron microscopy establishes a diagnosis of minimal change disease.
- In minimal change disease, proteinuria develops suddenly and can be massive.
- Minimal change disease is a relapsing and remitting disease.
- Prednisone, 60 mg on a daily or alternate-day basis for 4 weeks and then 40 mg/m^2 every other day for 4 weeks, is indicated to treat minimal change disease.
- Immunofluorescence microscopy in focal segmental glomerulosclerosis reveals coarse deposits of immunoglobulins, C3, and usually fibrin trapped in the segmentally involved glomeruli.
- In non-nephrotic patients with focal segmental glomerulosclerosis, angiotensin-converting enzyme inhibitors, angiotensin receptor blockers, or both is indicated.
- In patients with focal segmental glomerulosclerosis with persistent nephrotic syndrome, 16 weeks of daily or alternate-day prednisone, cyclosporine, or mycophenolate mofetil is indicated.
- Pulse corticosteroid therapy combined with cytotoxic therapy is effective in persistent nephrosis associated with membranous nephropathy.
- Cyclosporine is an appropriate alternative therapy for persistent nephrosis associated with membranous nephropathy, but the process returns when cyclosporine is discontinued.
- Membranoproliferative glomerulonephritis usually is associated with autoimmune diseases or infections.
- Cryoglobulin study specimens should be drawn in warm conditions and analyzed by an experienced laboratory.
- A footprint for the diagnosis of cryoglobulinemia in the setting of glomerulopathy is suggested by the presence of low C4 and low normal C3 levels.
- Membranoproliferative glomerulonephritis usually improves with successful treatment of the associated disease.

Secondary Causes of Glomerular Diseases

Diabetic Nephropathy

Diabetic nephropathy is characterized by proteinuria, hypertension, and a decline in the glomerular filtration rate (GFR) in patients with a longstanding history of type 1 diabetes mellitus or a 5- to 10-year history of type 2 diabetes. Diabetic nephropathy is the most common cause of progressive decline in renal function and end-stage renal disease.

The morphologic changes in the kidney associated with diabetes include glomerular enlargement; basement membrane thickening; mesangial expansion; glomerular epithelial cell foot process fusion; and, in advanced cases, sclerosis of glomeruli with tubular atrophy and interstitial fibrosis. Glomerulosclerosis leads to a decrease in filtration surface area, which results in a reduction in the GFR. The presence of Kimmelstiel–Wilson nodules is the most pathognomonic finding of diabetic nephropathy. However, these nodules develop in only 20% to 30% of patients with a clinical diagnosis of diabetic nephropathy.

Epidemiology

The prevalence of diabetic nephropathy is approximately 30% in patients with type 1 diabetes but varies in type 2 diabetes from 5% to 30% in different populations. Diabetic nephropathy and hypertension are present in 40% to 50% of patients with diabetes, and this prevalence increases with age and the duration of diabetes; at least 60% of patients who have had diabetes for >10 years have elevated blood pressure. Approximately 75% of patients with diabetes and hypertension require treatment with at least two hypertensive agents.

The familial and ethnic differences in the predisposition to diabetic nephropathy suggest involvement of metabolic and hemodynamic as well as genetic and environmental factors in the development of this condition. Diabetic nephropathy is much less prevalent in white patients compared with Native American, Mexican American, and black patients.

A family history of kidney disease and of hypertension are predictors of diabetic nephropathy. In Pima Indians, the incidence of proteinuria in offspring with diabetes is highest (46%) if both parents have diabetes and proteinuria. Identification of genes that confer susceptibility to diabetic nephropathy may help to reveal the risk for a given patient and identify those for whom intensive therapy may be most beneficial.

Pathophysiology

After an initial period of diabetes, usually exceeding 10 years, patients develop low-grade albuminuria or microalbuminuria, defined as a urinary albumin excretion >30 mg and >300 mg/24 h. Within 7 to 10 years, microalbuminuria progresses to macroalbuminuria (urinary albumin excretion >300 mg/24 h) or dipstick-positive proteinuria (urinary protein excretion >500 mg/24 h). A decline in renal function requiring dialysis or transplantation, usually within 5 to 10 years, characterizes this stage of overt diabetic nephropathy.

Screening

Because microalbuminuria precedes macroalbuminuria or clinical proteinuria and the decline in kidney function, particularly in patients with type 1 diabetes, screening for microalbuminuria is essential in patients with diabetes. To confirm the presence of persistent microalbuminuria, two out of three urine samples obtained within a 6-month period should reveal microalbuminuria.

Annual screening for microalbuminuria, usually by obtaining an albumin–creatinine ratio on an early morning urine sample, a random sample, or a timed urine collection, is recommended. Microalbuminuria is defined as a urine albumin (mg/dL)–urine creatinine (mg/dL) ratio of >0.03 (>30 mg albumin/g creatinine) and <0.3. However, the following factors may confound the assessment of microalbuminuria: urinary tract infection, heavy exercise, high dietary protein intake, congestive heart failure, acute febrile illness, menstruation, and vaginal discharge. Testing in the presence of these factors should be postponed.

Microalbuminuria is not only a major risk factor for the development of diabetic nephropathy but also a predictor for increased mortality from cardiovascular disease in patients with type 1 and type 2 diabetes and those without diabetes. The major goal of screening for microalbuminuria is to prevent the progression to clinical proteinuria and overt nephropathy.

Despite the prognostic significance of microalbuminuria, the frequency of annual screening for this condition in diabetes clinics is low. Furthermore, therapy with inhibitors of the renin–angiotensin system usually is not initiated even after microalbuminuria is detected.

Risk Factors

In diabetes, structural injury in the kidney is induced by hyperglycemia, systemic hypertension, intraglomerular hypertension, elaboration of cytokines and growth factors, and oxidative stress. Environmental and genetic factors modulate the likelihood of development of diabetic nephropathy. Patients with diabetic nephropathy also commonly have concomitant diabetic vascular complications, such as retinopathy, as well as macrovascular complications, including cardiovascular, cerebrovascular, and peripheral arterial disease.

Treatment

Glycemic control delays or prevents progression from normoalbuminuria to microalbuminuria, clinical proteinuria, and overt nephropathy. Hemoglobin A_{1c} levels correlate strongly with diabetic microvascular disease, both renal and retinal. Specific strategies to decrease microalbuminuria and proteinuria involve blocking the renin–angiotensin system and decreasing the blood pressure to ≤130/80 mm Hg in all patients with diabetes and to <125/75 mm Hg in patients with proteinuria >1g/24 h.

Use of ACE inhibitors or angiotensin receptor blockers slows the rate of GFR decline (4, 5, 6). Recent studies show that angiotensin II receptor blockers and ACE inhibitors have an equivalent renoprotective effect. These studies also reveal that the rate of cardiovascular events does not differ in patients treated with ACE inhibitors compared with angiotensin receptor blockers (7).

Protein restriction is beneficial particularly in patients with type 1 diabetes. Treatment of hyperlipidemia and of other cardiovascular risk factors, such as cessation of smoking, also helps to slow renal function decline and the associated increase in cardiovascular risk. Renal transplantation is the preferred modality to treat patients with end-stage renal disease secondary to diabetes. Diabetic nephropathy may recur or occur *de novo* in the transplanted kidney.

Dysproteinemias

Pathophysiology

Numerous dysproteinemias cause the nephrotic syndrome, including primary and secondary amyloidosis, LCDD in multiple myeloma, cryoglobulinemia, fibrillary glomerulonephritis, and immunotactoid glomerulonephritis. All of these lesions are associated with glomerular deposition of material visible on electron microscopy as microfibrils or microtubules that are extracellular and nonbranching and have no periodicity.

Amyloidosis

Amyloidosis is associated with extracellular deposition of an insoluble fibrillary protein that has a characteristic β-sheet configuration that is stained by Congo red dye. The most prevalent form of immunoglobulin light chain found in amyloid deposits are γ light chains. Amyloidosis is classified as primary, secondary, familial, or senile, depending on the nature of the deposited protein. Hereditary amyloidosis constitutes nearly 10% of cases of amyloidosis and usually occurs as an autosomal dominant pattern of inheritance with variable penetration. Related proteins include transthyretin, fibrinogen α chain and apolipoprotein I, or lysozyme.

The majority of amyloidosis is primary (AL) amyloidosis. Twenty percent of patients with AL amyloidosis develop multiple myeloma, whereas a slightly smaller percentage of patients with multiple myeloma develop AL amyloidosis. Many patients with amyloidosis develop the nephrotic syndrome and, eventually, renal insufficiency.

Of the major organ systems involved in AL amyloidosis, kidney involvement resulting in the nephrotic syndrome occurs in about 30% of affected patients and congestive heart failure occurs in 20% to 25%. Carpal tunnel syndrome, peripheral nephropathy, and orthostatic hypotension develop in 15% of patients. Patients with nephrotic syndrome from AL amyloidosis develop massive edema and frequently are hypotensive.

Secondary (AA) amyloidosis usually is associated with various chronic inflammatory disorders. The clinical presentations of this condition and AL amyloidosis are similar.

Treatment

Patient survival in amyloidosis remains poor. Mean survival in patients with the nephrotic syndrome is approximately 16 months. Therapies in AL amyloidosis include prednisone, melphalan, or cyclophosphamide, with or without colchicine. Numerous experimental approaches also have been examined, including stem-cell transplantation. This therapy may become the treatment of choice in less severely affected patients, such as those with proteinuria >1g/24 h, a left ventricular ejection fraction >40%, and a systolic blood pressure >85 mm Hg). A renal response with decreased proteinuria and improved renal function occurs in 70% of patients. Nonetheless, optimal therapy for AL amyloidosis has yet to be determined.

Multiple Myeloma

Myeloma-related kidney disorders that cause the nephrotic syndrome are usually LCDD or amyloidosis. Monoclonal immunoglobulin deposition in patients with multiple myeloma occurs as light-chain or, rarely, heavy-chain deposition disease. This plasma cell dyscrasia results in the extracellular deposition of a monoclonal immunoglobulin that is negative on Congo red staining of glomeruli, and the fibrillar deposits are not β-pleated. Proteinuria and renal insufficiency are frequently the first signs of LCDD, and renal biopsy may establish a diagnosis of plasma cell dyscrasia. End-stage renal disease is common in up to 50% of affected patients.

LCDD and amyloidosis affect men more frequently than women. LCDD typically is associated with circulating K light chains, whereas amyloidosis is more likely to have circulating λ light chains.

Kidney function abnormalities are common in multiple myeloma (8). Approximately 40% of patients with this condition have a creatinine level >1.5 mg/dL, and 20% of these patients have a creatinine level >2.0 mg/dL at the time of diagnosis. In myeloma-related kidney disorders, dipstick urinalysis does not reveal albuminuria, but the addition of sulfosalicylic acid to the urine precipitates all proteins, including light chains. Urine immunoelectrophoresis confirms the presence and type of light chains excreted in the urine. Kidney biopsy is recommended to confirm the diagnosis of multiple myeloma and/or if other kidney disorders are suspected.

Treatment

Treatment of myeloma-related kidney disorders includes systemic chemotherapy and stem-cell transplantation to resolve the underlying lymphoproliferative disorder (9). Treatment of concomitant hypercalcemia and alkalization of the urine to a pH >6 decreases the risk for intratubular cast formation and progressive renal failure.

Kidney function is one of the most important determinants of survival in multiple myeloma. Patients with a creatinine level <1.5 mg/dL have a 1-year survival rate of 80%, whereas those with a creatinine level >2.3 mg/dL have a 50% 1-year survival rate.

HIV-Associated Nephropathy
Pathophysiology
HIV-associated nephropathy (HIVAN) primarily affects black patients and may occur at any stage of clinical infection with HIV. There is no relationship among the duration of the HIV infection, the type of opportunistic infection, or patient age (10).

The kidney biopsy pattern in affected patients primarily resembles that in FSGS of the collapsing variety except for an additional characteristic microcystic tubular disease. Endothelial tuboreticular inclusions occur in this form of focal segmental sclerosis. However, other forms of glomerulopathy may develop in patients with HIV, including membranoproliferative glomerulonephritis, usually associated with hepatitis C; IgA nephropathy; lupus-like syndromes; and thrombotic microangiopathies, such as hemolytic uremic syndrome and thrombotic thrombocytopenic purpura.

HIVAN presents with heavy proteinuria, the nephrotic syndrome, renal insufficiency, and rapid progression to end-stage kidney disease. On ultrasonography, the kidneys are typically large and highly echogenic.

There are numerous therapies that attempt to slow the progress of HIVAN, including antiviral therapy, ACE inhibition, and immunosuppression. Highly active antiretroviral treatment (HAART) typically is administered.

KEY POINTS

- Diabetic nephropathy is characterized by proteinuria, hypertension, and a decline in the glomerular filtration rate in patients with a longstanding history of type 1 diabetes mellitus or a 5- to 10-year history of type 2 diabetes.

- Glomerulosclerosis leads to a decrease in filtration surface area, which results in a reduced glomerular filtration rate.

- Glycemic control delays or prevents progression from normoalbuminuria to microalbuminuria, clinical proteinuria, and overt nephropathy.

- Renal transplantation is the preferred intervention in patients with end-stage renal disease secondary to diabetes.

- In patients with myeloma-related kidney disorders, treatment of concomitant hypercalcemia and alkalization of the urine to a pH >6 decreases the risk for intratubular cast formation and progressive renal failure.

- Ultrasonography in patients with HIV-associated nephropathy typically reveals large, highly echogenic kidneys.

Diseases That Cause Glomerulonephritis

Numerous disorders that primarily affect the kidneys result in glomerulonephritis, including IgA nephropathy, poststreptococcal glomerulonephritis, anti-GBM antibody disease, and renal limited ANCA glomerulonephritis. However, most patients with glomerular disease have a widespread systemic illness.

Some patients have glomerulonephritis and dermal inflammation, including palpable purpura, necrosis, ulcers, and nodules. These renal–dermal syndromes include lupus, Henoch–Schönlein purpura, ANCA-associated vasculitis, and cryoglobulinemia. Pulmonary–renal syndromes also may develop in glomerulonephritis. Serologic analysis for anti-GBM antibodies, ANCA, and markers for immune complex diseases (such as antinuclear antibodies, anti–double-stranded DNA antibodies, cryoglobulins, anti–hepatitis B or C antibodies, and complement levels) may refine the appropriate diagnosis (**Table 46**).

Chronic glomerulonephritis leading to end-stage kidney disease also may develop. Many glomerular diseases progress with glomerular scarring and a progressive inexorable decline in kidney function. Glomerular disease is the third leading cause of end-stage kidney disease in the United States.

Some glomerular diseases are much more likely to rapidly progress to end-stage kidney disease, such as ANCA crescentic glomerulonephritis and anti-GBM antibody disease. Numerous other indolent glomerulopathies slowly progress to end-stage kidney disease. Chronic glomerulonephritis is the clinical consequence of almost all untreated glomerular diseases. These conditions are characterized by glomerular scarring, interstitial fibrosis, and arteriosclerosis.

IgA Nephropathy (Berger's Disease)
Pathophysiology
IgA nephropathy is a consequence of defective mucosal immunity where IgA molecules react to as yet unidentified antigens. These IgA antibodies are abnormally glycosylated so that the reticular endothelial system poorly removes them. Once deposited, these abnormally glycosylated, enriched immune complexes incite an inflammatory response that stimulates numerous circulating factors, including platelet-derived growth factor that results in mesangial cell proliferation and mesangial matrix expansion.

On kidney biopsy, IgA is the dominant type of immunoglobulin observed by immunofluorescence microscopy, hence the name of this condition, IgA nephropathy. Light microscopy reveals varying degrees of mesangial cell proliferation with areas of glomerular scarring in those glomeruli affected by episodes of relapsing and remitting disease.

Epidemiology
IgA nephropathy is the most common glomerulonephritic disease. In the United States, an estimated 5% of all kidney

TABLE 46 Clinical Associations of Autoantibodies

ANA

Associated with SLE and a variety of other conditions, including rheumatoid diseases, chronic active hepatitis, viral infections, and drug ingestion. Nucleolar pattern is associated with scleroderma, speckled pattern with MCTD, Sjögren's syndrome, SLE, and polymyositis.

Anti-dsDNA

A good marker for active lupus; titers may fluctuate with disease activity.

Anti-Sm

Virtually diagnostic of SLE, but only found in 25% of patients.

Antiphospholipid antibodies

Hypercoagulable state may be found in SLE and in other diseases but has no significance in others; present in thrombocytopenia and later-trimester abortions.

Antihistone antibodies

>95% in drug-related lupus; present in RA, SLE, and systemic sclerosis with pulmonary fibrosis.

ANCAs

Positive test results for ANCAs reveal one of two basic staining patterns: C-ANCA or P-ANCA staining. In small-vessel vasculitis, P-ANCAs and C-ANCAs usually are attributable to anti-MPO antibodies (MPO-ANCAs) and antibodies to PR3 (PR3-ANCAs), respectively. Markers for pauci-immune small-vessel vasculitis, including Wegener's granulomatosis, microscopic polyangiitis, Churg–Strauss syndrome, and some forms of necrotizing glomerulonephritis. Titers may correlate with disease activity.

ASO

Appears in serum after the onset of streptococcal infections; indicative of poststreptococcal disease, such as scarlet fever, rheumatic fever, or acute glomerulonephritis.

Anti-DNase B

Often done concurrently with ASO titer. Elevated in most patients with poststreptococcal glomerulonephritis or rheumatic fever.

Anti-GBM

Reactive with a highly restrictive portion of the noncollagenous domain of type IV collagen. Marker for Goodpasture's syndrome.

Anti-C3 neph

Associated with membranoproliferative glomerulonephritis and results in continuous activation of C3.

ANAs = antinuclear antibodies; MCTD = mixed connective tissue disease; SLE = systemic lupus erythematosus; anti-dsDNA = anti–double-stranded DNA; anti-Sm = anti-Smith; ANCAs = antineutrophil cytoplasmic antibodies; C-ANCA = cytoplasmic antineutrophil cytoplasmic antibody; P-ANCA = perinuclear antineutrophil cytoplasmic antibody; PR3 = proteinase 3; MPO = myeloperoxidase; ASO = antistreptolysin O; anti-DNase = anti-deoxyribonuclease; anti-GBM = anti–glomerular basement membrane; anti-C3 neph = antibodies to C3 nephritis factor.

biopsies and 10% of biopsies of patients with glomerulonephritis reveal IgA nephropathy. The prevalence of IgA nephropathy is much higher in Europe and Asia, where this condition may account for the diagnosis in almost 40% of all patients with glomerulonephritis. IgA nephropathy is rare in black individuals but common in Native Americans.

Genetic differences may affect the regional variations in disease prevalence, but renal biopsy practices in a particular locale also may be a contributing factor. For example, IgA nephropathy is detected more frequently if patients with minor urinary abnormalities undergo biopsy. In Japan, all school-aged children undergo routine screening for urinary abnormalities.

IgA nephropathy may have a genetic propensity, although the majority of cases of this condition are sporadic. Familial clustering has occurred in some regions of North America and in Asia. Ten-year actuarial survival rates were lowest in North America and highest in Europe, ranging from 61% to 95%. IgA nephropathy also typically affects middle-aged individuals.

IgA nephropathy may only involve the kidney or occur as part of a syndrome that includes skin disease, liver disease, inflammatory bowel disease, ankylosing spondylitis, and infections. IgA nephropathy also may develop in Henoch–Schönlein purpura.

Clinical Presentation

Patients with IgA nephropathy may present with one of several clinical disease patterns. Approximately 30% to 40% of affected patients present with an episodic macroscopic hematuria. The overt gross hematuria usually is associated with a simultaneous pharyngitic or gastrointestinal infection, such as synpharyngitic glomerulonephritis. Patients with episodic macroscopic hematuria in which all hematuria resolves have infrequent disease recurrence and excellent long-term prognosis with prolonged periods of disease quiescence.

Forty percent of patients with IgA nephropathy have persistent asymptomatic hematuria and proteinuria. In this setting, hypertension is much more common, renal function impairment develops over time, and remission is uncommon. Some patients with IgA nephropathy may present with the nephrotic syndrome as a consequence of diffuse proliferative glomerulonephritis due to glomerular scarring induced by previous illness, or the presence of a concomitant unrelated glomerulopathy, such as minimal change disease.

Over time, one third of all patients with IgA nephropathy achieve clinical remission with resolution of proteinuria and hematuria, one third develop a more benign disease course with urinary protein excretion <1 g/24 h, and one third have a progressive decline in renal function over the course of a decade or more. Generally, patients with normal renal function, normal blood pressure, and urinary protein excretion <1g/24 h have a positive prognosis.

Treatment

Patients with IgA nephropathy who have good prognostic indicators with minimal proteinuria and normal renal function should be managed conservatively with an ACE inhibitor, an angiotensin receptor blocker, or both. Patients with a more progressive disease who have elevated serum creatinine levels should receive pulse corticosteroid therapy or, if they have renal insufficiency, corticosteroids and an alkylating agent (11).

Poststreptococcal Glomerulonephritis

Poststreptococcal glomerulonephritis is an example of an acute nephritis marked by electron microscopy findings of subepithelial humps or deposits of the offending antigen between the glomerular epithelial cell and the GBM. The ensuing inflammation causes a membranoproliferative glomerulonephritic pattern resulting in proteinuria. The clinical disease begins with sudden development of edema, hematuria, and renal insufficiency 2 or 3 weeks after streptococcal pharyngitis or cellulitis presents.

Typical serologic findings in poststreptococcal glomerulonephritis include a low C3, low normal C4, and elevated antistreptolysin O (ASO) and positive anti-DNAse B antibody titers. In the setting of glomerulonephritis 2 to 3 weeks after pharyngitis or cellulitis, antistreptococcal antibodies are beneficial. The ASO titer is elevated in about 70% of affected patients, and titers of the more specific anti-DNAse B antibodies are elevated in approximately 90% of these patients. The combination of ASO and anti-DNAse B testing is the most effective method of diagnosis.

The hypertension and acute renal insufficiency associated with poststreptococcal glomerulonephritis may be alarming, but clinical manifestations of this condition rapidly resolve. Diuresis begins within 1 week, and kidney function returns to baseline after 3 or 4 weeks. Most patients, particularly children, achieve complete clinical resolution from the initial episode.

Some patients with severe glomerular damage have persistent proteinuria and hypertension that require long-term therapy. Repetitive episodes of poststreptococcal glomerulonephritis are rare and probably occur because of antibodies to the nephritogenic streptococcal antigen.

Lupus Nephritis

Pathophysiology

The kidney is commonly affected in lupus. One third to one half of patients presenting with lupus have an abnormal urinalysis or some degree of renal dysfunction. Within the first 3 years of diagnosis of lupus, whether a patient will develop kidney disease becomes evident.

TABLE 47 Classification of Lupus Nephritis
Class I
Characterized by minimal mesangial immune deposits and glomeruli that still appear normal on light microscopy.
Class II
A mesangioproliferative glomerulonephritis with expansion of mesangial cells and matrix visible on light microscopy.
Class III
A focal nephritis with <50% of glomeruli actively involved with inflammation on light microscopy. These lesions can be proliferative or necrotizing.
Class IV
A diffuse glomerulonephritis with <50% glomerular involvement with a proliferative response or necrotizing lesions. These lesions are usually associated with subendothelial deposits.
Class V
Characterized by the presence of subepithelial immune deposits that result in membranous nephropathy.
Class VI
The chronic form of disease in which >90% of the glomeruli are globally sclerotic. Chances of long-term renal failure are high.

The pathogenesis of glomerular injury in this setting relates to the deposition of immune complexes, either as a consequence of *in situ* localization of an antigen followed by antibody binding or the deposition of preformed circulating immune complexes that launch a cascade of inflammatory events. These events include activation of the complement and coagulation cascades and leukocyte recruitment.

The site of immune complex deposition correlates with the clinical phenotype of the disease. Immune complexes deposited in the mesangium or subendothelium result in a focal or diffuse proliferative glomerulonephritis. Deposits that bind in the subepithelial region or within the GBM manifest as membranous nephropathy. Deposits that line the subepithelial space usually manifest as proteinuria that is often in the nephrotic range.

The classification of lupus nephritis into pathologic categories recently has been modified (**Table 47**) (12).

Clinical Presentation

The clinical presentation of most patients with lupus nephritis mirrors the pattern of the histology. Patients with class I or II lupus nephritis typically have hematuria and/or proteinuria and usually do not have renal insufficiency. Those with class III or IV disease have acute nephritis with hematuria; proteinuria; typically erythrocyte casts; and, depending on the number of glomeruli involved, renal insufficiency. Patients with membranous nephropathy typically present with proteinuria, usually in the nephrotic range.

The following factors help to determine the outcome of patients with lupus nephritis: the presence of renal insufficiency at the time of biopsy, the severity of the renal histology, the presence of interstitial fibrosis indicating scarring, or the presence of crescents indicative of active and aggressive glomerulonephritis. Black race constitutes an independent predictor of end-stage kidney disease in patients with Class IV disease.

Treatment

Disease severity determines the treatment in lupus nephritis. Studies supported by the National Institutes of Health indicate that treatment with intravenous cyclophosphamide once monthly for 6 consecutive months, with additional cyclophosphamide therapy administered every 3 months for up to 2 years, provides long-term improvement in renal function. Prednisone alone does not provide the same degree of renal protection over 10 years.

The advent of mycophenolate mofetil therapy has recently challenged the status of cyclophosphamide as the mainstay of immunomodulatory therapy. An alternative to cyclophosphamide therapy has been investigated because of the substantial side effects of this agent, which include major infection; mutagenesis; and premature ovarian failure in women. As induction therapy, mycophenolate mofetil appears equivalent to intravenous cyclophosphamide in patients with diffuse proliferative glomerulonephritis (13).

A U.S. study revealed that a higher number of patients achieved complete remission with mycophenolate mofetil compared with intravenous cyclophosphamide. Mycophenolate mofetil has been shown to be superior to intravenous cyclophosphamide in maintaining disease remission when intravenous cyclophosphamide was used for 6 months for induction, followed by mycophenolate mofetil, azathioprine, or intravenous cyclophosphamide for a period of up to 48 months. Mycophenolate mofetil and azathioprine also were superior to intravenous cyclophosphamide in maintaining remission with fewer side effects (14).

It is uncertain whether these less-toxic therapies will prevent end-stage renal disease over decades of use. When mycophenolate mofetil therapy is discontinued, recrudescence of disease is much more common than with intravenous cyclophosphamide therapy.

Anti–Glomerular Basement Membrane Antibody Disease

Anti-GBM antibody disease (which involves only the kidney) and Goodpasture's syndrome (which involves the kidney and lung) are caused by antibodies to a noncollagenous portion of type IV collagen. The epitope of these conditions is limited to a specific region of approximately nine amino acids that cause the autoantigen response. The pathology is that of a necrotizing and crescentic glomerulonephritis affecting most if not all of the glomeruli. Immunofluorescence microscopy reveals linear staining of IgG lining the GBM.

Young men typically have kidney and lung disease, whereas older women typically have involvement of only the kidney. Rapidly progressive glomerulonephritis is the most common feature of anti-GBM antibody disease.

Patient and renal survival are largely contingent on the promptness of therapy and the serum creatinine level at the time of diagnosis. Patients who are dialysis dependent or who have a serum creatinine level between 5 mg/dL and 6 mg/dL have a much lower chance of renal survival than those with normal renal function.

Pulmonary hemorrhage is a medical emergency requiring immediate plasmapheresis to remove the offending antibody. Corticosteroid and cyclophosphamide therapy are then indicated to induce disease remission. Disease relapse is rare; therefore, cyclophosphamide may be discontinued after 3 to 6 months of therapy.

Approximately 30% of patients with Goodpasture's syndrome also have ANCA-associated vasculitis. These patients may present with vasculitis outside the lung and kidney. The clinical course in this setting is initially that of anti-GBM antibody disease, but, as in ANCA-associated vasculitis, this condition tends to relapse.

Small- and Medium-Vessel Vasculitis

Many forms of systemic vasculitis affect the kidneys. Large-vessel vasculitides, including giant-cell arteritis and Takayasu's arteritis, induce renal ischemia from a narrowed abdominal aorta or narrowed renal arteries. Middle-sized vasculopathies, including Kawasaki's disease and polyarteritis nodosa, similarly reduce renal blood flow because of renal artery or intrarenal artery narrowing resulting in infarction. Renal infarctions and renovascular hypertension are common.

The most common kidney involvement in systemic vasculitis is a necrotizing and crescentic glomerulonephritis that occurs because of small-vessel vasculitis. This lesion is associated with the systemic disorders microscopic polyangiitis, Wegener's granulomatosis, and the Churg–Strauss syndrome. These are pauci-immune complex deposition diseases, in contrast to the immune complex lupus nephritis or IgA diseases of Henoch–Schönlein purpura (**Table 48**).

Pauci-immune small-vessel vasculitis is associated with and most likely caused by ANCAs. These small-vessel vasculitides involve vessels that include postcapillary venules and arterioles and result primarily in glomerular and pulmonary capillaritis. The hallmark of these lesions in the acute phase is segmental fibrinoid necrosis with leukocyte infiltration. Crescentic glomerulonephritis develops with more aggressive inflammation. The presence of mononuclear leukocytes and glomerulus fibrosis characterizes the chronic phase of the glomerular lesion. As in all glomerulonephritides, once

TABLE 48 Names and Definitions Adopted by the Chapel Hill Consensus Conference on the Nomenclature of Systemic Vasculitis

Large-Vessel Vasculitis

Giant cell arteritis

Granulomatous arteritis of the aorta and its major branches, with a predilection for the extracranial branches of the carotid artery. Often involves the temporal artery. Usually occurs in patients >50 years of age and often is associated with polymyalgia rheumatica.

Takayasu's arteritis

Granulomatous inflammation of the aorta and its major branches. Usually occurs in patients <50 years of age.

Medium-Sized Vessel Vasculitis

Polyarteritis nodosa

Necrotizing inflammation of medium-sized or small arteries without glomerulonephritis or vasculitis in arterioles, capillaries, or venules.

Kawasaki's disease

Arteritis involving large, medium-sized, and small arteries and associated with mucocutaneous lymph node syndrome. Coronary arteries are often involved. Aorta and veins may be involved. Usually occurs in children.

Small-Vessel Vasculitis

Wegener's granulomatosis[§]

Granulomatous inflammation involving the respiratory tract and necrotizing vasculitis affecting small to medium-sized vessels.[†] Necrotizing glomerulonephritis is common.

Churg–Strauss syndrome[§]

Eosinophil-rich and granulomatous inflammation involving the respiratory tract and necrotizing vasculitis affecting small to medium-sized vessels. Associated with asthma and eosinophilia.

Microscopic polyangiitis[§]

Necrotizing vasculitis with few or no immune deposits affecting small vessels.[‡] Necrotizing arteritis involving small and medium-sized arteries may be present. Necrotizing glomerulonephritis is very common. Pulmonary capillarities often occur.

Henoch-Schönlein purpura

Vasculitis with IgA-dominant immune deposits affecting small vessels[‡]. Typically involves skin, gut, and glomeruli and is associated with arthralgias or arthritis.

Cryoglobulinemic vasculitis

Vasculitis with cryoglobulin immune deposits affecting small vessels* and associated with cryoglobulins in serum. Skin and glomeruli are often involved.

Cutaneous leukocytoclastic angiitis

Isolated cutaneous leukocytoclastic angiitis without systemic vasculitis or glomerulonephritis.

* "Large artery" refers to the aorta and the largest branches directed toward major body regions (the extremities and the head and neck); "medium-sized artery" refers to the main visceral arteries (renal, hepatic, coronary, and mesenteric arteries); and "small artery" refers to the distal arterial radicals that connect with arterioles. Note that large and medium-sized vessel vasculitides do not involve vessels other than arteries.

† Capillaries, venules, arterioles, and arteries.

‡ Capillaries, venules, and arteries.

§ Strongly associated with ANCAs.

Modified with permission from Jennette JC, Falk RJ, Andrassy K, Bacon PA, Churg J, Gross WL, et al. Nomenclature of systemic vasculitides. Proposal of an international consensus conference. Arthritis Rheum. 1994;37:187-92. PMID: 8129773

the glomerulus is involved, tubular interstitial damage occurs, as well.

Cytoplasmic ANCAs react with a serine proteinase called proteinase 3 (PR3), whereas perinuclear ANCAs react with myeloperoxidase (MPO) in necrotizing vasculitis. Patients with renal-limited, Wegener's, or microscopic polyangiitis may have either of these two ANCA serotypes. However, PR3 ANCAs are more common in Wegener's granulomatosis and MPO ANCAs are more common in microscopic polyangiitis.

The cause of ANCA-associated small-vessel vasculitis has been determined by *in vitro* data, which demonstrate that ANCAs react with their MPO or protein antigens released at the surface of cytokine-stimulated leukocytes. These leukocytes are then activated to marginate and degranulate along vessel walls, resulting in disease induction. The *in vivo* proof that anti-MPO antibodies cause vascular disease was demonstrated when antibodies to MPO were passively transferred to naïve recipients who developed a pauci-immune necrotizing glomerulonephritis.

Clinical Presentation

The presentation of patients with systemic vasculitis affecting the kidney is largely associated with the type of vessel involved. Most patients have systemic symptoms, including myalgias, arthralgias, and weight loss. Larger-vessel and middle-sized vessel vasculitis typically presents as an ischemic disease of the tissue supported by those vessels. ANCA-associated small-vessel vasculitides present with hematuria and proteinuria. Because of the aggressive nature of the disease, these conditions also frequently present as a rapidly progressive glomerulonephritis.

The majority of patients with these conditions develop a migratory polyarthropathy that may be accompanied by frank synovitis. In addition to the glomerulonephritides, any organ system may be involved, including the upper respiratory tract, which results in ear, nose, and throat disease. Fleeting pulmonary infiltrates, nodules, or cavities may cause pulmonary symptoms, whereas hemoptysis and frank pulmonary hemorrhage are the gravest consequences of pulmonary bleeding.

Leukocytoclastic angiitis in dermal vessels results in purpura; ecchymoses; and livedo reticularis, urticaria, and ulcers. Vasculitis involving the mesenteric vessels results in abdominal pain and mucosal and bowel wall infarctions. Mononeuritis multiplex causes peripheral nerve involvement. Ultimately, vasculitis may involve any part of the body.

The features cited above typically are associated with any kind of small-vessel vasculitis, but patients with Wegener's granulomatosis have necrotizing granulomatous inflammation that may involve the lung or ear, nose, and throat. This type of inflammation more commonly results in nodular lesions in the lung that can cavitate and bleed. Similarly, asthma and eosinophilia are characteristic of the Churg–Strauss syndrome.

Treatment

Methylprednisolone with tapering dosages of corticosteroids over a 16-week course is indicated for ANCA-associated small-vessel vasculitis. In addition, intravenous or oral cyclophosphamide is indicated for 3 to 6 months. After these treatment courses are completed, therapy may be discontinued or a trial of remission-maintaining agents including azathioprine or, more experimentally, mycophenolate mofetil may be beneficial. Plasmapheresis is indicated for pulmonary hemorrhage and perhaps for dialysis-dependent patients at the onset of therapy.

Relapse and remission characterize the long-term course of these diseases. Typically, patients with a PR3 ANCA or upper and/or lower respiratory tract disease are much more likely to relapse than patients without these features (15).

Therefore, treatment is tailored based on the propensity for relapse. Long-term therapy with azathioprine or mycophenolate mofetil is appropriate for patients likely to relapse, whereas discontinuation of therapy with very close follow-up is indicated for those with a low propensity for relapse.

KEY POINTS

- Light microscopy in IgA nephropathy reveals varying degrees of mesangial cell proliferation and possibly areas of glomerular scarring.
- An angiotensin-converting enzyme inhibitor, an angiotensin receptor blocker, or both are indicated for patients with IgA nephropathy who have good prognostic indicators with minimal proteinuria and normal renal function.
- Poststreptococcal glomerulonephritis usually manifests with the sudden development of edema, hematuria, and renal insufficiency 2 or 3 weeks after streptococcal pharyngitis or cellulitis presents.
- As induction therapy, mycophenolate mofetil appears equivalent to intravenous cyclophosphamide in patients with diffuse proliferative glomerulonephritis but is more commonly associated with disease recrudescence.
- Pauci-immune small-vessel vasculitis is associated with and most likely caused by antineutrophil cytoplasmic antibodies.
- Azathioprine or mycophenolate mofetil may help to maintain remission in antineutrophil cytoplasmic antibody–associated small-vessel vasculitis.
- In antineutrophil cytoplasmic antibody–associated small-vessel vasculitis, plasmapheresis is indicated for pulmonary hemorrhage and perhaps for dialysis-dependent patients at the onset of therapy.

References

1. Tryggvason K, Patrakka J, Wartiovaara J. Hereditary proteinuria syndromes and mechanisms of proteinuria. N Engl J Med. 2006;354:1387-401. [PMID: 16571882]
2. Troyanov S, Wall CA, Miller JA, Scholey JW, Cattran DC. Focal and segmental glomerulosclerosis: definition and relevance of a partial remission. J Am Soc Nephrol. 2005;16:1061-8. [PMID: 15716334]
3. Cattran D. Management of membranous nephropathy: when and what for treatment. J Am Soc Nephrol. 2005;16:1188-94. [PMID: 15800117]
4. Lewis EJ, Hunsicker LG, Clarke WR, Berl T, Pohl MA, Lewis JB, et al. Renoprotective effect of the angiotensin-receptor antagonist irbesartan in patients with nephropathy due to type 2 diabetes. N Engl J Med. 2001;345:851-60. [PMID: 11565517]
5. Lewis EJ, Hunsicker LG, Bain RP, Rohde RD. The effect of angiotensin-converting-enzyme inhibition on diabetic nephropathy. The Collaborative Study Group. N Engl J Med. 1993;329:1456-62. [PMID: 8413456]
6. Brenner BM, Cooper ME, de Zeeuw D, Keane WF, Mitch WE, Parving HH, et al. Effects of losartan on renal and cardiovascular outcomes in patients with type 2 diabetes and nephropathy. N Engl J Med. 2001;345:861-9. [PMID: 11565518]

7. **Barnett AH, Bain SC, Bouter P, Karlberg B, Madsbad S, Jervell J, et al.** Angiotensin-receptor blockade versus converting-enzyme inhibition in type 2 diabetes and nephropathy. N Engl J Med. 2004;351:1952-61. [PMID: 15516696]

8. **Blade J, Fernandez-Llama P, Bosch F, Montoliu J, Lens XM, Montoto S, et al.** Renal failure in multiple myeloma: presenting features and predictors of outcome in 94 patients from a single institution. Arch Intern Med. 1998;158:1889-93. [PMID: 9759684]

9. **Johnson WJ, Kyle RA, Pineda AA, O'Brien PC, Holley KE.** Treatment of renal failure associated with multiple myeloma. Plasmapheresis, hemodialysis, and chemotherapy. Arch Intern Med. 1990;150:863-9. [PMID: 2183734]

10. **Balow JE.** Nephropathy in the context of HIV infection [Editorial]. Kidney Int. 2005;67:1632-3. [PMID: 15780122]

11. **Pozzi C, Andrulli S, Del Vecchio L, Melis P, Fogazzi GB, Altieri P, et al.** Corticosteroid effectiveness in IgA nephropathy: long-term results of a randomized, controlled trial. J Am Soc Nephrol. 2004;15:157-63. [PMID: 14694168]

12. **Weening JJ, D'Agati VD, Schwartz MM, Seshan SV, Alpers CE, Appel GB, et al.** The classification of glomerulonephritis in systemic lupus erythematosus revisited. J Am Soc Nephrol. 2004;15:241-50. [PMID: 14747370]

13. **Ginzler EM, Dooley MA, Aranow C, Kim MY, Buyon J, Merrill JT, et al.** Mycophenolate mofetil or intravenous cyclophosphamide for lupus nephritis. N Engl J Med. 2005;353:2219-28. [PMID: 16306519]

14. **Contreras G, Tozman E, Nahar N, Metz D.** Maintenance therapies for proliferative lupus nephritis: mycophenolate mofetil, azathioprine and intravenous cyclophosphamide. Lupus. 2005;14 Suppl 1:s33-8. [PMID: 15803929]

15. **Hogan SL, Falk RJ, Chin H, Cai J, Jennette CE, Jennette JC, et al.** Predictors of relapse and treatment resistance in antineutrophil cytoplasmic antibody-associated small-vessel vasculitis. Ann Intern Med. 2005;143:621-31. [PMID: 16263884]

Self-Assessment Test

This self-assessment test contains one-best-answer multiple-choice questions. Please read these directions carefully before answering the questions. Answers, critiques, and bibliographies immediately follow these multiple-choice questions.

The American College of Physicians is accredited by the Accreditation Council for Continuing Medical Education (ACCME) to provide continuing medical education for physicians.

The American College of Physicians designates MKSAP 14® Nephrology for a maximum of 13 *AMA PRA Category 1 Credits*™. Physicians should only claim credit commensurate with the extent of their participation in the activity.

Separate answer sheets are provided for each book of the MKSAP program. Please use one of these answer sheets to complete the Nephrology self-assessment test. Indicate in Section H on the answer sheet the actual number of credits you earned, up to the maximum of 13, in ¼-credit increments. (One credit equals one hour of time spent on this educational activity.)

Credit is available from the publication date of December 29, 2006, until July 31, 2009. You may submit your answer sheets at any time during this period.

Self-Scoring Instructions:
Nephrology

Compute your percent correct score as follows:

Step 1: Give yourself 1 point for each correct response to a question.

Step 2: Divide your total points by the total number of questions: 105.

The result, expressed as a percentage, is your percent correct score.

	Example	Your Calculations
Step 1	89	
Step 2	89 ÷ 105	÷ 105
% Correct	85%	%

Directions

Item 1

A 50-year-old man is evaluated for poorly controlled hypertension. His blood pressure has been elevated for 12 years and remains between 150/105 mm Hg and 170/105 mm Hg despite the use of multiple medications. He also has poor exercise tolerance and fatigue and often falls asleep in the afternoon. Medications are atenolol, 50 mg/d; amlodipine, 10 mg/d; and hydrochlorothiazide, 25 mg/d.

On physical examination, blood pressure is 168/110 mm Hg. He is obese and appears plethoric. The remainder of the examination is normal.

Laboratory studies:

Glucose (fasting)	102 mg/dL (5.66 mmol/L)
Blood urea nitrogen	20 mg/dL (7.14 mmol/L)
Creatinine	1.4 mg/dL (123.79 μmol/L)
Sodium	140 meq/L (140 mmol/L)
Potassium	3.9 meq/L (3.9 mmol/L)
Bicarbonate	25 meq/L (25 mmol/L)
Cholesterol	220 mg/dL (5.69 mmol/L)
Triglycerides	190 mg/dL (2.15 mmol/L)
High-density lipoprotein cholesterol	37 mg/dL (0.96 mmol/L)

Which of the following is the most likely cause of this patient's resistant hypertension?

(A) Renovascular hypertension
(B) Primary hyperaldosteronism
(C) Pheochromocytoma
(D) Type 2 diabetes mellitus
(E) Sleep apnea syndrome

Item 2

A 60-year-old woman with a history of type 1 diabetes mellitus and stage 4 chronic kidney disease comes for a routine follow-up examination. She asks about modalities of renal replacement therapy.

Which of the following is the best option for this patient?

(A) 0-Antigen-mismatched deceased donor kidney transplantation
(B) Peritoneal dialysis
(C) Hemodialysis
(D) Living donor kidney transplantation after a course of dialysis
(E) Preemptive living donor kidney transplantation

Item 3

A 21-year-old woman is evaluated for facial and lower-extremity edema of 1 week's duration. For the past 3 weeks, she has had fatigue. She has no history of diabetes mellitus, cigarette smoking, or illicit drug use.

On physical examination, blood pressure is 90/55 mm Hg. Cardiac and pulmonary examinations are normal. There is periorbital edema. The abdomen is soft and without masses. There is 2+ lower-extremity edema.

Laboratory studies:

Creatinine	0.7 mg/dL (61.89 μmol/L)
Total cholesterol	325 mg/dL (8.4 mmol/L)
Albumin	2.9 g/dL (29 g/L)
C3 and C4	Normal
Urinalysis	Specific gravity 1.026, 3+ protein, 0–1 erythrocytes/hpf, numerous oval fat bodies/hpf
24-Hour urinary protein excretion	15 g/24 h

Which of the following is the most likely diagnosis?

(A) Minimal change glomerulopathy
(B) Membranous nephropathy
(C) Focal segmental glomerulosclerosis
(D) Membranoproliferative glomerulonephritis
(E) Systemic lupus erythematosus nephritis

Item 4

A 30-year-old woman who is 25 weeks pregnant is evaluated for a sore throat. On physical examination, temperature is 38.5 °C (101.3 °F), pulse rate is 110/min, and blood pressure is 100/70 mm Hg. The lungs are clear to auscultation. The pharynx is erythematous. Abdominal examination reveals a gravid abdomen.

Laboratory studies:

Hematocrit	34%
Leukocyte count	7500/μL (7.5 × 10^9/L)
Platelet count	275,000/μL (275 × 10^9/L)

Blood urea nitrogen	8 mg/dL (2.86 mmol/L)
Creatinine	0.6 mg/dL (53.05 μL)
Sodium	134 meq/L (134 mmol/L)
Potassium	3.7 meq/L (3.7 mmol/L)
Chloride	100 meq/L (100 mol/L)
Bicarbonate	22 meq/L (22 mmol/L)

In addition to pharyngitis, which of the following is also present in this patient?

(A) Sepsis
(B) Volume depletion
(C) Syndrome of inappropriate antidiuretic hormone secretion
(D) Normal pregnancy

Item 5

A 59-year-old man with end-stage renal disease comes to the emergency department for the acute onset of progressively severe abdominal pain. He has been on chronic hemodialysis for the past 2 years and is compliant with his treatment schedule; his most recent treatment was yesterday. He has type 2 diabetes mellitus, hypertension, atrial fibrillation, and asthma. Medications are enalapril, 20 mg twice daily; glipizide, 5 mg twice daily; and aspirin, 325 mg twice daily.

Physical examination is significant only for an irregularly irregular heart rate, a slightly distended abdomen that is diffusely tender, and trace lower-extremity edema. A stool specimen is positive for occult blood.

Laboratory studies:

Glucose	212 mg/dL (11.77 mmol/L)
Blood urea nitrogen	54 mg/dL (19.28 mmol/L)
Creatinine	8.3 mg/dL (733.89 μmol/L)
Sodium	134 meq/L (134 mmol/L)
Potassium	6.9 meq/L (6.9 mmol/L)
Chloride	96 meq/L (96 mmol/L)
Bicarbonate	13 meq/L (13 mmol/L)
Calcium	9.1 mg/dL (2.27 mmol/L)
Phosphorus	6.6 mg/dL (2.13 mmol/L)

Lactic acid	9.3 mg/dL (1.03 mmol/L)
Albumin	3.8 g/dL (38 g/L)

Which of the following is the most likely cause of this patient's hyperkalemia?

(A) Inadequate dialysis therapy
(B) Insulin deficiency
(C) Tissue ischemia
(D) Enalapril
(E) Catecholamine deficiency

Item 6

A 17-year-old man is evaluated for the abrupt onset of a lower-extremity rash and intermittent episodes of mild abdominal pain. He is otherwise asymptomatic.

On physical examination, respiratory rate is 18/min, pulse rate is 78/min, and blood pressure is 140/90 mm Hg. Cardiac, pulmonary, and abdominal examinations are normal. There are lesions resembling palpable purpura on the extremities.

Laboratory studies:

Blood urea nitrogen	16 mg/dL (5.71 mmol/L)
Creatinine	0.9 mg/dL (79.58 μmol/L)
C3	100 mg/dL (1000 mg/L)
C4	31 mg/dL (310 mg/L)
Urinalysis	1+ protein, 12 dysmorphic erythrocytes and 1 erythrocyte cast/hpf

Which of the following is the most likely diagnosis?

(A) Systemic lupus erythematosus glomerulonephritis
(B) Antineutrophil cytoplasmic autoantibody–associated small-vessel vasculitis
(C) Cryoglobulinemic vasculitis
(D) Henoch–Schönlein purpura
(E) Postinfectious glomerulonephritis

Item 7

A 62-year-old woman with type 2 diabetes mellitus, cerebrovascular disease, and chronic kidney disease develops nonoliguric acute renal failure after a left femoral–popliteal bypass. During the surgery, intra- or postoperative hypotension did not develop. Preoperatively, she began cefazolin therapy for wound prophylaxis. For the first 48 hours postoperatively, she received hydration with dextran 40, followed by half-normal saline (0.45%). Over the first 3 days of hospitalization, her creatinine level increased to 5.4 mg/dL (477.47 μmol/L); her creatinine level had been between 1.6 mg/dL (141.47 µmol/L) and 1.8 mg/dL (159.16 µmol/L) over the past year. Regular medications are ramipril; atenolol; and clopidogrel, which was discontinued 5 days preoperatively and has not been reinitiated.

On physical examination, temperature is 36.7 °C (98.1 °F), pulse rate is 86/min, and blood pressure is 132/80 mm Hg. Cardiac examination is unremarkable except for a murmur of aortic sclerosis. The lungs are clear to auscultation. There is trace pretibial edema bilaterally. The operative site shows no erythema or drainage.

Complete blood count is normal without peripheral eosinophilia. C3 and C4 levels are normal. Urinalysis shows 1+ protein, many monomorphic erythrocytes, and no cellular casts. Ultrasound shows symmetric echogenic kidneys without hydronephrosis.

Which of the following is the most likely diagnosis?

(A) Osmotic tubular injury
(B) Ischemic tubular epithelial cell injury
(C) Angiotensin-converting enzyme inhibitor–induced acute renal failure
(D) Thrombotic microangiopathy

Item 8

A 52-year-old woman with type 2 diabetes mellitus and hypertension comes for a routine office visit. She has a 30-pack-year history of cigarette smoking. Her mother had diabetes and was on hemodialysis. Medications are insulin; metoprolol, 100 mg/d; fosinopril, 40 mg/d; hydrochlorothiazide, 50 mg/d; atorvastatin, 40 mg/d; and aspirin, 81 mg/d.

On physical examination, blood pressure is 165/95 mm Hg. There are retinal microaneurysms. Cardiac examination reveals a regular rhythm with an S4. The lungs are clear to auscultation. There is no jugular venous distention. There is 1+ pedal edema. The distal pulses are absent in both feet.

Laboratory studies:

Hemoglobin A_{1C}	7.2%
Glucose	180 mg/dL (9.99 mmol/L)
Creatinine	1.2 mg/dL (106.1 µmol/L)
24-Hour urinary protein excretion	1.8 g/24 h

Which of the following factors is most likely to cause this patient's chronic kidney disease to rapidly progress to end-stage renal disease?

(A) Poorly controlled diabetes
(B) Family history
(C) Poorly controlled hypertension
(D) Proteinuria
(E) Cigarette smoking

Item 9

A 51-year-old man with a history of chronic lymphocytic leukemia with transformation to prolymphocytic leukemia is hospitalized for chemotherapy with R-CHOP (cyclophosphamide doxorubicin vincristine prednisone rituximab). Before initiation of chemotherapy, he receives allopurinol and normal saline at a rate of 250 mL/h. One day later, his creatinine level is 2.3 mg/dL (203.37 µmol/L) (baseline creatinine is 0.8 mg/dL [70.74 µmol/L]) and his urine output over the past 12 hours is 200 mL despite continued saline hydration.

On physical examination, he is afebrile, pulse rate is 98/min, respiratory rate is 16/min, and blood pressure is 134/78 mm Hg. There is lymphadenopathy involving the cervical and submental chains and supraclavicular areas bilaterally, as well as bulky axillary and inguinal lymphadenopathy. Cardiac and pulmonary examinations are normal. The spleen is palpable approximately 3 cm to 4 cm below the left costal margin, and there is no hepatomegaly. There is no edema, cyanosis, or clubbing of the extremities.

Laboratory studies:

Hematocrit	22%
Leukocyte count	72,000/µL (72 × 10^9/L)
Platelet count	19,000/µL (19 × 10^9/L)
Blood urea nitrogen	63 mg/dL (22.5 mmol/L)
Uric acid	19 mg/dL (1.13 mmol/L)
Creatinine	2.3 mg/dL (203.37 µmol/L)
Potassium	5.5 meq/L (5.5 mmol/L)
Bicarbonate	17 meq/L (17 mmol/L)
Albumin	4.2 g/dL (42 g/L)
Calcium	7.5 mg/dL (1.87 mmol/L)
Phosphorus	11 mg/dL (3.55 mmol/L)
Urinalysis	pH 5, numerous finely granular casts/hpf, no uric acid crystals

Which of the following is the most appropriate next step in this patient's management?

(A) Switch intravenous hydration to sodium bicarbonate
(B) Start furosemide
(C) Start rasburicase
(D) Start hemodialysis
(E) Start probenecid

Item 10

A 54-year-old woman is evaluated for a creatinine level of 1.3 mg/dL (114.95 µmol/L); 18 months ago, this value was 0.9 mg/dL (79.58 µmol/L). She has a 5-year history of type 2 diabetes mellitus; hyperlipidemia; and hypertension well controlled with lisinopril, hydrochlorothiazide, and atenolol. She also uses glipizide and simvastatin. Laboratory studies reveal a normal hemoglobin level.

Which of the following diagnostic studies is most appropriate for this patient?

(A) 24-Hour urine collection for proteinuria
(B) Kidney ultrasonography
(C) Measurement of urine microalbumin
(D) Serum protein electrophoresis
(E) Measurement of hemoglobin A_{1c}

Item 11

A 55-year-old man with hypertension and diabetic nephropathy comes for a follow-up visit. He was diagnosed with type 2 diabetes mellitus 10 years ago. He has no shortness of breath or edema. Medications are glipizide, 5 mg twice daily; pioglitazone, 30 mg/d; metoprolol, 100 mg/d; fosinopril, 80 mg/d; hydrochlorothiazide, 25 mg/d; atorvastatin, 40 mg/d; and aspirin, 81 mg/d.

On physical examination, pulse rate is 55/min and blood pressure is 145/85 mm Hg. He is obese. Retinal microaneurysms are present. On cardiac examination, there is a regular sinus rhythm with no murmurs. The lungs are clear to auscultation. There is trace pedal edema.

Laboratory studies:

Creatinine	1.0 mg/dL (88.42 µmol/L)
Sodium	140 meq/L (140 mmol/L)
Potassium	4.0 meq/L (4.0 mmol/L)
Chloride	106 meq/L (106 mmol/L)
Bicarbonate	24 meq/L (24 mmol/L)
24-Hour urine protein excretion	6 g/24 h
Urinalysis	4+ protein, 1–2 erythrocytes and 8 leukocytes/hpf

On abdominal ultrasound, the right kidney is 12 cm and the left kidney is 12.2 cm. There is normal echogenicity and no hydronephrosis, masses, or stones.

Which of the following is the most appropriate next step in this patient's management?

(A) Increase hydrochlorothiazide dose to 50 mg/d
(B) Add amlodipine
(C) Add prazosin
(D) Increase metoprolol dose to 150 mg/d
(E) Add losartan

Item 12

An 18-year-old man with hepatitis C virus infection is evaluated in the emergency department for nausea, vomiting, anorexia, hiccups, hemoptysis, and itching. He felt well until 4 weeks ago, when he developed an upper respiratory tract infection.

On physical examination, pulse rate is 90/min and blood pressure is 170/100 mm Hg. The conjunctivae are pale. Cardiac examination reveals a grade 2/6 systolic murmur along the left sternal border. There are diffuse crackles in both lung bases. The abdomen is soft and nontender with no masses. There is 1+ edema in the extremities.

Laboratory studies:

Hemoglobin	8.5 g/dL (85 g/L)
Leukocyte count	10,500/µL (10.5 × 10^9/L)
Platelet count	250,000/µL (250 × 10^9/L)
Blood urea nitrogen	70 mg/dL (25 mmol/L)
Creatinine	4.3 mg/dL (380.21 µmol/L)
Albumin	3.5 g/dL (35 g/L)
C3	140 mg/dL (1400 mg/L)
C4	35 mg/dL (350 mg/L)
Antinuclear antibodies	Negative
Urinalysis	15–20 dysmorphic erythrocytes and 1 erythrocyte cast/hpf

Chest radiograph reveals bilateral fluffy pulmonary infiltrates.

Which of the following assays is most likely to be positive in this patient?

(A) Antistreptolysin O and anti-DNAse B antibody
(B) Anti–double-stranded DNA antibody
(C) Antiphospholipid antibody
(D) Anti–glomerular basement membrane antibody
(E) Cryoglobulins

Item 13

A 45-year-old woman is referred for evaluation for a blood pressure measurement of 150/94 mm Hg. Her husband is a nurse and regularly measures her blood pressure at home. Her usual home blood pressure measurement is between 110/76 mm Hg and 120/80 mm Hg. She does not smoke cigarettes. Her mother has hypertension.

On physical examination, her average blood pressure is 148/98 mm Hg. Results of laboratory studies, including the creatinine level, are normal.

In addition to counseling regarding lifestyle modifications, which of the following is the most appropriate management for this patient?

(A) Begin hydrochlorothiazide
(B) Begin enalapril
(C) Perform ambulatory blood pressure monitoring
(D) Continue home blood pressure measurement

Item 14

A 23-year-old man with HIV infection comes for a follow-up examination. He was hospitalized 1 week ago with *Pneumocystis jiroveci* (formerly *Pneumocystis carinii*) pneumonia, which is being treated with trimethoprim–sulfamethoxazole and a prednisone taper. During his hospitalization, he was diagnosed with hyponatremia. He feels well, and his condition has significantly improved since his discharge 3 days ago.

On physical examination, temperature is 36.6 °C (97.8 °F), pulse rate is 84/min, respiratory rate is 12/min, and blood pressure is 110/60 mm Hg. He appears thin and in no apparent distress. Cardiac examination is normal. The lungs are clear to auscultation. There is no peripheral edema.

Laboratory studies:

CD4 cell count	87/µL (0.087 × 10^9/L)
Glucose	182 mg/dL (10.1 mmol/L)
Blood urea nitrogen	12 mg/dL (4.29 mmol/L)
Creatinine	0.7 mg/dL (61.89 µmol/L)
Sodium	111 meq/L (111 mmol/L)
Potassium	3.6 meq/L (3.6 mmol/L)
Chloride	96 meq/L (96 mmol/L)
Bicarbonate	22 meq/L (22 mmol/L)
Albumin	3.3 g/dL (33 g/L)
Phosphorus	2.6 mg/dL (0.84 mmol/L)
Serum osmolality	246 mosm/kg H_2O (246 mmol/kg)
Urine sodium	117 meq/L (117 mmol/L)
Urine potassium	24 meq/L (24 mmol/L)
Urine osmolality	453 mosm/kg (453 mmol/kg)

Which of the following is the most likely cause of this patient's hyponatremia?

(A) Syndrome of inappropriate antidiuretic hormone secretion
(B) Volume depletion
(C) Adrenal insufficiency
(D) Pseudohyponatremia
(E) Psychogenic polydipsia

Item 15

A 38-year-old woman is evaluated in the emergency department for generalized itching, an erythematous skin rash, and joint pain. She initially tried over-the-counter diphenhydramine but her itching and rash did not improve. She was diagnosed with a sinus infection 2 weeks ago that was treated with a course of amoxicillin. Her sinus drainage and cough have improved. However, her joint pain remains and her temperature has been between 37.5 °C (99.5 °F) and 37.8 °C (100 °F). She states that she has otherwise been healthy and takes no additional medications.

On physical examination, temperature is 37.3 °C (99.2 °F), pulse rate is 88/min, and blood pressure is 122/68 mm Hg. There is a diffuse erythematous macular papular skin rash involving her trunk, arms, and upper thighs.

Laboratory studies:

Hemoglobin	12.5 g/dL (125 g/L)
Leukocyte count	9800/µL (9.8 × 10^9/L) (10% eosinophils)
Platelet count	325,000/µL (325 × 10^9/L)
Blood urea nitrogen	36 mg/dL (12.86 mmol/L)
Creatinine	2.6 mg/dL (229.89 µmol/L)
Sodium	138 meq/L (138 mmol/L)
Potassium	4.4 meq/L (4.4 mmol/L)
Bicarbonate	26 meq/L (26 mmol/L)
Urinalysis	pH 5, specific gravity 1.020, 2+ blood, trace protein, 4+ leukocyte esterase, 20–25 leukocytes and several leukocyte casts/hpf, 3–5 intact erythrocytes/hpf, Hansel stain shows eosinophils

Which of the following is the most likely diagnosis in this patient?

(A) Thrombotic thrombocytopenic purpura
(B) Antineutrophil cytoplasmic autoantibody–associated vasculitis

(C) Acute tubular necrosis

(D) Acute interstitial nephritis

(E) Membranous glomerulopathy

Item 16

A 65-year-old man is evaluated for hypoalbuminemia, hyperlipidemia, and slowly progressive proteinuria that have developed over 1 year. One year ago, he underwent squamous cell lung cancer resection.

On physical examination, blood pressure is 150/90 mm Hg. Cardiac examination reveals a normal S1 and S2 without rubs or gallops. Pulmonary examination shows decreased breath sounds in the right lower lobe consistent with his previous surgery. Abdominal examination is normal. There is 3+ edema of the lower extremities.

Laboratory studies:

Blood urea nitrogen	17 mg/dL (6.07 mmol/L)
Creatinine	1.0 mg/dL (88.42 µmol/L)
Urinalysis	Specific gravity 1.020, numerous granular casts and oval fat bodies/hpf
24-Hour urinary protein excretion	15 g/24 h

Chest radiograph reveals a new 1-cm nodule in the left upper lobe.

Which of the following is the most likely cause of this patient's renal symptoms?

(A) Minimal change glomerulopathy

(B) Focal segmental glomerulosclerosis

(C) Membranous nephropathy

(D) IgA glomerulonephritis

(E) Antineutrophil cytoplasmic autoantibody–associated vasculitis

Item 17

A 62-year-old man with chronic kidney disease, long-standing type 2 diabetes mellitus, and hypertension is hospitalized for a 2-week history of progressive leg edema and dyspnea on exertion. Two weeks ago, he came to the emergency department for left shoulder pain and began therapy with propoxyphene and ibuprofen; his other medications are aspirin, simvastatin, pioglitazone, glipizide, atenolol, furosemide, clopidogrel, glargine insulin, metolazone, and omeprazole.

On admission, his creatinine level is 3.0 mg/dL (265.26 µmol/L); 2 months ago, this value was 1.6 mg/dL (141.47 µmol/L). A urinary bladder catheter is placed and initially yields 120 mL of blood-tinged urine; his urine output on the first day of admission is 1200 mL. Intravenous furosemide therapy is initiated.

On physical examination, he is afebrile, pulse rate is 54/min, respiratory rate is 18/min, and blood pressure is 110/46 mm Hg. Funduscopic examination shows proliferative changes and microaneurysms. The jugular venous pressure is 8 cm H_2O. On cardiac examination, an S4 gallop is present. Pulmonary examination reveals bibasilar crackles. There is 1+ leg edema bilaterally.

Laboratory studies 1 day later:

Hemoglobin	7.6 g/dL (76 × 10^9/L)
Leukocyte count	2100/µL (12.1 × 10^9/L)
Platelet count	476,000/µL (476 × 10^9/L)
Blood urea nitrogen	96 mg/dL (34.28 mmol/L)
Creatinine	5.0 mg/dL (442.1 µmol/L)
Sodium	140 meq/L (140 mmol/L)
Potassium	5.3 meq/L (5.3 mmol/L)
Chloride	100 meq/L (100 mmol/L)
Bicarbonate	17 meq/L (17 mmol/L)
Total protein	7.1 g/dL (71 g/L)
Albumin	3.5 g/dL (35 g/L)
Calcium	8.6 mg/dL (2.15 mmol/L)
Phosphorus	6 mg/dL (1.94 mmol/L)
Urinalysis	Specific gravity 1.010, trace leukocyte esterase, 1+ protein, trace blood, leukocyte casts
Urine sodium	20 meq/L (20 mmol/L)
Urine creatinine	100 mg/dL (8842 µmol/L)

Renal ultrasonography reveals that both kidneys are 11.6 cm in length. There is no hydronephrosis, perinephric fluid collection, or nephrolithiasis.

Which of the following is the most appropriate next step in this patient's management?

(A) Initiate ciprofloxacin

(B) Perform renal biopsy

(C) Discontinue ibuprofen

(D) Initiate dialysis

(E) Initiate prednisone

Item 18

A 49-year-old man with a history of gouty arthritis comes for a follow-up evaluation. One week ago, he was evaluated in the emergency department for left-sided flank pain and hematuria.

A plain abdominal radiograph is unremarkable. After radiography is performed, the patient urinates debris and his pain is immediately relieved.

Laboratory studies obtained in the emergency department:

Blood urea nitrogen	12 mg/dL (4.29 mmol/L)
Uric acid	9.0 mg/dL (0.54 mmol/L)
Creatinine	1.0 mg/dL (88.42 µmol/L)
Sodium	138 meq/L (138 mmol/L)
Potassium	4.6 meq/L (4.6 mmol/L)
Bicarbonate	26 meq/L (26 mmol/L)
Albumin	4.0 mg/dL (40 g/L)
Calcium	10.1 mg/dL (2.52 mmol/L)
Phosphorus	2.1 mg/dL (0.68 mmol/L)
Urinalysis	pH 5, 3+ blood, 10–15 erythrocytes/hpf

He has had no further symptoms.

Which of the following is the most likely diagnosis?

(A) Calcium oxalate stones
(B) Uric acid stones
(C) Calcium phosphorous stones
(D) Struvite calculi
(E) Cystine stones

Item 19

A 50-year-old woman with type 2 diabetes mellitus and progressive chronic kidney disease comes for a follow-up visit. She has had leg swelling but does not have nausea, vomiting, chest pain, shortness of breath, orthopnea, paroxysmal nocturnal dyspnea, or dysuria. She follows a 0.8 mg/kg/d dietary protein restriction and takes lisinopril, 80 mg/d.

On physical examination, blood pressure is 130/70 mm Hg. There are retinal microaneurysms. Cardiac examination reveals a regular sinus rhythm with an S4 and a grade 2/6 systolic murmur at the base. The lungs are clear to auscultation. There is jugular vein distension. The abdomen is large with normal bowel sounds. There is no pedal edema. Pinprick and vibratory sensation are absent in both feet.

Laboratory studies:

Hematocrit	35%
Hemoglobin	11 g/dL (110 g/L)
Iron	45 µg/dL (8.06 µmol/L)

Ferritin	<12 ng/mL
Iron-binding capacity	290 µg/dL (51.91 µmol/L)
Creatinine	2.0 mg/dL (176.84 µmol/L)
Sodium	138 meq/L (138 mmol/L)
Potassium	5.0 meq/L (5 mmol/L)
Chloride	106 meq/L (106 mmol/L)
Bicarbonate	22 meq/L (22 mmol/L)
Albumin	3.5 g/dL (35 g/L)
24-Hour urinary protein excretion	3 g/24 h

An electrocardiogram is normal.

Which of the following is the most appropriate next step in this patient's management?

(A) Refer for permanent vascular access
(B) Restrict protein intake to 0.6 g/kg/d
(C) Start erythropoietin treatment
(D) Add diltiazem, 120 mg/d

Item 20

An 85-year-old woman is evaluated for resistant hypertension. She has a longstanding history of hypertension that had been well controlled with β-blocker therapy. Her physician recently passed away, and results of blood pressure measurement performed in the office by her new physician have been high. Records from her previous physician show that office blood pressure measurements were always normal. She also has fatigue, weakness, and dizziness, particularly after standing up. She has been unable to tolerate angiotensin-converting enzyme inhibitor, angiotensin receptor blocker, and dihydropyridine calcium antagonist therapy. Current medications are metoprolol, 50 mg/d, and hydrochlorothiazide, 25 mg/d.

On physical examination, pulse rate is 60/min and blood pressure in the supine and standing positions is 170/70 mm Hg. The remainder of the examination is normal.

Laboratory studies:

Glucose	78 mg/dL (4.33 mmol/L)
Blood urea nitrogen	18 mg/dL (6.43 mmol/L)
Creatinine	0.8 mg/dL (70.74 µmol/L)
Sodium	136 meq/L (136 mmol/L)
Potassium	3.6 meq/L (3.6 mmol/L)
Bicarbonate	26 meq/L (26 mmol/L)

Which of the following is the most appropriate next step in this patient's management?

(A) Perform a magnetic resonance angiography of the renal arteries

(B) Increase the hydrochlorothiazide to 50 mg/d

(C) Discontinue metoprolol

(D) Perform ambulatory blood pressure monitoring

Item 21

A 25-year-old woman who is a new patient is evaluated for elevated blood pressure. She is 14 weeks pregnant, and this is her first pregnancy. She has a family history of hypertension and type 2 diabetes mellitus.

On physical examination, blood pressure is 150/90 mm Hg. BMI is 28. The remainder of her examination is unremarkable.

Laboratory studies:

Blood urea nitrogen	16 mg/dL (5.71 mmol/L)
Creatinine	1.5 mg/dL (132.63 µmol/L)
Sodium	136 meq/L (136 mmol/L)
Potassium	3.8 meq/L (3.8 mmol/L)
Chloride	100 meq/L (100 mmol/L)
Bicarbonate	24 meq/L (24 mmol/L)
Urinalysis	2+ protein, no leukocytes or erythrocytes

Which of the following is the most likely diagnosis?

(A) Preeclampsia

(B) Chronic essential hypertension

(C) Chronic glomerulopathy

(D) Gestational hypertension

Item 22

A 56-year-old woman with a history of membranous nephropathy and renal cell carcinoma treated with a right nephrectomy is evaluated for a 2-day history of left-sided flank pain, fever, and gross hematuria. On physical examination, temperature is 38.1 °C (100.5 °F), pulse rate is 96/min, and blood pressure is 170/105 mm Hg. She is in moderate distress from flank pain. Cardiac and pulmonary examinations are unremarkable. There is left costovertebral angle tenderness and 2+ leg edema bilaterally.

Laboratory studies 6 weeks ago:

Creatinine	1.3 mg/dL (114.95 µmol/L)
24-Hour urine protein	6 g/24 h
Creatinine clearance	68 mL/min

Laboratory studies today:

Hemoglobin	11.5 g/dL (7.14 mmol/L)
Leukocyte count	11,500/µL (11.5 × 10⁹/L)
Platelet count	156,000/µL (156 × 10⁹/L)
Creatinine	2.5 mg/dL (221.05 µmol/L)
Sodium	132 meq/L (132 mmol/L)
Potassium	5.6 meq/L (5.6 mmol/L)
Chloride	106 meq/L (106 mmol/L)
Bicarbonate	18 meq/L (18 mmol/L)
Lactate dehydrogenase	765 U/L (12.75 ukat/L)
Urinalysis	2+ blood, 2+ protein, isomorphic erythrocytes too numerous to count

Renal ultrasound shows no hydronephrosis.

Which of the following studies is most likely to establish a definitive diagnosis?

(A) Fractional excretion of sodium

(B) Renal arteriography

(C) Renal biopsy

(D) Abdominal magnetic resonance venography

Item 23

A 54-year-old woman comes for a follow-up examination. She was discharged from the hospital 7 days ago after hospitalization for severe shortness of breath. During her hospitalization, a large pleural effusion was found and pleurodesis was performed. At today's visit, she feels tired. She has not had nausea, headache, or irritability and has not vomited. She was diagnosed with metastatic small-cell lung carcinoma 13 months ago and was treated with palliative chemotherapy with a good response. Previous surgeries include two cesarean sections. She also has a 75-pack-year history of cigarette smoking.

On physical examination, her temperature is 36.8 °C (98.2 °F), pulse rate is 84/min, respiratory rate is 18/min, and blood pressure is 126/84 mm Hg. She appears cachectic. Cardiac examination is normal. On pulmonary examination, there are diminished breath sounds in the right base and the left side is clear to auscultation. There is no pedal edema.

Laboratory studies:

Glucose	114 mg/dL (6.33 mmol/L)
Blood urea nitrogen	10 mg/dL (3.57 mmol/L)

Creatinine	0.6 mg/dL (53.05 µmol/L)
Sodium	112 meq/L (112 mmol/L)
Potassium	3.2 meq/L (3.2 mmol/L)
Chloride	84 meq/L (84 mmol/L)
Bicarbonate	21 meq/L (21 mmol/L)
Phosphorus	3.1 mg/dL (1 mmol/L)
Albumin	3.2 g/dL (32 g/L)
Serum osmolality	243 mosm/kg H_2O (243 mmol/kg)
Urine sodium	120 meq/L (120 mmol/L)
Urine potassium	24 meq/L (24 mmol/L)
Urine osmolality	542 mosm/kg H_2O (542 mmol/kg)

Which of the following is the most appropriate therapy at this time?

(A) 3% saline via infusion pump
(B) Demeclocycline
(C) Fluid restriction <1 L/d
(D) Sodium chloride tablets, 2 g three times daily
(E) Hydrochlorothiazide

Item 24

A 34-year-old asymptomatic black man is evaluated for peripheral edema of several months' duration. Medical history is unremarkable.

On physical examination, pulse rate is 79/min and blood pressure is 140/90 mm Hg. He is in excellent health and appears muscular. There is 2+ lower-extremity edema. The remainder of the examination is normal.

Laboratory studies:

Blood urea nitrogen	5.1 mg/dL (1.82 mmol/L)
Creatinine	1.8 mg/dL (159.16 µmol/L)
Albumin	3.0 g/dL (30 g/L)
Urinalysis	3+ proteinuria, several oval fat bodies/hpf
Urinary protein–creatinine ratio	3 mg/g

Which of the following is the most likely diagnosis?

(A) Membranous nephropathy
(B) Focal segmental glomerulosclerosis
(C) Minimal change disease
(D) Membranoproliferative glomerulonephritis
(E) Focal proliferative lupus nephritis

Item 25

A 38-year-old man with advanced AIDS is hospitalized for respiratory distress, fever, and hypoxemia. He is diagnosed with community-acquired pneumonia and initially improves after initiation of levofloxacin therapy. Over the next 2 weeks, his creatinine level progressively increases from 0.8 mg/dL (70.74 µmol/L) to 3.7 mg/dL (327.15 µmol/L). Over the past 3 days, his urine output has decreased to 500 mL/24 h. He has previously been treated for pulmonary tuberculosis and polysubstance abuse.

On physical examination, temperature is 37.8 °C (100.1 °F), pulse rate is 110/min, and blood pressure is 110/60 mm Hg. He is thin and in mild respiratory distress. There are scattered petechiae and ecchymoses across his skin, and he has spontaneous gingival bleeding. Pulmonary examination reveals crackles at the right base. The point of maximal impulse is laterally displaced. The abdomen is soft without organomegaly. There is no edema. On neurologic examination, he is lethargic and able to answer only simple questions.

Laboratory studies:

Hemoglobin	7.6 g/dL (76 g/L)
Leukocyte count	9400/µL (9.4 × 10^9/L)
Platelet count	18,000/µL (18 × 10^9/L)
Blood urea nitrogen	75 mg/dL (26.78 mmol/L)
Creatinine	3.5 mg/dL (309.47 µmol/L)
Sodium	129 meq/L (129 mmol/L)
Potassium	3.2 meq/L (3.2 mmol/L)
Chloride	88 meq/L (88 mmol/L)
Bicarbonate	30 meq/L (30 mmol/L)
Lactate dehydrogenase	7483 U/L (124.74 µkat/L)
Urinalysis	1+ leukocyte esterase, 1+ protein, trace blood, 5–10 dysmorphic erythrocytes/hpf

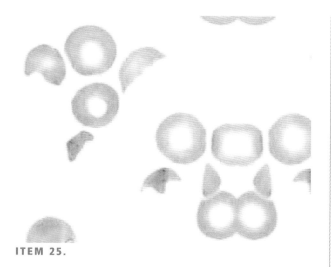

ITEM 25.

A peripheral blood smear is shown (Figure).

Which of the following is the most appropriate next step in this patient's management?

(A) Cryoprecipitate infusions
(B) Renal biopsy
(C) Plasmapheresis and antiretroviral therapy
(D) Oral corticosteroids

Item 26

A 71-year-old man is hospitalized after a seizure that developed after 1 week of intermittent fevers and headaches. He underwent deceased donor kidney transplantation 7 years ago. Medications are cyclosporine, mycophenolate mofetil, prednisone, simvastatin, aspirin, metoprolol, and enalapril.

On physical examination, temperature is 38.3 °C (100.9 °F). There is no papilledema. The neck is rigid. On neurologic examination, the patient is obtunded and able to move all extremities.

Cerebrospinal fluid examination shows the following:

Cell count	45 total nucleated cells/μL (75% neutrophils)
Protein	81 mg/dL (810 g/L)
Glucose	55 mg/dL (3.05 mmol/L)
Gram stain	Many polymorphonuclear leukocytes and gram-positive bacilli

CT of the brain is unremarkable.

Which of the following is the most appropriate therapy for this patient?

(A) Vancomycin and ceftriaxone
(B) Vancomycin and gentamicin
(C) Ampicillin and gentamicin
(D) Ceftriaxone

Item 27

A 25-year-old man with a history of active Crohn's disease with several small-bowel resections is evaluated for recurrent calcium oxalate kidney stones. He typically passes three to four stones each year and he becomes incapacitated during acute attacks. He requests further therapy for stone prevention.

A plain abdominal radiograph is obtained in the office and reveals no calcifications in the genitourinary tract.

Laboratory studies:

Uric acid	6.8 mg/dL (0.4 mmol/L)
Blood urea nitrogen	10 mg/dL (3.57 mmol/L)
Creatinine	0.8 mg/dL (70.74 μmol/L)
Sodium	139 meq/L (139 mmol/L)
Potassium	4.3 meq/L (4.3 mmol/L)
Bicarbonate	25 meq/L (25 mmol/L)
Calcium	9.9 mg/dL (2.47 mmol/L)
Phosphorus	2.2 mg/dL (0.71 mmol/L)
Urinalysis	pH 5.0, no blood or protein

In addition to increasing fluid intake, which of the following recommendations is warranted?

(A) Calcium intake >1 g/d
(B) A high-sodium diet
(C) A high-protein diet
(D) Furosemide, 40 mg/d

Item 28

A 64-year-old man is admitted to the intensive care unit with pneumonia and septic shock. Over the past 4 days, he has had increasing shortness of breath and fever. He has hypertension. Surgical history is significant for a previous cholecystectomy. Medications are amlodipine and hydrochlorothiazide.

On physical examination, temperature is 38.8 °C (98.8 °F), pulse rate is 110/min, respiratory rate is 22/min, and blood pressure is 85/50 mm Hg. Cardiac examination reveals a grade 2/6 systolic murmur. On pulmonary examination, there are crackles over the entire right lung field. There is trace pedal edema.

Laboratory studies on admission:

Glucose	115 mg/dL (6.38 mmol/L)
Blood urea nitrogen	22 mg/dL (7.86 mmol/L)
Creatinine	1.4 mg/dL (123.79 μmol/L)

Sodium	135 meq/L (135 mmol/L)
Potassium	4.8 meq/L (4.8 mmol/L)
Chloride	103 meq/L (103 mmol/L)
Bicarbonate	10 meq/L (10 mmol/L)
Albumin	3.8 g/dL (38 g/L)

Arterial blood gas studies (with the patient breathing room air):

pH	6.94
P_{CO_2}	48 mm Hg
P_{O_2}	51 mm Hg

Which of the following conditions is most likely present in this patient?

(A) Anion gap metabolic acidosis
(B) Mixed non–anion gap metabolic acidosis and respiratory acidosis
(C) Mixed anion gap metabolic acidosis and respiratory alkalosis
(D) Mixed anion gap metabolic acidosis and respiratory acidosis
(E) Mixed non–anion gap metabolic acidosis and respiratory alkalosis

Item 29

A 53-year-old man with stage 4 chronic kidney disease secondary to type 1 diabetes mellitus comes for a follow-up visit. He underwent coronary bypass surgery 2 years earlier. Physical examination is normal except for the presence of diabetic retinopathy. His estimated glomerular filtration rate is 25 mL/min/1.73 m^2.

Which of the following treatment options is associated with the best chance of survival and highest quality of life in this clinical scenario?

(A) Peritoneal dialysis
(B) Clinic hemodialysis
(C) Renal transplantation
(D) Home hemodialysis

Item 30

A 65-year-old woman is evaluated for resistant hypertension. Despite use of antihypertensive therapy for over 20 years, her blood pressure usually is approximately 160/90 mm Hg. For several years she has been taking amlodipine, 10 mg/d, and metoprolol, 100 mg/d. However, her regimen recently was changed to lisinopril, 20 mg/d, and sustained-release verapamil, 180 mg/d.

On physical examination, pulse rate is 68/min and blood pressure is 178/100 mm Hg. On cardiac examination, the point of maximal impulse is prominent and dis-

placed laterally. The lungs are clear to auscultation. The remainder of the examination is normal.

Laboratory studies:

Blood urea nitrogen	18 mg/dL (6.43 mmol/L)
Creatinine	0.9 mg/dL (79.58 μmol/L)
Sodium	147 meq/L (147 mmol/L)
Potassium	3.3 meq/L (3.3 mmol/L)
Chloride	100 meq/L (100 mmol/L)
Bicarbonate	28 meq/L (28 mmol/L)

An echocardiogram reveals increased left ventricular mass.

Which of the following is the most appropriate next step in this patient's management?

(A) Magnetic resonance angiography
(B) Hydrochlorothiazide, 25 mg/d
(C) Aldosterone–renin ratio
(D) CT scanning

Item 31

A 58-year-old man is brought to the emergency department after he was unable to arise from a chair due to muscle pain and weakness, which he has had for 2 to 3 weeks. He was recently diagnosed with high cholesterol and began therapy with simvastatin, 20 mg/d. He takes no other medications and does not use illicit drugs.

On physical examination, temperature is 37.3 °C (99.2 °F), pulse rate is 105/min, and blood pressure is 178/98 mm Hg. Fundoscopic examination shows no retinal hemorrhages or papilledema. Cardiac examination reveals a grade 2/6 systolic ejection murmur. There is bilateral lower-extremity proximal muscle weakness.

Laboratory studies:

Hemoglobin	11.8 g/dL (118 g/L)
Leukocyte count	9100/μL (9.1 × 10^9/L)
Blood urea nitrogen	38 mg/dL (13.57 mmol/L)
Creatinine	2.6 mg/dL (229.89 mmol/L)
Sodium	132 meq/L (132 mmol/L)
Potassium	5.6 meq/L (5.6 mmol/L)
Bicarbonate	18 meq/L (18 mmol/L)

Calcium	8.8 mg/dL (2.2 mmol/L)
Phosphorus	8.0 mg/dL (2.58 mmol/L)
Urinalysis	pH 5.5, specific gravity 1.015, 3+ blood, trace protein, occasional hyaline casts/hpf

Renal ultrasound shows normal-sized kidneys and no hydronephrosis.

Which of the following is the most likely cause of this patient's kidney failure?

(A) Acute glomerulonephritis
(B) Hypertensive nephrosclerosis
(C) Acute rhabdomyolysis
(D) Acute interstitial nephritis

Item 32

A 66-year-old woman is evaluated 5 days after total hip and knee replacement for osteoarthritis. She has a history of type 2 diabetes mellitus, hypertension, and a seizure disorder. She has no known kidney disease. The surgery was uneventful, and her hospital course has been unremarkable. Since the surgery, she has been receiving subcutaneous heparin, 5000 U twice daily; promethazine, 12.5 mg as needed for nausea and vomiting; and meperidine, 25 mg as needed for pain. Outpatient medications are insulin, metformin, atenolol, hydrochlorothiazide, and phenytoin.

Her preoperative chemistry studies were normal.

Laboratory studies:

Glucose	181 mg/dL (10.05 mmol/L)
Blood urea nitrogen	16 mg/dL (5.71 mmol/L)
Creatinine	1.2 mg/dL (106.1 μmol/L)
Sodium	139 meq/L (139 mmol/L)
Potassium	5.6 meq/L (5.6 mmol/L)
Chloride	103 meq/L (103 mmol/L)
Bicarbonate	28 meq/L (28 mmol/L)

Which of the following agents is most likely causing this patient's hyperkalemia?

(A) Metformin
(B) Phenytoin
(C) Heparin
(D) Meperidine
(E) Atenolol

Item 33

A 42-year-old woman is evaluated for minimal edema and a urinary protein excretion of 5 g/24 h. As a child and young adult, she frequently developed urinary tract infections, and she underwent a surgical procedure to reimplant the ureters in order to prevent urinary reflux.

On physical examination, blood pressure is 140/95 mm Hg. There is trace pretibial edema. The remainder of the examination is normal.

Laboratory studies:

Creatinine	1.5 mg/dL (132.63 μmol/L)
Total cholesterol	300 mg/dL (7.76 mmol/L)
Albumin	3.4 g/dL (34 g/L)
Urinalysis	3+ protein, several oval fat bodies/hpf

Chest radiograph is unremarkable. Abdominal ultrasound reveals that the left kidney is normal, but the right kidney is small and difficult to visualize.

Which of the following is most likely causing this patient's proteinuria?

(A) Minimal change disease
(B) Membranous nephropathy
(C) Focal segmental glomerulosclerosis
(D) Membranoproliferative glomerulonephritis

Item 34

A 61-year-old woman is hospitalized for a 5-day history of nausea and vomiting and a 2-day history of postural lightheadedness. Her creatinine level is 7 mg/dL (618.94 μmol/L) (baseline creatinine 1 month ago was 1 mg/dL [88.42 μmol/L]). She has a history of hypertension and type 2 diabetes mellitus. Medications include aspirin, atenolol, glipizide, enalapril, and chlorthalidone.

On physical examination, pulse rate is 68/min and blood pressure is 85/60 mm Hg. She is not in distress. Skin turgor is decreased. Cardiac and pulmonary examinations are normal. There is no peripheral edema. On neurologic examination, she is alert and oriented.

Laboratory studies:

Glucose	56 mg/dL (3.11 mmol/L)
Blood urea nitrogen	85 mg/dL (30.35 mmol/L)
Creatinine	8 mg/dL (707.36 μmol/L)
Sodium	120 meq/L (120 mmol/L)
Potassium	3.7 meq/L (3.7 mmol/L)
Chloride	86 meq/L (86 mmol/L)
Bicarbonate	26 meq/L (26 mmol/L)

Urinalysis	Several hyaline casts/hpf
Urine creatinine	40 mg/dL (3536.8 µmol/L)
Urine sodium	40 meq/L (40 mmol/L)

Which of the following is the next best step in this patient's management?

(A) Intravenous sodium chloride (3%), 100 mL
(B) Bolus therapy with 1000 mL of normal saline (0.9%)
(C) Dialysis
(D) Fluid restriction
(E) Dopamine titrated to maintain a mean arterial pressure >60 mm Hg

Item 35

A 75-year-old man with a 6-month history of the nephrotic syndrome is evaluated for the sudden onset of flank pain and hematuria of 18 hours' duration. Three months ago, his creatinine level was 1 mg/dL (88.42 µmol/L) and 24-hour urinary protein excretion was 3 g/24 h. At that time, he began treatment with an angiotensin-converting enzyme inhibitor to decrease his proteinuria. His loop diuretic dose also was increased to treat worsening peripheral edema.

On physical examination, his blood pressure is 170/90 mm Hg with no orthostatic drop. Cardiac examination reveals an S4 and a normal S1 to S2 with a systolic murmur at the base. The lungs are clear to auscultation and percussion. Ophthalmologic examination reveals hypertensive retinopathy. The abdomen is soft with no masses.

Laboratory studies:

Blood urea nitrogen	38 mg/dL (13.57 mmol/L)
Creatinine	2.0 mg/dL (176.84 µmol/L)
Cholesterol	300 mg/dL (7.76 mmol/L)
Urinalysis	5 erythrocytes and numerous oval fat bodies/hpf; no leukocytes
24-Hour urinary protein excretion	15 g/24 h

Which of the following most likely precipitated this patient's renal insufficiency?

(A) Overaggressive diuresis
(B) Renal artery stenosis
(C) Renal vein thrombosis
(D) Kidney stones

Item 36

A 56-year-old woman is evaluated for recurrent urinary tract infections. Three weeks ago, she had a urinary tract infection with *Klebsiella*, and she has had four previous *Proteus* urinary tract infections over the past 6 months.

Physical examination is unremarkable. Urinalysis is significant for leukocyte esterase and 2+ blood, and urine pH is 7.5. Abdominal CT reveals a 5-cm staghorn calculus in the left kidney.

In addition to increasing fluid intake, which of the following is the most appropriate therapy in this setting?

(A) Potassium citrate
(B) Allopurinol
(C) Antibiotics
(D) Low-calcium diet

Item 37

A 49-year-old man with an 8-year history of type 2 diabetes mellitus and hypertension comes for a routine examination. Medications are glyburide, 5 mg twice daily; subcutaneous insulin, 15 U at bedtime; and hydrochlorothiazide, 25 mg/d. On physical examination, blood pressure is 135/75 mm Hg. His hemoglobin A_{1C} level is 6% and creatinine is 0.9 mg/dL (79.58 µmol/L). On urinalysis, there is no microalbuminuria.

Which of the following agents should be added to this patient's regimen?

(A) Verapamil
(B) Terazosin
(C) Nifedipine
(D) Trandolapril

Item 38

A 68-year-old woman with a longstanding history of poorly controlled hypertension is evaluated for primary aldosteronism. On physical examination, blood pressure is 176/105 mm Hg. Cardiac examination reveals an S3 gallop. The lungs are clear to auscultation. Plasma renin activity is 0.06 ng/mL (0.06 µg/L) per hour and 24-hour urine aldosterone excretion is 18 µg (49.93 nmol/d).

An adrenal CT scan reveals a 1.5-cm solitary nodule in the left adrenal gland. The right adrenal gland appears normal but may be slightly enlarged.

Which of the following is the most appropriate next step in this patient's management?

(A) Laparoscopic left adrenalectomy
(B) Adrenal vein sampling for aldosterone and cortisol
(C) Renal arteriography
(D) Dexamethasone suppression test

Item 39

A 34-year-old woman who underwent elective laparoscopic bilateral tubal ligation 1 day ago develops severe headache and nausea the next morning. During the surgery, 5% dextrose in 1/4 strength normal saline therapy is initiated and maintained at 125 mL/h. She remains in recovery until late in the afternoon because she is too sedated to be discharged. Intravenous meperidine is administered with adequate relief of her pain.

Laboratory studies:

Glucose	115 mg/dL (6.38 mmol/L)
Blood urea nitrogen	12 mg/dL (4.29 mmol/L)
Creatinine	1.0 mg/dL (88.42 µmol/L)
Sodium	126 meq/L (126 mmol/L)
Potassium	3.9 meq/L (3.9 mmol/L)
Chloride	96 meq/L (96 mmol/L)
Bicarbonate	22 meq/L (22 mmol/L)

Which of the following is the most appropriate next step in the management of this patient?

(A) Discontinue 5% dextrose in 1/4 strength normal saline; begin 3% saline via infusion pump
(B) Discontinue 5% dextrose in 1/4 strength normal saline; begin intravenous 0.9% saline at 200 mL/h
(C) Emergent CT scan of the head
(D) Administer naloxone
(E) Switch meperidine to fentanyl

Item 40

A 74-year-old woman is evaluated for a 2-month history of dysphonia, anorexia, and dry eyes. She was previously well, uses no medications, and does not use over-the-counter or herbal preparations.

On physical examination, temperature is 37.2 °C (99 °F) and blood pressure is 150/92 mm Hg. There is no rash. The mucous membranes of the oropharynx are dry but without ulcers. Cardiac and pulmonary examinations are normal. There is no peripheral edema.

Laboratory studies:

Hemoglobin	10 g/dL (100 g/L)
Leukocyte count	6900/µL (6.9 × 10^9/L)
Platelet count	204,000/µL (204 × 10^9/L)
Glucose	80 mg/dL (4.44 mmol/L)
Blood urea nitrogen	22 mg/dL (7.86 mmol/L)
Creatinine	1.7 mg/dL (150.31 µmol/L) (2 months ago creatinine was 0.7 mg/dL [61.89 mmol/L])
Sodium	141 meq/L (141 mmol/L)

Potassium	4.4 meq/L (4.4 mmol/L)
Chloride	105 meq/L (105 mmol/L)
Bicarbonate	28 meq/L (28 mmol/L)
Albumin	3.5 g/dL (35 g/L)
Total protein	9.6 g/dL (96 g/L)
C3	Normal
C4	Normal
Urinalysis	pH 6.5, specific gravity 1.009, trace protein, 5–8 leukocytes/hpf, occasional leukocyte casts

Which of the following is the most likely diagnosis?

(A) Systemic lupus erythematosus
(B) Scleroderma
(C) Sjögren's syndrome
(D) Myeloma cast nephropathy

Item 41

A 29-year-old black man with HIV infection comes for a routine examination. He has a history of numerous opportunistic infections and was recently treated with a course of intravenous acyclovir. He also is positive for the hepatitis C antibody.

On physical examination, there is 2+ pitting edema to the knees. The remainder of the examination is normal.

Laboratory studies:

Blood urea nitrogen	30 mg/dL (10.71 mmol/L)
Creatinine	1.8 mg/dL (159.16 µmol/L) (6 months ago, creatinine was 0.9 mg/dL [79.58 µmol/L])
Albumin	2.8 g/dL (28 g/L)
Urinalysis	No hematuria, 4+ proteinuria, abundant oval fat bodies in microscopic examination, no other formed cellular elements, no glycosuria, no amino aciduria, no granular casts
C3	110 mg/dL (1100 mg/L)
C4	35 mg/dL (350 mg/L)
CD4 cell count	180 cells/µL (0.18 × 10^9/L)

HIV RNA viral load   5000 copies/mL

Renal ultrasound reveals echogenic kidneys.

Which of the following is the most likely cause of this patient's renal dysfunction?

(A) Trimethoprim–sulfamethoxazole
(B) Pentamidine
(C) Collapsing focal segmental glomerulosclerosis
(D) Postinfectious membranoproliferative glomerulonephritis

Item 42

A 43-year-old woman with advanced cirrhosis secondary to hepatitis C is hospitalized for tense ascites and leg edema. She undergoes therapeutic paracentesis with removal of 4 L of ascitic fluid and begins treatment with intravenous furosemide, 40 mg three times daily. Her usual dose of spironolactone is continued.

Over the next 3 days, she has a net diuresis of 3 kg during which the creatinine level increases from a baseline level of 0.8 mg/dL (70.74 µmol/L) to 1.6 mg/dL (141.47 µmol/L). Her urine output decreases to 480 mL/24 h.

On physical examination, blood pressure is 96/40 mm Hg. There is scleral icterus. Pulmonary examination reveals decreased breath sounds at lung bases. She has modest ascites and no edema.

Laboratory studies:

INR	2.2
Prothrombin time	27.8 s
Blood urea nitrogen	20 mg/dL (7.14 mmol/L)
Creatinine	1.6 mg/dL (141.47 µmol/L)
Sodium	117 meq/L (117 mmol/L)
Potassium	3.6 meq/L (3.6 mmol/L)
Chloride	80 meq/L (80 mmol/L)
Bicarbonate	28 meq/L (28 mmol/L)
Total bilirubin	21 mg/dL (359.1 µmol/L)
Albumin	2.3 g/dL (23 g/L)
Urinalysis	Several granular and epithelial casts/hpf
Urine sodium	12 meq/L (12 mmol/L)

In addition to discontinuing spironolactone and furosemide, which of the following is the most appropriate next step in this patient's management?

(A) Initiate octreotide and midodrine
(B) Place a transjugular intrahepatic portosystemic shunt

(C) Repeat large-volume paracentesis
(D) Infuse 1.5 L of normal saline over the next 24 hours

Item 43

An 86-year-old woman with a history of type 2 diabetes mellitus and chronic kidney disease is brought to the emergency department for shortness of breath. She has a history of advanced multi-infarct dementia, left parietal stroke, and ischemic cardiomyopathy with an estimated ejection fraction of 20%. She has resided in a nursing home for 2 years after falling several times at home and sustaining a right hip fracture. Since that time, her functional status has declined and she has been confined to bed. A stage II sacral decubitus ulcer has developed. Her family notes that her appetite has declined over the past 2 months.

On physical examination, respiratory rate is 26/min and blood pressure is 180/70 mm Hg. BMI is 17. On cardiac examination, a grade 2/6 holosystolic murmur is present and is heard best at the apex. Jugular venous pressure is 10 cm H_2O. There are crackles halfway up both lung fields posteriorly. There is 2+ edema.

Laboratory studies:

Hemoglobin	9.6 g/dL (96 g/L)
Leukocyte count	5600/µL (5.6 × 10^9/L)
Platelet count	343,000/µL (343 × 10^9/L)
Blood urea nitrogen	50 mg/dL (17.85 mmol/L)
Creatinine	5.2 mg/dL (459.78 µmol/L)
Sodium	130 meq/L (130 mmol/L)
Potassium	6.3 meq/L (6.3 mmol/L)
Chloride	107 meq/L (107 mmol/L)
Bicarbonate	16 meq/L (16 mmol/L)
Calcium	7.4 mg/dL (1.85 mmol/L)
Phosphorus	6.7 mg/dL (2.16 mmol/L)
Urinalysis	pH 5.3, specific gravity 1.011, 3+ protein, trace hemoglobin, broad waxy casts

Renal ultrasound shows echogenic kidneys measuring 10 cm with thin cortices.

Which of the following is the most appropriate treatment for this patient?

(A) Hemodialysis
(B) Peritoneal dialysis

(C) Low-protein diet

(D) Palliative care

Item 44

A 44-year-old man with a history of nephrolithiasis requests nonpharmaceutical interventions for stone prevention. His last symptomatic kidney stone was 2 years ago. He does not recall the exact type of stone that he formed but believes that it contained calcium. Previous laboratory studies have showed normal renal function and normal levels of calcium, phosphorus, and uric acid. A plain abdominal radiograph performed 1 year ago revealed no genitourinary calcifications. He does not have a family history of nephrolithiasis but wishes to reduce his chances of developing further kidney stones.

In addition to increasing fluid intake to >2 L/d, which of the following is the best initial therapy for this patient?

(A) Increase dietary calcium intake

(B) Decrease dietary sources of citrate

(C) Increase dietary animal protein intake

(D) Increase dietary sodium intake

Item 45

A 35-year-old woman who is pregnant with her third child is evaluated for right upper quadrant abdominal pain. She has no significant medical history. Her father died of cerebral aneurysm. She takes no medication.

On physical examination, temperature is normal, pulse rate is 88/min, and blood pressure is 140/90 mm Hg. Cardiac and pulmonary examinations are normal. Abdominal examination is unremarkable. There is no edema. Creatinine level is 0.8 mg/dL (70.74 µmol/L).

On abdominal ultrasound, the right kidney is 14 cm and the left kidney is 13 cm. There are multiple cysts in both kidneys and the liver. No hydronephrosis, solid masses, or stones are present.

Which of the following is the most likely diagnosis in this patient?

(A) Autosomal recessive polycystic kidney disease

(B) Acquired cystic kidney disease

(C) Autosomal dominant polycystic kidney disease

(D) Nephronophthisis

Item 46

A 38-year-old man recently diagnosed with pheochromocytoma comes to the office for medical evaluation in anticipation of surgery. On physical examination, his blood pressure is 190/105 mm Hg. The remainder of the examination is unremarkable.

Therapy with which of the following is indicated in preparation for surgery in this patient?

(A) A calcium-channel blocker

(B) Phenoxybenzamine

(C) Labetalol

(D) Atenolol

(E) Hydrochlorothiazide

Item 47

A 44-year-old woman comes for a routine examination. She has a history of antineutrophil cytoplasmic antibody–associated small-vessel vasculitis, sinusitis, nasal crusting, purpuric vasculitic rash, pulmonary nodules, and a pauci-immune necrotizing and crescentic glomerulonephritis. She is currently in remission and feels well. Medications are maintenance prednisone and azathioprine. She asks about discontinuing immunosuppressive therapy. Physical examination is unremarkable except for evidence of nasal scarring.

Laboratory studies:

Hemoglobin	12.9 g/dL (129 g/L)
Leukocyte count	5700/µL (5.7 × 10^9/L)
Platelet count	315,000/µL (315 × 10^9/L)
Creatinine	1.5 mg/dL (132.63 µmol/L)
Proteinase-3 antinuclear antibodies	Titer of 70 (upper limits of normal <20 IU)
Urinalysis	No hematuria or proteinuria

Chest CT is unremarkable.

Which of the following factors best predicts a relapse of this patient's condition if present at the time of diagnosis?

(A) Respiratory and renal dysfunction

(B) Lower and upper respiratory tract disease and proteinase-3 antinuclear cytoplasmic antibody positivity

(C) Renal dysfunction and proteinase-3 antinuclear cytoplasmic antibody positivity

(D) Upper respiratory tract and skin vasculitis

(E) Renal dysfunction; ear, nose and throat disease; and skin disease

Item 48

A 73-year-old woman is brought to the emergency department after falling at home. Her family states that she has been very confused and disoriented over the past 2 days and that she began therapy with a new medication 1 week ago. She also has type 2 diabetes mellitus.

On physical examination, temperature is 37 °C (98.6 °F), pulse rate is 68/min, respiratory rate is 12/min, and blood pressure is 115/65 mm Hg. She is confused and unable to appropriately answer questions. Cardiac examination is normal. The lungs are clear to auscultation. There is no edema.

Laboratory studies:

Glucose	94 mg/dL (5.22 mmol/L)
Blood urea nitrogen	17 mg/dL (6.07 mmol/L)
Creatinine	1.1 mg/dL (97.26 μmol/L)
Sodium	107 meq/L (107 mmol/L)
Potassium	2.9 meq/L (2.9 mmol/L)
Chloride	76 meq/L (76 mmol/L)
Bicarbonate	21 meq/L (21 mmol/L)

Therapy with which of the following agents was most likely recently started in this patient?

(A) Furosemide
(B) Acetazolamide
(C) Spironolactone
(D) Hydrochlorothiazide
(E) Amiloride

Item 49

A 42-year-old man is evaluated for a 2-month history of rash on his lower extremities and a 6-month history of cold-induced acral cyanosis and discomfort. He also has a 2-month history of alcohol abuse.

On physical examination, pulse rate is 78/min and blood pressure is 150/90 mm Hg. Cardiac and pulmonary examinations are unremarkable. On abdominal examination, the liver is 3 cm below the right costal margin. A spleen tip is not felt. There is 1+ lower-extremity edema. A purpuric rash also is present on the lower extremities.

Laboratory studies:

Hemoglobin	11.4 g/dL (114 g/L)
Platelet count	120,000/μL (120 × 10⁹/L)
Creatinine	1.7 mg/dL (150.31 μmol/L)
C3	86 mg/dL (860 mg/L)
C4	5 mg/dL (50 mg/L)
Aspartate aminotransferase	57 U/L
Alanine aminotransferase	75 U/L
Urinalysis	3+ hematuria, 1+ protein, 7–10 dysmorphic erythrocytes/hpf

Which of the following is most likely causing this patient's renal abnormalities?

(A) Systemic lupus erythematosus glomerulonephritis
(B) Henoch–Schönlein purpura glomerulonephritis
(C) Cryoglobulinemic glomerulonephritis
(D) Antineutrophil cytoplasmic antibody–associated small-vessel vasculitis
(E) Anti–glomerular basement membrane glomerulonephritis

Item 50

A 75-year-old woman is hospitalized for blood-streaked sputum, lower-extremity edema, and accelerated hypertension. She has a 3-year history of diet-controlled type 2 diabetes mellitus, atrial fibrillation with pacemaker implantation, hypertension, and osteoporosis. Several weeks ago, she was evaluated in the emergency department after developing an acute onset of lower back pain after a fall. She was diagnosed with three lumbar vertebral compression fractures and was treated symptomatically with oxycodone three times daily.

On physical examination, she is afebrile, pulse rate is 60/min, respiratory rate is 25/min, and blood pressure is 138/76 mm Hg. Cardiac examination reveals a grade 2/6 systolic murmur at the lower left sternal border and no gallops. There is no jugular venous distention. Pulmonary examination reveals bibasilar crackles. The point of maximal impulse is not displaced. There is 4+ edema in the bilateral lower extremities.

Laboratory studies:

Leukocyte count	6600/μL (6.6 × 10⁹/L)
Hemoglobin	12.2 g/dL (122 g/L)
Hematocrit	37.6
Platelet count	294,000/μL (294 × 10⁹/L)
Blood urea nitrogen	21 mg/dL (7.5 mmol/L)
Creatinine	1.7 mg/dL (150.31 μmol/L)
Sodium	134 meq/L (134 mmol/L)
Potassium	3.6 meq/L (3.6 mmol/L)
Chloride	100 meq/L (100 mmol/L)
Bicarbonate	26 meq/L (26 mmol/L)
Albumin	3.2 mg/dL (32 g/L)
Urinalysis	pH 5.0, specific gravity 1.015, 1+ blood, 4+ protein, 5–10 erythrocytes and several erythrocyte casts/hpf

Urinary protein–creatinine ratio	3.5 mg/g

Renal ultrasound reveals small bilateral 1-cm simple cysts, normal-sized kidneys, and no hydronephrosis. Chest radiograph shows bilateral infiltrates and a normal cardiac silhouette.

Which of the following is the most appropriate next step in the management of this patient's kidney disease?

(A) Echocardiography
(B) Kidney biopsy
(C) Corticosteroids
(D) Antibiotics

Item 51

A 66-year-old man with a history of coronary artery disease and hypertension is evaluated for abdominal pain, low-grade fever, myalgias, nausea, and generalized weakness. His creatinine level is 6 mg/dL (530.52 µmol/L) (baseline creatinine is 1.4 mg/dL [123.79 µmol/L]). Two weeks ago, he was hospitalized for anginal chest pain. Cardiac catheterization at that time showed a 30% left anterior descending artery stenosis and a 90% right coronary artery lesion. A right coronary artery stent was placed.

On physical examination today, temperature is 37.8 °C (100.1 °F) and blood pressure is 140/96 mm Hg. On cardiac examination, a right carotid bruit and S4 gallop are present. On pulmonary examination, the lungs are clear to auscultation. Findings of funduscopic examination are shown (Figure). Abdominal examination is unremarkable. There is trace pretibial edema bilaterally, and the distal pulses are not palpable. A netlike violaceous rash is visible over the legs, and the right great toe is cool and cyanotic.

Laboratory studies:

Hemoglobin	8.3 g/dL (83 g/L)
Leukocyte count	6700/µL (6.7 × 10^9/L) (67% neutrophils, 22% lymphocytes, 1% monocytes, 8% eosinophils, 2% basophils)
Platelet count	434,000/µL (434 × 10^9/L)
C3	Low
C4	Normal
Urinalysis	1+ blood, 1+ protein, 3–5 leukocytes/hpf, 5–10 erythrocytes/hpf

Which of the following is the most likely diagnosis?

(A) Radiocontrast nephropathy
(B) Prerenal acute renal failure
(C) Acute interstitial nephritis
(D) Microscopic polyangiitis
(E) Atheroembolic disease

Item 52

A 64-year-old woman comes for a follow-up visit after an episode of kidney stones 2 weeks ago. During the episode, she went to the emergency department and was treated with nonsteroidal anti-inflammatory drugs and fluids. Spiral abdominal CT performed at that time revealed a 3-mm nonobstructing calculus in the midleft ureter. She also has osteoporosis.

Laboratory studies:

Blood urea nitrogen	21 mg/dL (7.5 mmol/L)
Uric acid	5.1 mg/dL (0.3 mmol/L)
Creatinine	1.6 mg/dL (141.47 µmol/L)
Sodium	137 meq/L (137 mmol/L)
Potassium	3.8 meq/L (3.8 mmol/L)
Chloride	105 meq/L (105 mmol/L)
Bicarbonate	24 meq/L (24 mmol/L)
Albumin	4.1 mg/dL (41 g/L)
Calcium	11.5 mg/dL (2.87 mmol/L)
Phosphorus	1.2 mg/dL (0.39 mmol/L)
Urinalysis	pH 5.5 , 1+ blood

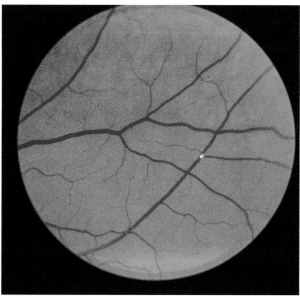

ITEM 51.

Which of the following is the most appropriate management for this patient's kidney stones?

(A) Decrease dietary calcium to <1 g/d
(B) Refer for parathyroidectomy
(C) Refer for stone removal
(D) Initiate potassium citrate therapy
(E) Observe

Item 53

A 30-year-old man is evaluated for hematuria and increasing creatinine levels. He has had persistent hematuria since early childhood but for the past 2 months has noticed gross hematuria. He does not have back pain, fever, or chills. His grandfather was deaf and developed end-stage renal disease at 40 years of age. The patient takes no medication.

On physical examination, temperature is 37.4 °C (99.3 °F), pulse rate is 80/min, and blood pressure is 150/90 mm Hg. The pupils are equal. Cardiac and pulmonary examinations are normal. There is no costovertebral angle tenderness, and no masses are palpable on abdominal examination. There is ankle edema.

Laboratory studies:

Hematocrit	34%
Platelets	110,000/µL (110 x 10^9/L)
Creatinine	2.2 mg/dL (194.52 µmol/L)
Sodium	140 meq/L (140 mmol/L)
Potassium	5 meq/L (5 mmol/L)
Chloride	106 meq/L (106 mmol/L)
Bicarbonate	20 meq/L (20 mmol/L)
C3	120 mg/dL (1200 mg/L)
C4	28 mg/dL (280 mg/L)
Urinalysis	Specific gravity 1.015, 3+ blood, 3+ protein, no acanthocytes or cellular casts

Abdominal ultrasound shows that the right kidney is 9.2 cm and the left kidney is 9 cm. There is cortical thinning and increased echogenicity. No hydronephrosis or stones are present.

Which of the following is the most likely diagnosis?

(A) IgA nephropathy
(B) Thin basement membrane disease
(C) Membranoproliferative glomerulonephritis
(D) Alport's syndrome

Item 54

A 36-year-old man is evaluated in the emergency department after being trapped for 20 hours under a collapsed concrete wall. On physical examination, pulse rate is 100/min and blood pressure is 112/50 mm Hg. On pulmonary examination, breath sounds are equal bilaterally. There are scattered abrasions, and he is conscious. Neurologic examination is normal. He has fractures of the pelvis and ribs and an open fracture of the right femur. He has no evidence of compartment syndrome.

Laboratory studies:

Hemoglobin	12.4 g/dL (7.7 mmol/L)
Leukocyte count	11,000/µL (11 × 10^9/L)
Platelet count	434,000/µL (434 × 10^9/L)
Creatine kinase	86,000 U/L
Blood urea nitrogen	43 mg/dL (15.36 mmol/L)
Creatinine	1.6 mg/dL (141.47 µmol/L)
Sodium	134 meq/L (134 mmol/L)
Potassium	6.2 meq/L (6.2 mmol/L)
Chloride	107 meq/L (107 mmol/L)
Bicarbonate	20 meq/L (20 mmol/L)
Urinalysis	pH 5.7, specific gravity 1.016, trace protein, 3+ hemoglobin, 2–3 erythrocytes/hpf, many hyaline casts/hpf

Which of the following is the most appropriate management for this patient?

(A) Isotonic saline
(B) Dopamine, 2 µg/kg/min to 5 µg/kg/min
(C) Prophylactic fasciotomy
(D) Mannitol
(E) Acetazolamide

Item 55

A 79-year-old man is evaluated for poorly controlled hypertension. He has had hypertension for 30 years, but his condition has become more difficult to control during the past 2 years. Over the last 6 months, his blood pressure measurements have ranged from 150/70 mm Hg to 170/90 mm Hg. Medications are atenolol, 50 mg/d; enalapril, 20 mg twice daily; and hydrochlorothiazide, 25 mg/d.

On physical examination, pulse rate is 66/min and blood pressure is 168/80 mm Hg; these results were the same on two previous office visits. Cardiac examination reveals a faint midline abdominal bruit and a left femoral bruit. Creatinine level is 1.1 mg/dL (97.26 µmol/L), which has not changed for 2 years. Low-density lipoprotein cholesterol level is 160 mg/dL (4.14 mmol/L).

Which of the following is the most appropriate management at this time?

(A) Renal angiography
(B) Amlodipine
(C) Plasma renin activity measurement
(D) Renal vein renin sampling
(E) Magnetic resonance angiography of the renal arteries

Item 56

A 46-year-old man is hospitalized for severe necrotizing pancreatitis. He has a history of alcoholism, hepatitis C, and chronic liver disease. He was given nothing by mouth overnight and received 6 L of normal saline. Twenty-four hours after admission, his abdominal pain worsens and nasogastric suction is initiated. He continues to have nothing by mouth. At this time, his sodium level is 145 meq/L (145 mmol/L).

Over the next 24 hours, his urine output increases and isotonic saline is continued at 100 mL/h. Total parenteral nutrition is initiated with a total volume of 2 L, 120 meq (120 mmol) of sodium, and a high amino acid content. Findings of chemistry and urine studies 48 hours after admission are listed.

Laboratory studies on admission:

Sodium	138 meq/L (138 mmol/L)
Potassium	3.4 meq/L (3.4 mmol/L)
Chloride	103 meq/L (103 mmol/L)
Bicarbonate	22 meq/L (22 mmol/L)
Blood urea nitrogen	25 mg/dL (8.93 mmol/L)
Creatinine	1.4 mg/dL (123.79 µmol/L)
Urine output	45 mL/h

Laboratory studies 48 hours after admission:

Sodium	153 meq/L (153 mmol/L)
Potassium	3.0 meq/L (3.0 mmol/L)
Chloride	112 meq/L (112 mmol/L)
Bicarbonate	24 mmol/L (24 mmol/L)
Blood urea nitrogen	49 mg/dL (17.5 mmol/L)

Creatinine	1.1 mg/dL (97.26 µmol/L)
Urine output	200 mL/h
Urine sodium	50 meq/L (50 mmol/L)
Urine potassium	20 meq/L (50 mmol/L)
Urine osmolality	620 mosm/kg H_2O (620 mmol/kg H_2O)

Which of the following is the most likely cause of this patient's polyuria?

(A) Solute diuresis
(B) Central diabetes insipidus
(C) Nephrogenic diabetes insipidus
(D) Postobstructive diuresis
(E) Urinary tract infection

Item 57

A 72-year-old man with hypertension comes for a follow-up examination. Three repeat urinalyses have shown 1+ to 2+ blood over the past 6 months. He is hesitant to begin further evaluation because he does not feel sick and does not see blood in his urine. He has a 20-year history of cigarette smoking. Medications are hydrochlorothiazide, 25 mg/d, and simvastatin, 20 mg/d.

Renal ultrasound reveals a right kidney 10.5 cm in diameter with a 1-cm simple cyst in the upper pole. The left kidney is 11.1 cm in diameter with a 3.5-cm complex cyst in the lower pole without associated hydronephrosis.

Which of the following is the most appropriate management for this patient?

(A) Repeat renal ultrasonography in 6 months
(B) Reassurance
(C) MRI of the abdomen
(D) Cystoscopy

Item 58

A 75-year-old man is evaluated for a 6-month history of fatigue, malaise, and anorexia. He also has a 2-week history of peripheral edema.

On physical examination, sitting blood pressure is 110/75 mm Hg and standing blood pressure is 90/55 mm Hg with little change in the pulse rate. Cardiac examination reveals a normal S1 and S2, a grade 2/6 systolic murmur at the base without radiation, and a positive S4. The lungs are clear to auscultation. On abdominal examination, the liver spans 12 cm. The spleen is not palpable. There is 2+ peripheral edema of the extremities. The remainder of the examination is unremarkable.

Laboratory studies:

Hemoglobin	12.9 g/dL (129 g/L)

Blood urea nitrogen	25 mg/dL (8.93 mmol/L)
Creatinine	1.3 mg/dL (114.95 µmol/L)
Total cholesterol	300 mg/dL (7.76 mmol/L)
Albumin	3 g/dL (30 g/L)
Urinalysis	No hematuria, several oval fat bodies and fatty casts/hpf
Urinary protein–creatinine ratio	3 mg/g

Chest radiograph reveals normal lung fields and a slightly enlarged heart.

Which of the following is the most likely diagnosis?

(A) Light-chain nephropathy
(B) Focal segmental glomerulosclerosis
(C) Membranoproliferative glomerulonephritis
(D) Membranous nephropathy

Item 59

A 60-year-old man with a 10-year history of hypertension is hospitalized for shortness of breath. Two weeks before admission, he developed headache and dyspnea on exertion. Medications include metoprolol and hydrochlorothiazide.

Physical examination on admission reveals a blood pressure of 180/120 mm Hg. Laboratory studies at that time showed a potassium level of 4.2 meq/L (4.2 mmol/L) and a creatinine level of 1.5 mg/dL (132.63 µmol/L).

Over the next 2 weeks, the blood pressure gradually normalizes after enalapril, 5 mg once daily, and amlodipine, 5 mg once daily, are added to his regimen. On follow-up examination, his blood pressure is 132/76 mm Hg. Funduscopic examination shows arteriolar tortuosity. The point of maximal impulse is laterally displaced. Cardiac examination reveals a right femoral systolic bruit. Distal pulses are 1+ bilaterally, and there is no peripheral edema.

Laboratory studies:

Blood urea nitrogen	45 mg/dL (16.07 mmol/L)
Creatinine	3.5 mg/dL (309.47 µmol/L)
Sodium	140 meq/L (140 mmol/L)
Potassium	5.1 meq/L (5.1 mmol/L)
Chloride	105 meq/L (105 mmol/L)
Bicarbonate	20 meq/L (20 mmol/L)
Urinalysis	Trace protein; several hyaline casts/hpf

Which of the following is the most appropriate initial step in this patient's management?

(A) Perform renal biopsy
(B) Decrease the enalapril dose to 2.5 mg/d
(C) Perform magnetic resonance angiography of the renal arteries
(D) Discontinue enalapril
(E) Switch enalapril to losartan

Item 60

A 41-year-old woman is evaluated for increased fatigue and weakness. Her breathing is more labored when she walks to get her mail at the end of her driveway. She also has increased redness of her eyes and a skin rash over her nose and cheeks. She has a history of osteoarthritis and hypertension. Medications are amlodipine and intermittent acetaminophen.

On physical examination, blood pressure is 135/80. She has perilimbal injection (ciliary flush) and a scaly purplish rash across her nose and cheeks. Cardiac examination reveals a soft holosystolic ejection murmur at the lower left sternal border. There is no jugular venous pressure or gallops. Pulmonary examination is unremarkable. There is no lower-extremity edema.

Laboratory studies:

Hemoglobin	10.5 g/dL (105 g/L)
Blood urea nitrogen	24 mg/dL (8.57 mmol/L)
Creatinine	1.8 mg/dL (159.16 µmol/L)
Sodium	137 meq/L (137 mmol/L)
Potassium	5.1 meq/L (5.1 mmol/L)
Chloride	105 meq/L (105 mmol/L)
Bicarbonate	22 meq/L (22 mmol/L)
Glucose (fasting)	113 mg/dL (6.27 mmol/L)
Albumin	4 mg/dL (40 g/L)
Calcium	11.1 mg/dL (2.77 mmol/L)
Phosphorus	2.4 mg/dL (0.77 mmol/L)
Urinalysis	1+ protein, 1+ blood, 10–15 leukocytes/hpf, 3–5 nondysmorphic erythrocytes/hpf

Results of serum protein electrophoresis are normal. Chest radiograph reveals hilar lymphadenopathy. Renal ultrasound reveals a right kidney 8.9 cm in diameter and a left kidney 9.5 cm in diameter with bilateral increased echogenicity.

Which of the following is the most likely cause of this patient's kidney disease?

(A) Acute glomerulonephritis
(B) Membranous glomerulopathy
(C) Interstitial nephritis
(D) Myeloma kidney

Item 61

A 46-year-old black man is evaluated for hypertension. He was told several years previously at an employee health fair that his blood pressure was elevated. Therapy with an unknown antihypertensive agent was initiated at that time but was discontinued after 3 months because of negative side effects. He has since been checking his blood pressure at local grocery stores; his blood pressure typically is approximately 160/90 mm Hg. He currently takes no medications.

On physical examination, pulse rate is 64/min and resting blood pressure is 158/88 mm Hg. Funduscopic examination reveals hypertensive retinopathy. There is 1+ lower-extremity edema.

Laboratory studies:

Hemoglobin	11.8 g/dL (118 g/L)
Blood urea nitrogen	34 mg/dL (12.14 mmol/L)
Uric acid	8.2 mg/dL (0.49 mmol/L)
Creatinine	1.9 mg/dL (168 µmol/L)
Sodium	142 meq/L (142 mmol/L)
Potassium	3.9 meq/L (3.9 mmol/L)
Chloride	110 meq/L (110 mmol/L)
Bicarbonate	22 meq/L (22 mmol/L)
Calcium	10.1 mg/dL (2.52 mmol/L)
Phosphorus	4.0 mg/dL (1.29 mmol/L)
Urinalysis	2+ protein, no blood

Urinary protein–creatinine ratio 0.45 mg/g

Renal ultrasound reveals a right kidney 9.2 cm in diameter and a left kidney 9.1 cm in diameter with two simple cysts.

Which of the following is the most appropriate treatment of this patient's hypertension?

(A) Ramipril
(B) Metoprolol
(C) Amlodipine
(D) Terazosin

Item 62

A 44-year-old woman with cirrhosis secondary to autoimmune hepatitis is hospitalized for a progressively worsening 2-day history of fever and abdominal pain. She is currently on the orthotopic liver transplantation list and has been clinically stable for the past month. She has previously undergone transjugular intrahepatic portosystemic shunt placement and a cholecystectomy. Medications are oral spironolactone, 100 mg twice daily; furosemide, 80 mg twice daily; and oral lactulose, 30 mL twice daily.

On physical examination, temperature is 38.2 °C (100.8 °F), pulse rate is 72/min, respiratory rate is 24/min, and blood pressure is 74/55 mm Hg. She appears cachectic. Cardiac and pulmonary examinations are normal. The abdomen is distended, and there is diffuse tenderness. There is 1+ pitting edema in the lower extremities. Spontaneous bacterial peritonitis is suspected, and she is admitted to the hospital.

Laboratory studies:

Glucose	84 mg/dL (4.66 mmol/L)
Blood urea nitrogen	20 mg/dL (7.14 mmol/L)
Creatinine	1.3 mg/dL (114.95 µmol/L)
Sodium	128 meq/L (128 mmol/L)
Potassium	5.1 meq/L (5.1 mmol/L)
Chloride	104 meq/L (104 mmol/L)
Bicarbonate	12 meq/L (12 mmol/L)
Albumin	1.4 g/dL (14 g/L)

Arterial blood gas studies (with the patient breathing room air):

pH	7.25
P_{CO_2}	28 mm Hg
P_{O_2}	78 mm Hg

Which of the following is the most likely diagnosis in this clinical scenario?

(A) Mixed anion gap metabolic acidosis and respiratory alkalosis
(B) Mixed anion gap metabolic acidosis and respiratory acidosis
(C) Mixed non–anion gap metabolic acidosis and respiratory acidosis
(D) Anion gap metabolic acidosis
(E) Non–anion gap metabolic acidosis

Item 63

An 83-year-old male nursing home resident with a history of dementia is evaluated in the emergency department for abdominal pain. According to the nursing home staff, he had become increasingly agitated over the past day.

On physical examination, temperature is 36.7 °C (98 °F), pulse rate is 96/min, and blood pressure is 150/92 mm Hg. The patient appears frail and confused and is clutching his abdomen and writhing in pain. He is unable to answer questions. Pulmonary examination reveals crackles at both lung bases. Skin turgor is normal. There is suprapubic tenderness. The prostate is smooth, enlarged, and has an estimated mass of 40 g. There is trace ankle edema bilaterally.

Laboratory studies:

Blood urea nitrogen	63 mg/dL (22.5 mmol/L)
Creatinine	3.6 mg/dL (318.31 µmol/L)
Sodium	137 meq/L (137 mmol/L)
Potassium	6.2 meq/L (6.2 mmol/L)
Chloride	107 meq/L (107 mmol/L)
Bicarbonate	18 meq/L (18 mmol/L)
Urinalysis	Specific gravity 1.014, trace protein, 2–3 leukocytes/hpf, 3–5 erythrocytes/hpf

Which of the following is most likely to establish a diagnosis?

(A) Response to normal saline
(B) Blood urea nitrogen–creatinine ratio
(C) Fractional excretion of sodium
(D) Placement of a urinary bladder catheter

Item 64

A 19-year-old man is evaluated for gross hematuria. Two days ago, he was diagnosed with pharyngitis. A similar episode occurred approximately 1 year ago.

On physical examination, blood pressure is 150/90 mm Hg. The remainder of the examination is normal except for a resolving pharyngitis.

Laboratory studies:

Blood urea nitrogen	14 mg/dL (5 mmol/L)
Creatinine	0.9 mg/dL (79.58 µmol/L)
C3	130 mg/dL (1300 mg/L)
C4	30 mg/dL (300 mg/L)
Urinalysis	No proteinuria, numerous dysmorphic erythrocytes and 1 erythrocyte cast/hpf

Which of the following is the most likely diagnosis?

(A) Systemic lupus erythematosus
(B) Antineutrophil cytoplasmic antibody–associated small-vessel vasculitis
(C) Postinfectious glomerulonephritis
(D) Cryoglobulinemic glomerulonephritis
(E) IgA glomerulonephritis

Item 65

A 21-year-old man is evaluated in the emergency department for severely diminished mental status. He has a 3-day history of nausea and has been unable to eat well. This morning, he vomited several times.

On physical examination, temperature is 37.4 °C (99.3 °F), pulse rate is 105/min, respiratory rate is 28/min, and blood pressure is 122/57 mm Hg. He is thin and appears in moderate distress. Cardiac and pulmonary examinations are normal. The abdomen is soft and nontender. A stool specimen is negative for occult blood.

During the examination, he begins to vomit large amounts, aspirates a significant amount of his stomach contents, and develops respiratory failure. He is intubated and started on mechanical ventilation.

Laboratory studies 1 hour after initiation of mechanical ventilation:

Glucose	980 mg/dL (54.39 mmol/L)
Blood urea nitrogen	11 mg/dL (3.93 mmol/L)
Creatinine	1.7 mg/dL (150.31 µmol/L)
Sodium	138 meq/L (138 mmol/L)
Potassium	3.7 meq/L (3.7 mmol/L)
Chloride	91 meq/L (91 mmol/L)
Bicarbonate	16 meq/L (16 mmol/L)

Arterial blood gas studies (with the patient breathing oxygen):

pH	7.53
P_{CO_2}	19 mm Hg
P_{O_2}	67 mm Hg

Which of the following is the most likely acid–base disturbance present in this patient?

(A) Mixed anion gap metabolic acidosis/non–anion gap metabolic acidosis/respiratory acidosis
(B) Mixed anion gap metabolic acidosis/metabolic alkalosis/respiratory alkalosis
(C) Mixed anion gap metabolic acidosis with respiratory alkalosis
(D) Mixed metabolic alkalosis with respiratory acidosis

Item 66

A 45-year-old woman is evaluated for newly diagnosed hypertension. She has a family history of essential hypertension, and both her parents have type 2 diabetes mellitus.

On physical examination, blood pressure is 150/95 mm Hg. BMI is 32. The remainder of the examination is normal.

Laboratory studies:

Blood urea nitrogen	Normal
Creatinine	Normal
Electrolytes	Normal
Glucose (fasting)	90 mg/dL (5 mmol/L)
Total cholesterol	220 mg/dL (5.69 mmol/L)
High-density lipoprotein cholesterol	35 mg/dL (0.91 mmol/L)
Low-density lipoprotein cholesterol	140 mg/dL (3.62 mmol/L)
Triglycerides (fasting)	250 mg/dL (2.82 mmol/L)

In addition to repeating blood pressure measurement to confirm the diagnosis of hypertension and counseling regarding lifestyle modification, therapy with which of the following agents is indicated for this patient?

(A) Hydrochlorothiazide
(B) Doxazosin
(C) Atenolol
(D) Irbesartan

Item 67

A 42-year-old man is evaluated for intermittent claudication. He has hypertension, type 2 diabetes mellitus, chronic kidney disease, and peripheral arterial disease. Medications are metformin, 1000 mg twice daily; rosiglitazone, 8 mg/d; fosinopril, 80 mg/d; furosemide, 40 mg/d; and atorvastatin, 40 mg/d.

On physical examination, pulse rate is 60/min and blood pressure is 130/70 mm Hg. There are retinal microaneurysms. Cardiac examination reveals regular rhythm with an S4 and a grade 2/6 systolic ejection murmur at the base but no S3 or rub. Bowel sounds are normal. The peripheral pulses are absent in both feet. There is 1+ pedal edema.

Laboratory studies:

Creatinine	1.6 mg/dL (141.47 μmol/L)
Sodium	140 meq/L (140 mmol/L)
Potassium	4.0 meq/L (4.0 mmol/L)
Chloride	106 meq/L (106 mmol/L)
Bicarbonate	24 meq/L (24 mmol/L)

Angiography of the legs is scheduled.

In addition to initiating therapy with 0.9% saline at 1 mL/kg 12 hours before the procedure, which of the following additional strategies is indicated?

(A) Begin oral *N*-acetylcysteine
(B) Begin intravenous mannitol
(C) Begin fenoldopam
(D) Discontinue metformin
(E) Begin intravenous mannitol and furosemide

Item 68

A 66-year-old woman is evaluated for fatigue, decreased exercise tolerance of 1 month's duration, and new-onset dyspnea on exertion. Therapy with over-the-counter ibuprofen was unsuccessful, and she discontinued its use. She has a history of hypertension and was diagnosed with type 2 diabetes mellitus that is controlled by diet 2 years ago. Medications are lisinopril, 20 mg/d, and hydrochlorothiazide, 25 mg/d.

On physical examination, pulse rate is 74/min and blood pressure is 148/86 mm Hg. The conjunctivae are pale. Cardiac examination reveals a grade 2/6 systolic ejection murmur. There is 1+ lower-extremity edema.

Laboratory studies:

Hemoglobin	7.2 g/dL (72 g/L)
Leukocyte count	7100/μL (7.1 × 10^9/L)
Platelet count	125,000/μL (125 × 10^9/L)
Blood urea nitrogen	64 mg/dL (22.85 mmol/L)
Creatinine	5.2 mg/dL (459.78 μmol/L)
Sodium	133 meq/L (133 mmol/L)
Potassium	4.1 meq/L (4.1 mmol/L)
Chloride	110 meq/L (110 mmol/L)
Bicarbonate	19 meq/L (19 mmol/L)
Glucose	142 mg/dL (7.88 mmol/L)
Albumin	4.0 mg/dL (40 g/L)
Calcium	11.0 mg/dL (2.74 mmol/L)

Phosphorus	5.4 mg/dL (1.74 mmol/L)
Urinalysis	pH 5.0, specific gravity 1.015, no blood, 1+ protein, 5–10 leukocytes/hpf
Urinary protein–creatinine ratio	2.5 mg/g

Which of the following is the most likely cause of this patient's renal failure?

(A) Chronic interstitial nephritis
(B) Hypertensive nephrosclerosis
(C) Acute interstitial nephritis
(D) Myeloma kidney
(E) Diabetic nephropathy

Item 69

A 55-year-old man with chronic kidney disease presumed secondary to diabetic nephropathy comes for an evaluation before a planned débridement of his left great toe for a chronic nonhealing diabetic foot ulcer. His creatinine level is 2.4 mg/dL (212.21 µmol/L). Medications are lisinopril, atenolol, furosemide, and glyburide. In addition, he is currently taking a 14-day course of amoxicillin–clavulanate.

On physical examination, pulse rate is 72/min and blood pressure is 148/68 mm Hg. Cardiac examination reveals a normal S1 and S2 and a grade 2/6 systolic murmur radiating to his axilla. Pulmonary examination is normal. There is a 7-mm ulcer extending across the left great toe with purulent drainage.

Which of the following is recommended to determine the stage of this patient's chronic kidney disease?

(A) 24-Hour urine for creatinine clearance
(B) ^{125}I-iothalamate radionuclide scanning
(C) Cystatin C measurement
(D) Renal ultrasonography
(E) Mathematical formula for estimation of the glomerular filtration rate

Item 70

A 64-year-old man with a history of coronary artery disease, peripheral vascular disease, chronic cigarette smoking, chronic kidney disease, and uncontrolled hypertension comes for a follow-up office visit. He was recently hospitalized for acute pulmonary edema. His estimated glomerular filtration rate is 45 mL/min. Renal ultrasound performed during his hospitalization revealed a left kidney of 8.5 cm and a right kidney of 11 cm and increased echogenicity of the kidneys. He states that he has been compliant with his diet restrictions. Medications are aspirin, 81 mg/d; simvastatin, 40 mg/d; carvedilol, 25 mg twice daily; furosemide, 40 mg twice daily; digoxin, 0.125 mg once daily; losartan, 100 mg/d; amlodipine, 5 mg/d; and clonidine, 0.2 mg twice daily.

On physical examination, pulse rate is 62/min and blood pressure is 186/72 mm Hg. Cardiac examination reveals an S4 gallop. An abdominal bruit is heard. There is 1+ bilateral lower-extremity edema.

Which of the following is the most appropriate next step in managing this patient's hypertension?

(A) Increase amlodipine to 10 mg/d
(B) Perform magnetic resonance angiography of the abdomen
(C) Discontinue carvedilol
(D) Add lisinopril
(E) Perform CT of the abdomen with intravenous contrast

Item 71

A 70-year-old woman with hypertension and chronic kidney disease comes for a follow-up visit. On physical examination, pulse rate is 80/min and blood pressure is 140/80 mm Hg. BMI is 21. Cardiac examination reveals a regular sinus rhythm with no murmur. The lungs are clear to auscultation. Bowel sounds are normal. There is 1+ pedal edema.

Laboratory studies:

Blood urea nitrogen	30 mg/dL (10.71 mmol/L)
Creatinine	2.5 mg/dL (221.05 µmol/L)
Sodium	140 meq/L (140 mmol/L)
Potassium	5 meq/L (5.0 mmol/L)
Chloride	105 meq/L (105 mmol/L)
Bicarbonate	20 meq/L (20 mmol/L)
Phosphorus	7 mg/dL (2.26 mmol/L)
Calcium	9 mg/dL (2.25 mmol/L)
Albumin	3.5 g/dL (35 g/L)

Which of the following is the most likely cause of this patient's hyperphosphatemia?

(A) Primary hyperparathyroidism
(B) High phosphorus intake
(C) Vitamin D deficiency
(D) Glomerular filtration rate decrease
(E) Hypocalcemia

Item 72

An 80-year-old woman is evaluated for resistant hypertension and fatigue. Home blood pressure measurements are typically approximately 180/70 mm Hg. Medications are metoprolol, 50 mg/d; lisinopril, 20 mg/d; and hydrochlorothiazide, 12.5 mg/d.

On physical examination, pulse rate is 72/min and blood pressure is 180/70 mm Hg.

Laboratory studies:

Blood urea nitrogen	12 mg/dL (4.29 mmol/L)
Creatinine	0.9 mg/dL (79.58 µmol/L)
Sodium	132 meq/L (132 mmol/L)
Potassium	3.3 meq/L (3.3 mmol/L)
Chloride	99 meq/L (99 mmol/L)
Bicarbonate	26 meq/L (26 mmol/L)
Plasma renin activity	0.36 ng/mL per hour (0.36 µg/L per hour)

Which of the following is the most appropriate next step in this patient's management?

(A) Double the dose of hydrochlorothiazide
(B) Double the dose of metoprolol
(C) Double the dose of lisinopril
(D) Discontinue hydrochlorothiazide; add spironolactone, 25 mg/d

Item 73

A 68-year-old man is brought to the emergency department after an intentional toxic ingestion. He has a history of hypertension and gout. Two years ago, coronary artery bypass graft surgery was performed. He smokes cigarettes but does not use alcohol or illicit drugs.

On physical examination, temperature is 36.7 °C (98 °F), pulse rate is 79/min, respiratory rate is 32/min, and blood pressure is 156/80 mm Hg. He is lethargic and weak, in moderate respiratory distress, and oriented only to place and person. Cardiovascular examination is normal. Pulmonary examination reveals no wheezing.

Laboratory studies:

Glucose	128 mg/dL (7.1 mmol/L)
Blood urea nitrogen	21 mg/dL (7.5 mmol/L)
Creatinine	1.2 mg/dL (106.1 µmol/L)
Sodium	141 meq/L (141 mmol/L)
Potassium	3.9 meq/L (3.9 mmol/L)
Chloride	103 meq/L (103 mmol/L)

Bicarbonate	11 meq/L (11 mmol/L)

Arterial blood gas studies (with the patient breathing room air):

pH	7.49
P_{CO_2}	15 mm Hg
P_{O_2}	67 mm Hg

Measurement of which of the following is most likely to establish a diagnosis in this patient?

(A) Serum osmolality
(B) Ethylene glycol
(C) Methanol
(D) Salicylate
(E) Urinary hippurate

Item 74

A 60-year-old man develops acute renal failure after a radical perineal prostatectomy for localized prostate cancer. The surgery was performed in the exaggerated lithotomy position under general anesthesia, and intraoperative hypotension did not develop. A bowel injury prolonged the operative time to 4 hours, 30 minutes. Blood loss was estimated at 400 mL, and urine output during the surgery was 300 mL. Preoperatively, the patient received 1 dose of levofloxacin.

On postoperative day 1, the patient developed severe low back pain and intravenous morphine was administered. Urine output was maintained at 1500 mL during the initial 24 hours postoperatively.

On physical examination, temperature is 37.2 °C (99 °F) and blood pressure is 160/92 mm Hg. The patient is in distress due to low back pain. There is diffuse tenderness and spasm in the lumbar paraspinal muscles. The remainder of the examination is unremarkable.

Laboratory studies:

Blood urea nitrogen	23 mg/dL (8.21 mmol/L)
Creatinine	1.6 mg/dL (141.47 µmol/L) (preoperative creatinine was 1.2 mg/dL [106.1 µmol/L])
Creatine kinase	546,000 U/L
Sodium	140 meq/L (140 mmol/L)
Potassium	6.3 meq/L (6.3 mmol/L)
Chloride	104 meq/L (104 mmol/L)
Bicarbonate	18 meq/L (18 mmol/L)
Calcium	6.2 mg/dL (1.55 mmol/L)

Phosphorus	7.8 mg/dL (2.52 mmol/L)
Bilirubin	Normal
Aspartate aminotransferase	1200 U/L
Alanine aminotransferase	204 U/L
Alkaline phosphatase	Normal
γ-Glutamyltransferase	Normal
Urinalysis	Specific gravity 1.012, 1+ protein, 2+ blood, 3–5 leuko-cytes/hpf, 2–3 monomorphic ery-throcytes/hpf, numerous hyaline and dark granular casts/hpf
Urine creatinine	32 mg/dL (2829.44 μmol/L)
Urine sodium	70 meq/L (70 mmol/L)
Urine myoglobin	Elevated

Renal ultrasound shows normal-sized kidneys without hydronephrosis.

Which of the following is the most likely diagnosis?

(A) Ischemic acute tubular necrosis
(B) Prerenal failure
(C) Urinary tract obstruction
(D) Pigment nephropathy
(E) Allergic interstitial nephritis

Item 75

A 29-year-old man with a 10-year history of IgA glomeru-lonephritis is evaluated for persistent microscopic hema-turia. He strictly maintains a sodium-restricted diet. His only medication is the maximal dose of an angiotensin-converting enzyme inhibitor. One year ago, the pro-tein/creatinine ratio was 1 mg/g.

On physical examination, the blood pressure is 138/85 mm Hg. The cardiac, pulmonary, and abdominal examinations are unremarkable. There is no peripheral edema or rash.

Laboratory studies:

Creatinine	1 mg/dL (88.42 μmol/L) (1 year ago, creatinine was 1 mg/dL)
Albumin	3.8 g/dL (38 g/L)
Urinary protein–creatinine ratio	2 mg/g

Which of the following is the most appropriate next step in the management of this patient's IgA glomeru-lonephritis?

(A) Tonsillectomy
(B) A diuretic

(C) Oral corticosteroids
(D) An angiotensin receptor blocker
(E) A calcium-channel blocker

Item 76

A 49-year-old man comes to the office for evaluation before cystoscopy because of a 20-year history of micro-scopic hematuria. He feels well and has no intercurrent dis-eases. Two previous CT scans have excluded renal mass; the most recent CT scan was performed 5 years ago. Find-ings of a cystoscopy 10 years ago were unremarkable. His mother has a history of microscopic hematuria.

On physical examination, pulse rate is 70/min and regular, and blood pressure is 90/70 mm Hg. The remain-der of the examination is unremarkable.

Creatinine is 0.7 mg/dL (61.89 μmol/L). Urinalysis reveals no proteinuria and 7 to 10 dysmorphic erythro-cytes/hpf.

Which of the following is the most likely diagnosis?

(A) Bladder cancer
(B) Polycystic kidney disease
(C) Thin basement membrane disease
(D) Renal cell carcinoma
(E) Recurrent urinary tract infection

Item 77

A 56-year-old man with a history of alcoholism is found lying on the street with impaired consciousness. On arrival at the emergency department, he is unresponsive and is intubated.

On physical examination, temperature is 36.1 °C (97 °F), pulse rate is 70/min, and blood pressure is 126/80 mm Hg. Funduscopic examination shows no papilledema. Cardiac, pulmonary, and abdominal exami-nations are normal. There is no peripheral edema.

Laboratory studies:

Glucose	86 mg/dL (4.77 mmol/L)
Blood urea nitrogen	45 mg/dL (16.07 mmol/L)
Creatinine	2.8 mg/dL (247.58 μmol/L)
Sodium	138 meq/L (138 mmol/L)
Potassium	5.4 meq/L (5.4 mmol/L)
Chloride	94 meq/L (94 mmol/L)
Bicarbonate	14 meq/L (14 mmol/L)
Arterial blood gas studies (with the patient breathing oxygen) obtained 15 minutes after intubation:	
pH	7.28
Pco2	29 mm Hg

P_{O_2}	108 mm Hg
Plasma osmolality	316 mosm/kg H_2O
Urinalysis	Calcium oxalate crystals

Renal ultrasonography reveals normal-sized kidneys with no obstruction or hydronephrosis.

Which of the following is the most appropriate treatment for this patient?

(A) Fomepizole and hemodialysis
(B) Bicarbonate supplementation
(C) Ethanol drip
(D) Hemodialysis
(E) Fomepizole and ethanol drip

Item 78

A 67-year-old man with a history of osteoarthritis, benign prostatic hyperplasia, and hyperlipidemia is evaluated for new-onset joint pain in his shoulders and wrists accompanied by lower-extremity swelling. Three months ago, his baseline kidney function was normal. Medications are acetaminophen, tamsulosin, and simvastatin. He also took two to three naproxen pills when the swelling first started.

On physical examination, pulse rate is 65/min and blood pressure is 132/68 mm Hg. The conjunctivae are pale. Cardiac examination shows an S3 gallop. Jugular venous pressure is 7 cm H_2O. Pulmonary examination reveals bilateral decreased breath sounds at both bases. There is 3+ lower-extremity edema. His rectal examination shows an enlarged prostate without masses or nodules.

Laboratory studies:

Hemoglobin	8.2 g/dL (82 g/L)
Leukocyte count	8100/μL (8.1 × 10^9/L)
Platelet count	132,000/μL (132 × 10^9/L)
Blood urea nitrogen	68 mg/dL (24.28 mmol/L)
Creatinine	5.6 mg/dL (495.15 μmol/L)
Sodium	131 meq/L (131 mmol/L)
Potassium	3.5 meq/L (3.5 mmol/L)
Chloride	110 meq/L (110 mmol/L)
Bicarbonate	18 meq/L (18 mmol/L)
Albumin	3.0 mg/dL (30 g/L)
Calcium	10.5 mg/dL (2.62 mmol/L)
Phosphorus	5.4 mg/dL (1.74 mmol/L)

Urinalysis	pH 5, specific gravity 1.015, no blood, 2+ protein
Urinary protein–creatinine ratio	5 mg/g

Which of the following studies is most likely to confirm the cause of this patient's kidney failure?

(A) Antinuclear cytoplasmic antibody assay
(B) Serum protein electrophoresis/urine protein electrophoresis
(C) Urine eosinophil measurement
(D) Hepatitis C antibody assay
(E) Kidney ultrasonography

Item 79

A 60-year-old woman with hypertension, type 2 diabetes mellitus, obesity, and chronic kidney disease comes for a routine office visit. She follows a renal diet. Medications are glipizide, 10 mg twice daily; pioglitazone, 30 mg/d; atenolol, 100 mg/d; benazepril, 80 mg/d; furosemide, 40 mg twice daily; simvastatin, 40 mg/d; and aspirin, 81 mg/d.

Laboratory studies:

Creatinine	2.3 mg/dL (203.37 μmol/L)
Sodium	140 meq/L (140 mmol/L)
Potassium	5.0 meq/L (5.0 mmol/L)
Chloride	106 meq/L (106 mmol/L)
Bicarbonate	23 meq/L (23 mmol/L)
Calcium	9.7 mg/dL (2.42 mmol/L)
Phosphorus	6.9 mg/dL (2.23 mmol/L)
Albumin	4 g/dL (40 g/L)

Which of the following should be started to most appropriately treat this patient?

(A) Aluminum hydroxide
(B) Sevelamer
(C) Vitamin D
(D) Hemodialysis

Item 80

A 50-year-old black man is evaluated for inadequately controlled hypertension. He currently takes hydrochlorothiazide, 25 mg/d.

On physical examination, blood pressure is 150/90 mm Hg. BMI is 28, and he appears well. The remainder of the examination is normal.

Laboratory studies:

Glucose	90 mg/dL (5 mmol/L)
Creatinine	1.3 mg/dL (114.95 µmol/L)
Potassium	3.6 meq/L (3.6 mmol/L)
Spot urine albumin–creatinine ratio	10 mg/g

Which of the following is the most appropriate treatment for this patient?

(A) Increase the diuretic dose
(B) Add atenolol
(C) Add an angiotensin-converting enzyme inhibitor
(D) Add a dihydropyridine calcium-channel blocker

Item 81

A 35-year-old woman who is 15 weeks pregnant is referred for evaluation of hypertension. She discontinued her antihypertensive regimen when she learned that she was pregnant.

On physical examination, pulse rate is 90/min and blood pressure is 160/98 mm Hg. Cardiac and pulmonary examinations are normal. There is trace ankle edema.

Laboratory studies:

Blood urea nitrogen	6 mg/dL (2.14 mmol/L)
Creatinine	0.6 mg/dL (53.05 µmol/L)
Sodium	136 meq/L (136 mmol/L)
Potassium	3.7 meq/L (3.7 mmol/L)
Bicarbonate	23 meq/L (23 mmol/L)

Treatment with which of the following agents is most appropriate for this patient?

(A) Hydrochlorothiazide
(B) Lisinopril
(C) Losartan
(D) Labetalol
(E) Atenolol

Item 82

A 66-year-old man with type 2 diabetes mellitus and hypertension is evaluated for an 8-day history of severe diarrhea, abdominal pain, and decreased food intake. His intake of liquids has been adequate. He believes that he became sick after babysitting his grandson, who had similar symptoms. Three years ago, he underwent coronary artery bypass graft surgery. Medications are enalapril, 20 mg twice daily; aspirin, 81 mg/d; atenolol, 25 mg/d; hydrochlorothiazide, 25 mg/d; and metformin, 1 g twice daily. He drinks alcoholic beverages occasionally and does not smoke cigarettes or use illicit drugs.

On physical examination, temperature is 37.1 °C (98.8 °F), pulse rate is 66/min with no orthostatic changes, and respiratory rate is 26/min. A stool specimen is positive for occult blood.

Laboratory studies:

Glucose	128 mg/dL (7.1 mmol/L)
Blood urea nitrogen	21 mg/dL (7.5 mmol/L)
Creatinine	1.2 mg/dL (106.1 µmol/L)
Sodium	136 meq/L (136 mmol/L)
Potassium	3.9 meq/L (3.9 mmol/L)
Chloride	114 meq/L (114 mmol/L)
Bicarbonate	13 meq/L (13 mmol/L)
Albumin	4.0 g/dL (40 g/L)
Urine pH	6
Urine sodium	32 meq/L (32 mmol/L)
Urine potassium	21 meq/L (21 mmol/L)
Urine chloride	80 meq/L (80 mmol/L)

Arterial blood gas studies (with the patient breathing room air):

pH	7.27
P_{CO_2}	30 mm Hg
P_{O_2}	90 mm Hg

Which of the following is most likely responsible for this patient's acid–base disorder?

(A) Metformin
(B) Diarrhea
(C) Type 4 renal tubular acidosis
(D) Type 1 renal tubular acidosis
(E) Enalapril

Item 83

A 23-year-old woman is evaluated for a 1-year history of slowly progressive high-frequency hearing loss. There is no history of trauma. The patient listens to soft, classical music. An older sister has a similar condition.

On physical examination, the blood pressure is 140/95 mm Hg. Otologic examination and audiometry reveal high-frequency hearing loss. The remainder of the examination is normal except for trace edema in the extremities.

Laboratory studies:

Blood urea nitrogen	15 mg/dL (5.36 mmol/L)
Creatinine	0.9 mg/dL (79.58 µmol/L)
Albumin	3.2 g/dL (32 g/L)
Urinalysis	2+ blood, 10 dysmorphic erythrocytes/hpf
Urinary protein–creatinine ratio	1.2 mg/g

Renal ultrasound reveals a small simple cyst.

Which of the following is the most likely diagnosis?

(A) Polycystic kidney disease
(B) Fabry's disease
(C) Alport's syndrome
(D) Familial benign hematuria

Item 84

A 74-year-old man is evaluated for a 5-month history of sinusitis and intermittent otitis media. He also has lost 4.1 kg (9 lbs) and had occasional monoarthritis migrating from joint to joint. He has been afebrile.

On physical examination, he is afebrile. Cardiac examination reveals a grade 2/6 early systolic murmur at the left sternal border. Pulmonary examination demonstrates occasional rhonchi. There is crusting in his right nares and an opaque right tympanic membrane. He has mild bilateral maxillary sinus tenderness. The abdomen is soft and nontender with no masses. There is 2+ edema of the extremities.

Laboratory studies:

Hemoglobin	11.5 g/dL (115 g/L)
Leukocyte count	10,800/µL (10.8 × 10⁹/L)
Blood urea nitrogen	28 mg/dL (10 mmol/L)
Creatinine	1.6 mg/dL (141.47 µmol/L)
Albumin	3.8 g/dL (38 g/L)
C3	100 mg/dL (1000 mg/L)
C4	32 mg/dL (320 mg/L)
Urinalysis	18 dysmorphic erythrocytes and 1 erythrocyte cast/hpf

Chest radiograph reveals a nodule in the right upper lobe and a hazy density in the left lower lobe.

Which of the following assays is most likely to establish a diagnosis?

(A) Antinuclear antibody
(B) Anti–glomerular basement membrane antibody
(C) Myeloperoxidase antineutrophil cytoplasmic antibody
(D) Proteinase-3 antineutrophil cytoplasmic antibody
(E) Anti–double-stranded DNA antibody

Item 85

A 64-year-old woman is evaluated for progressive weakness, nausea, dyspnea, and acute renal failure of several weeks' duration. Her creatinine level is 4.6 mg/dL (406.73 µmol/L) (baseline creatinine is 1.3 mg/dL [114.95 µmol/L]). She has a history of type 2 diabetes mellitus and hypertension treated with metoprolol and hydrochlorothiazide. Other medications include aspirin and glipizide.

On physical examination, the blood pressure is 110/70 mm Hg. Funduscopic examination reveals arteriovenous nicking but no evidence of diabetic retinopathy. Cardiac examination shows a laterally displaced point of maximal impulse and a grade I holosystolic murmur at the apex. On pulmonary examination, the lungs are clear to auscultation. There is no pedal edema.

Laboratory studies:

Hemoglobin	12.8 g/dL (128 g/L)
Leukocyte count	8000/µL (8 × 10⁹/L)
Platelet count	311,000/µL (311 × 10⁹/L)
Blood urea nitrogen	48 mg/dL (17.14 mmol/L)
Uric acid	11.6 mg/dL (0.69 mmol/L)
Creatinine	4.6 mg/dL (406.73 µmol/L)
Sodium	140 meq/L (140 mmol/L)
Potassium	4.3 meq/L (4.3 mmol/L)
Chloride	110 meq/L (110 mmol/L)
Bicarbonate	26 meq/L (26 mmol/L)
Total protein	8.4 g/dL (84 g/L)
Albumin	3.8 g/dL (38 g/L)
Calcium	10.5 mg/dL (2.62 mmol/L)
Phosphorus	5.6 mg/dL (1.81 mmol/L)
Lactate dehydrogenase	634 U/L (10.57 ukat/L)
Urinalysis	pH 6.5, trace protein, trace blood, 2 leukocytes/hpf, amorphous crystals
Urine sodium	60 meq/L (60 mmol/L)

Urine creatinine	90 mg/dL (7957.8 μmol/L)
Urine protein–creatinine ratio	3

Renal ultrasound shows enlarged hyperechoic kidneys bilaterally measuring 14 cm in length. Chest radiograph reveals mild cardiomegaly but is otherwise unremarkable.

Which of the following is the most likely diagnosis?

(A) Uric acid nephropathy
(B) Thiazide-induced acute renal failure
(C) Primary amyloidosis
(D) Myeloma cast nephropathy
(E) Lymphomatous infiltration of the kidneys

Item 86

A 55-year-old woman has a 1-week history of progressive shortness of breath and cough productive of blood-streaked sputum. She has no history of asthma.

On physical examination, pulse rate is 100/min and regular, respiratory rate is 28/min and shallow, and blood pressure is 170/100 mm Hg. Cardiac examination reveals a grade 2/6 systolic murmur along the left sternal border. Pulmonary examination shows bilateral crackles in both lung bases and in the midlung zones. The abdomen is soft and nontender, and there are no overt masses. There is 2+ edema of the extremities, and there is a palpable petechial rash on the extremities.

Laboratory studies:

Hemoglobin	7.5 g/dL (75 g/L)
Differential leukocyte count	90% polymorphonuclear cells, 6% lymphocytes, 3% monocytes, no eosinophils, 1% basophils
Platelet count	340,000/μL (340 × 10⁹/L)
Blood urea nitrogen	60 mg/dL (21.43 mmol/L)
Creatinine	4.5 mg/dL (397.89 μmol/L)
Sodium	130 meq/L (130 mmol/L)
Potassium	5.1 meq/L (5.1 mmol/L)
Chloride	96 meq/L (96 mmol/L)
Bicarbonate	28 meq/L (28 mmol/L)
Albumin	3.5 g/dL (35 g/L)
C3	121 mg/dL (1210 mg/L)
C4	38 mg/dL (380 mg/L)

Urinalysis	Mostly dysmorphic erythrocytes too numerous to count, several erythrocyte casts/hpf

Chest radiograph reveals bilateral pulmonary infiltrates.

Which of the following is the most likely diagnosis?

(A) Henoch–Schönlein purpura
(B) Cryoglobulinemic vasculitis
(C) Systemic lupus erythematosus
(D) Microscopic polyangiitis
(E) Churg–Strauss syndrome

Item 87

A 56-year-old man with a history of end-stage renal disease due to type 1 diabetes mellitus is hospitalized for fever, night sweats, nausea, emesis of coffee-ground material, and abdominal pain. More than 1 week before admission, he also had dark, tarry stools. Six months ago, he underwent renal transplantation. Before transplantation, a cytomegalovirus antibody assay was positive and an Epstein–Barr virus (EBV) antibody assay was negative. The kidney donor had evidence of previous Epstein–Barr virus infection but no cytomegalovirus antibodies. Medications are tacrolimus, mycophenolate mofetil, and prednisone. Two days before admission, the patient also took several doses of ibuprofen for fever.

On physical examination, temperature is 37.8 °C (100.1 °F), pulse rate is 80/min, and blood pressure is 136/80 mm Hg. Cardiac and pulmonary examinations are normal. There is bulky lymphadenopathy in the axillary and inguinal chains bilaterally. The liver is enlarged and spans 14 cm, and a spleen tip is palpable. There is no peripheral edema.

Laboratory studies:

Hemoglobin	9.2 mg/dL (5.71 mmol/L)
Leukocyte count	5100/μL (5.1 × 10⁹/L)
Platelet count	240,000/μL (240 × 10⁹/L)
Creatinine	1.6 mg/dL (141.47 μmol/L)
Lactate dehydrogenase	682 U/L (11.37 ukat/L)
Cytomegalovirus viral load	<50 copies/mL

Esophagogastroduodenoscopy shows multiple duodenal ulcers without active hemorrhage.

Which of the following is the most likely diagnosis?

(A) *Helicobacter pylori*–induced peptic ulcer disease
(B) Cytomegalovirus-induced mucosal injury

(C) Nonsteroidal anti-inflammatory drug–induced peptic ulcer disease

(D) Post-transplant lymphoproliferative disease

Item 88

A 32-year-old man comes to the office after being told at a health fair screening that he had blood in his urine. He states that he has never seen gross blood in his urine and has not passed any kidney stones. He does not smoke cigarettes and takes no medications.

On physical examination, pulse rate is 72/min and blood pressure is 138/78 mm Hg.

Laboratory studies:

Hemoglobin	13.8 g/dL (138 g/L)
Leukocyte count	6800/µL (6.8 × 10⁹/L)
Platelet count	325,000/µL (325 × 10⁹/L)
Blood urea nitrogen	12 mg/dL (4.29 mmol/L)
Creatinine	1.1 mg/dL (97.26 µmol/L)
Sodium	138 meq/L (138 mmol/L)
Potassium	4.2 meq/L (4.2 mmol/L)
Bicarbonate	25 meq/L (25 mmol/L)
Calcium	10.1 mg/dL (2.52 mmol/L)
Phosphorus	4.2 mg/dL (1.36 mmol/L)
Urinalysis	pH 5.0, specific gravity 1.010, 2+ blood, 2+ protein, 5–10 dysmorphic erythrocytes/hpf
Urinary protein–creatinine ratio	1.5 mg/g

Which of the following is the most likely cause of this patient's hematuria?

(A) Genitourinary tract malignancy
(B) Urinary tract infection
(C) Nephrolithiasis
(D) Glomerulonephritis

Item 89

A 42-year-old man with obesity is evaluated for hypertension. He feels well and has no shortness of breath, hematuria, or leg swelling. Medical history is insignificant. There is a family history of obesity, hyperlipidemia, and hypertension. He takes no medications.

Ophthalmologic examination is normal. Cardiac examination reveals normal rhythm and no murmurs or gallops. The lungs are clear to auscultation. There is no jugular venous distension. The abdomen is large and soft. There is no edema.

Laboratory studies:

Glucose (fasting)	110 mg/dL (6.11 mmol/L)
Creatinine	1.6 mg/dL (141.47 µmol/L)
Urinalysis	3+ protein, no hematuria
24-Hour urinary protein	2.8 g/24 h

Kidney biopsy is performed.

Which of the following is the most likely diagnosis?

(A) Membranous glomerulonephritis
(B) Glomerulopathy with secondary focal segmental glomerulosclerosis
(C) IgA nephropathy
(D) Minimal change disease
(E) Membranous nephropathy

Item 90

A 60-year-old man with type 2 diabetes mellitus is evaluated for chest pain, abnormal stress test results, and hypertension. Medications are metformin, a β-blocker, an angiotensin-converting enzyme inhibitor, aspirin, and a statin.

On physical examination, blood pressure is 160/90 mm Hg. There is evidence of early diabetic retinopathy.

Laboratory studies:

Blood urea nitrogen	15 mg/dL (5.36 mmol/L)
Creatinine	1.1 mg/dL (97.26 µmol/L)
Potassium	5.2 meq/L (5.2 mmol/L)

Spot urinary albumin–creatinine ratio   175 mg/g

Cardiac catheterization reveals mild-to-moderate diffuse triple-vessel disease that is not amenable to revascularization.

Which of the following agents is indicated to treat this patient's hypertension?

(A) An angiotensin receptor blocker
(B) A thiazide diuretic
(C) An α-blocker
(D) A potassium-sparing diuretic

Item 91

A 19-year-old woman is evaluated for sudden-onset periorbital and pretibial edema. Three weeks ago, she was diagnosed with an upper respiratory tract infection that has since resolved.

On physical examination, blood pressure is 150/100 mm Hg. Cardiac examination reveals a normal S1 to S2 with a soft S3. There are crackles in both lung bases. Abdominal examination reveals a tender, swollen liver. There is bilateral pitting tibial edema. There are no rashes.

Laboratory studies:

Hemoglobin	13.5 g/dL (135 g/L)
Leukocyte count	10,500/μL (10.5 × 10^9/L)
Platelet count	200,000/μL (200 × 10^9/L)
Blood urea nitrogen	30 mg/dL (10.71 mmol/L)
Creatinine	1.5 mg/dL (132.63 μmol/L)
Albumin	3.8 g/dL (38 g/L)
C3	15 mg/dL (150 mg/L)
C4	48 mg/dL (480 mg/L)
Urinalysis	1+ protein; several erythrocytes, dysmorphic erythrocytes, and erythrocyte casts/hpf

Which of the following is the most likely diagnosis?

(A) IgA glomerulonephritis
(B) Goodpasture's syndrome
(C) Antineutrophil cytoplasmic antibody–associated small-vessel vasculitis
(D) Postinfectious glomerulonephritis
(E) Systemic lupus erythematosus nephritis

Item 92

A 44-year-old man diagnosed with cryptogenic cirrhosis 2 years ago is hospitalized for a fractured left hip sustained after a car accident. He is asymptomatic except for pain in his hip. He has felt well recently and is currently on the liver transplant list. He smokes 1 pack of cigarettes daily and does not drink alcoholic beverages or use illicit drugs. Medications are spironolactone, 50 mg twice daily; lactulose, 30 mL twice daily; oral propranolol, 20 mg twice daily; and furosemide, 20 mg twice daily.

On physical examination, temperature is 36 °C (96.8 °F), pulse rate is 72/min, respiratory rate is 18/min, and blood pressure is 98/55 mm Hg. He is cachectic. There is scleral icterus. He has normal mentation, and no asterixis is noted. Cardiac examination reveals no murmurs or rubs, and his lungs are clear to auscultation. The abdomen is distended but nontender. There is 2+ peripheral edema and palmar erythema.

Laboratory studies:

Glucose	88 mg/dL (4.88 mmol/L)
Blood urea nitrogen	14 mg/dL (5 mmol/L)

Creatinine	0.9 mg/dL (79.58 μmol/L)
Sodium	130 meq/L (130 mmol/L)
Potassium	3.3 meq/L (3.3 mmol/L)
Chloride	107 meq/L (107 mmol/L)
Bicarbonate	18 meq/L (18 mmol/L)
Albumin	2.6 g/dL (26 g/L)

Arterial blood gas studies (with the patient breathing room air):

pH	7.48
P_{CO_2}	25 mm Hg
P_{O_2}	92 mm Hg

Which of the following is the most likely cause of this patient's acid–base disorder?

(A) Renal tubular acidosis
(B) Impaired hepatic conversion of lactate
(C) Lactulose-induced diarrhea
(D) Reduced acid buffering capacity of the blood
(E) Increased minute ventilation

Item 93

A 37-year-old male with longstanding alcoholism is admitted to the intensive care unit with severe pancreatitis. His friends state that for the last several weeks he has been drinking beer all day and has been eating very little except for salty snacks. Over the next 3 days, he develops sepsis and a pancreatic abscess that requires drainage. Two days later, he remains on mechanical ventilation and vasopressor support.

Laboratory studies obtained on hospital day 6:

Glucose	96 mg/dL (5.33 mmol/L)
Blood urea nitrogen	5 mg/dL (1.79 mmol/L)
Creatinine	0.7 mg/dL (61.89 μmol/L)
Sodium	136 meq/L (136 mmol/L)
Potassium	4.3 meq/L (4.3 mmol/L)
Chloride	105 meq/L (105 mmol/L)
Bicarbonate	22 meq/L (22 mmol/L)
Albumin	2.9 g/dL (29 g/L)
Calcium	7.1 mg/dL (1.77 mmol/L)
Phosphorus	2.4 mg/dL (0.77 mmol/L)
Magnesium	2.2 mg/dL (0.91 mmol/L)

He is started on total parenteral nutrition therapy with 2000 total calories, 20% from fat; 120 meq (120 mmol) of sodium; and 80 meq (80 mmol) of potassium. The total volume is 2 L.

Which of the following conditions does this patient have high risk for after total parenteral nutrition therapy is started?

(A) Rhabdomyolysis
(B) Leukopenia
(C) Torsade des pointes
(D) Cerebral edema
(E) Fulminant liver failure

Item 94

A 23-year-old woman is evaluated for a 3-week history of nausea, malaise, and anorexia. She has had two spontaneous abortions. During her third pregnancy, she also developed preeclampsia at 24 weeks gestation.

On physical examination, pulse rate is 85/min and blood pressure is 150/100 mm Hg. There is a faintly evident malar rash. Cardiac and pulmonary examinations are unremarkable. The abdomen is soft and nontender with no masses. She has an acral ulcer on the index finger of her right hand and the third finger of her left hand. There is 1+ edema of the extremities.

Laboratory studies:

Hemoglobin	9.8 g/dL (98 g/L)
Leukocyte count	5400/μL (5.4 × 10^9/L)
Platelet count	50,000/μL (50 × 10^9/L)
Creatinine	2.5 mg/dL (221.05 μmol/L)
Albumin	4 g/dL (40 g/L)
C3	105 mg/dL (1050 mg/L)
C4	30 mg/dL (300 mg/L)
Double-stranded DNA antibodies	Titer of 1:80
Urinalysis	1+ protein; 3–5 erythrocyte casts/hpf, no casts
Urinary protein–creatinine ratio	0.8 mg/g

A peripheral blood smear reveals rare schistocytes.

Which of the following is the most likely diagnosis?

(A) Lupus nephritis characterized by a focal proliferative glomerulonephritis
(B) Postinfectious membranoproliferative glomerulonephritis
(C) Lupus nephritis characterized with a thrombotic microangiopathy
(D) Lupus nephritis with a membranous pattern

Item 95

A 74-year-old man with stage V chronic kidney disease due to diabetic nephropathy is hospitalized for crampy right lower quadrant abdominal pain. His wife noted that he had been intermittently confused for several weeks previously. He has been maintained on peritoneal dialysis for the last 5 years but 2 days ago inadvertently disconnected his cycler tubing and reconnected it without notifying dialysis personnel. He also has peripheral vascular disease and coronary heart disease.

On physical examination, temperature is 36.9°C (98.4 °F), pulse rate is 108/min, respiration rate is 20/min, and blood pressure is 160/74 mm Hg. Cardiac and pulmonary examinations are unremarkable. Abdominal examination shows diffuse tenderness but no rebound. The dialysis catheter exit site appears normal. There is trace peripheral edema.

Laboratory studies:

Hemoglobin	10.7 g/dL (6.64 mmol/L)
Leukocyte count	2400/μL (2.4 × 10^9/L)
Platelet count	365,000/μL (365 × 10^9/L)
Blood urea nitrogen	39 mg/dL (13.93 mmol/L)
Creatinine	6.8 mg/dL (601.26 μmol/L)
Sodium	131 meq/L (131 mmol/L)
Potassium	2.8 meq/L (2.8 mmol/L)
Chloride	80 meq/L (80 mmol/L)
Bicarbonate	27 meq/L (27 mmol/L)
Glucose	244 mg/dL (13.54 mmol/L)
Gram stain of dialysis fluid	1+ polymorphonuclear leukocytes, no organisms
Peritoneal fluid cell count	156 total nucleated cells/μL (90% neutrophils)

Which of the following is the most appropriate therapy for this patient?

(A) Start cefazolin and ceftazidime
(B) Start metronidazole and piperacillin–tazobactam
(C) Start vancomycin
(D) Remove the peritoneal dialysis catheter

Item 96

A 44-year-old man with a history of nephrolithiasis is hospitalized for lethargy and confusion. His wife reports that he had taken approximately 80 propoxyphene–acetaminophen tablets for renal colic 3 days ago. In the emergency department, he develops worsening hypoxemia and increased respiratory distress, and intubation and mechanical ventilation are required.

On physical examination, temperature is 37.3 °C (99.1 °F), pulse rate is 120/min, and blood pressure is 158/79 mm Hg. Pupils are equal, round, and reactive to light and accommodation. Cardiac examination reveals tachycardia. On pulmonary examination, there are decreased breath sounds at both lung bases. The abdomen is slightly distended with no organomegaly. Bowel sounds are hypoactive. There is no peripheral edema.

Laboratory studies:

Hemoglobin	15.3 g/dL (153 g/L)
Leukocyte count	8300/µL (8.3 × 10^9/L)
Platelet count	232,000/µL (232 × 10^9/L)
INR	1.1
Prothrombin time	12.2 s
Activated partial thromboplastin time	34.8 s
Glucose	78 mg/dL (4.33 mmol/L)
Blood urea nitrogen	69 mg/dL (34.28 mmol/L)
Creatinine	5 mg/dL (442.1 µmol/L)
Sodium	140 meq/L (140 mmol/L)
Potassium	4.6 meq/L (4.6 mmol/L)
Chloride	106 meq/L (106 mmol/L)
Bicarbonate	20 meq/L (20 mmol/L)
Calcium	6.9 mg/dL (1.72 mmol/L)
Magnesium	2.4 mg/dL (0.99 mmol/L)
Phosphorus	4.8 mg/dL (1.55 mmol/L)
Total bilirubin	1.9 mg/dL (32.49 mmol/L)
Aspartate aminotransferase	1456 U/L
Alanine aminotransferase	1877 U/L
γ-Glutamyltransferase	40 U/L
Urine creatinine	25 mg/dL (2210.5 µmol/L)
Urine sodium	70 meq/L (70 mmol/L)

Arterial blood gas studies (with the patient breathing oxygen):

pH	7.28
P_{CO_2}	41 mm Hg
P_{O_2}	92.2 mm Hg
Urinalysis	pH 5.5, specific gravity 1.0152, 1+ leukocyte esterase, 2+ protein, 1+ glucose, 1+ ketones, 2 leukocytes/hpf, 55 erythrocytes/hpf, many hyaline casts/hpf, scattered dark granular casts
Urinary protein–creatinine ratio	1.2

Chest radiograph shows an endotracheal tube in place and bilateral lower-lobe infiltrates.

Which of the following is the most likely diagnosis?

(A) Hepatorenal syndrome
(B) Ischemic acute tubular necrosis
(C) Interstitial nephritis
(D) Prerenal acute renal failure
(E) Thrombotic microangiopathy

Item 97

A 60-year-old woman with a history of stage IV chronic kidney disease is anticipated to require dialysis therapy within the next year. She has a history of longstanding hypertension and Crohn's disease. She has undergone multiple bowel resections and has had one small-bowel obstruction. Medications are enalapril, 10 mg/d; furosemide, 60 mg/d; aspirin, 81 mg/d; and sevelamer, 800 mg three times daily.

On physical examination, pulse rate is 80/min and blood pressure is 130/80 mm Hg. Cardiac and pulmonary examinations are normal. Radial, femoral, dorsalis pedis, and posterior tibial pulses are 2+. Cephalic veins measuring approximately 5 mm in diameter are present in both forearms. There is trace pretibial edema.

Which of the following is the most appropriate management for this patient?

(A) Placement of a tunneled central venous catheter when dialysis is needed
(B) Placement of a polytetrafluoroethylene graft now
(C) Creation of an arteriovenous fistula now
(D) Placement of a peritoneal dialysis catheter when dialysis is needed

Item 98

A 69-year-old man is evaluated during a routine physical examination. He has a history of hypertension, hyperlipidemia, osteoarthritis of the knees, and cigarette smoking. Medications are hydrochlorothiazide, 25 mg/d; atenolol, 25 mg/d; simvastatin, 20 mg/d; and acetaminophen as needed. Six months ago, a urinalysis performed by another physician during evaluation for an upper respiratory infection revealed 2+ blood without proteinuria; previous urinalyses were normal. His physical examination is unremarkable.

Laboratory studies:

Blood urea nitrogen	12 mg/dL (4.29 mmol/L)
Creatinine	1.1 mg/dL (97.26 µmol/L)
Sodium	138 meq/L (138 mmol/L)
Potassium	4.2 meq/L (4.2 mmol/L)
Bicarbonate	25 meq/L (25 mmol/L)
Urinalysis	pH 5.0, specific gravity 1.015, 2+ blood, 5–10 intact erythrocytes/hpf without casts

Spiral CT of the abdomen reveals a 2.5-cm simple cyst in the upper pole of the right kidney and no hydronephrosis.

Which of the following is the most appropriate next step in the evaluation of this patient's hematuria?

(A) Repeat urinalysis in 6 months
(B) Cystoscopy
(C) Ciprofloxacin
(D) Kidney biopsy

Item 99

An 80-year-old man is evaluated for a routine examination. He has a history of hypertension and was diagnosed with chronic osteoarthritis 20 years ago. Medications are atenolol, 50 mg/d, and hydrochlorothiazide, 25 mg/d. One year ago, he began ibuprofen, 250 mg four times daily.

On physical examination, pulse rate is 60/min and blood pressure is 180/90 mm Hg without orthostatic changes. There is trace peripheral edema.

Laboratory studies:

Blood urea nitrogen	40 mg/dL (14.28 mmol/L)
Creatinine	1.5 mg/dL (132.63 µmol/L)
Sodium	134 meq/L (134 mmol/L)
Potassium	4.9 meq/L (4.9 mmol/L)

Which of the following treatment strategies is indicated for this patient?

(A) Increase the atenolol dose
(B) Increase the hydrochlorothiazide dose

(C) Add lisinopril
(D) Discontinue ibuprofen

Item 100

A 68-year-old woman is admitted to a rehabilitation hospital 1 week after a total hip arthroplasty. Her postoperative course has been uncomplicated. She has hypertension, type 2 diabetes mellitus, and closed-angle glaucoma. Current medications are oral warfarin, 3 mg twice daily; oral enalapril, 5 mg twice daily; atenolol, 50 mg/d; oral acetazolamide, 250 mg twice daily; oral pioglitazone, 30 mg twice daily; and oral glipizide, 10 mg twice daily.

On physical examination, temperature is 37.3 °C (99.1 °F), pulse rate is 66/min, respiratory rate is 22/min, and blood pressure is 146/80 mm Hg. She is moderately obese. The remainder of the examination is normal except for a well-healing surgical wound over her hip.

Laboratory studies:

Glucose	152 mg/dL (8.44 mmol/L)
Blood urea nitrogen	13 mg/dL (4.64 mmol/L)
Creatinine	0.8 mg/dL (70.74 µmol/L)
Sodium	141 meq/L (141 mmol/L)
Potassium	4.2 meq/L (4.2 mmol/L)
Chloride	117 meq/L (117 mmol/L)
Bicarbonate	14 meq/L (14 mmol/L)
Albumin	3.8 g/dL (38 g/L)

Arterial blood gas studies (with the patient breathing room air):

pH	7.29
P_{CO_2}	30 mm Hg
P_{O_2}	70 mm Hg

Which of the following agents is most likely contributing to this patient's acid–base disturbance?

(A) Warfarin
(B) Atenolol
(C) Pioglitazone
(D) Glipizide
(E) Acetazolamide

Item 101

A 29-year-old black woman comes for a routine examination. She has a 3-year history of systemic lupus erythematosus. She recently was diagnosed with a progressive kidney disease characterized by glomerular hematuria with dysmorphic erythrocytes and proteinuria. Over the past 3 weeks, her creatinine level has risen from 0.9 mg/dL to 1.4 mg/dL.

Laboratory studies:

C3	60 mg/dL (600 mg/L)
C4	8 mg/dL (80 mg/L)
Double-stranded DNA antibody	Positive
Antinuclear antibodies	Positive

Kidney biopsy reveals diffuse proliferative immune complex–laden glomerulonephritis with endothelial tubular reticular inclusion bodies.

In addition to corticosteroid therapy, which of the following is the most appropriate treatment for this patient?

(A) Intravenous cyclophosphamide followed by maintenance intravenous cyclophosphamide
(B) Intravenous cyclophosphamide followed by maintenance mycophenolate mofetil
(C) Oral cyclophosphamide
(D) Intravenous cyclophosphamide

Item 102

A 62-year-old man with a longstanding history of type 2 diabetes mellitus is evaluated for increasing anginal chest pain of 2 weeks' duration. For the past 6 weeks, he also has had intermittent dark, tarry stools.

On physical examination, respiratory rate is 16/min and blood pressure is 140/90 mm Hg. Funduscopic examination shows proliferative changes and microaneurysms. Jugular venous pressure is 5 cm H_2O. Cardiac examination shows no murmur or gallop. On pulmonary examination, the lung fields are clear to auscultation. There is trace pretibial edema. Rectal examination shows no masses or nodules. A stool specimen is positive for occult blood.

Laboratory studies:

Hemoglobin	8.6 g/dL (86 g/L)
Glucose	277 mg/dL (15.37 mmol/L)
Blood urea nitrogen	31 mg/dL (11.07 mmol/L)
Creatinine	2.1 mg/dL (185.68 µmol/L)
Albumin	2.6 g/dL (26 g/L)
Urinalysis	pH 6.5, specific gravity 1.005, 2+ protein, 3+ glucose, 2 leukocytes/hpf, several oval fat bodies and hyaline and fatty casts/hpf

A cardiac catheterization is scheduled.

Which of the following is most likely to decrease this patient's risk for developing radiocontrast nephropathy?

(A) 0.45% saline
(B) N-acetylcysteine
(C) Theophylline
(D) Fenoldopam
(E) 0.9% saline

Item 103

A 49-year-old woman with end-stage renal disease is evaluated for painful ulcers involving both legs. Approximately 6 months ago, she noted nodular lesions on the right thigh and then the left. These lesions became progressively more painful and developed into ulcerative lesions over several months. She also has type 2 diabetes mellitus, atrial fibrillation, and hypertension. She has been maintained on chronic in-center hemodialysis for the past 6 years. Medications are warfarin; aspirin, 81 mg/d; enalapril; metoprolol; atorvastatin; calcium carbonate; calcitriol; and erythropoietin.

On physical examination, pulse rate is 86/min and irregular and blood pressure is 140/90 mm Hg. She is obese. There are necrotic ulcers covering most of the thighs bilaterally. Cardiac examination shows an irregularly irregular rhythm. The lungs are clear to auscultation. Abdominal examination is unremarkable. There is no peripheral edema.

Laboratory studies:

Hemoglobin	11.6 g/dL (7.2 mmol/L)
Leukocyte count	15,000/µL (15 × 10⁹/L)
Platelet count	326,000/µL (326 × 10⁹/L)
INR	2.6
Sodium	136 meq/L (136 mmol/L)
Potassium	5.3 meq/L (5.3 mmol/L)
Chloride	105 meq/L (105 mmol/L)
Bicarbonate	19 meq/L (19 mmol/L)
Calcium	10.1 mg/dL (2.52 mmol/L)
Phosphorus	8.8 mg/dL (2.84 mmol/L)

Which of the following is the most likely diagnosis?

(A) Calcinosis cutis
(B) Necrobiosis lipoidica diabetoricum
(C) Calcific uremic arteriolopathy
(D) Venous stasis ulcers
(E) Warfarin-induced skin necrosis

Item 104

A 16-year-old man is evaluated before joining a high school athletic team. His medical history is unremarkable and he takes no medications. Family history is significant for breast cancer in his maternal grandmother and hypertension in his father.

On physical examination, pulse rate is 55/min and blood pressure is 106/62 mm Hg.

Results of laboratory studies including a complete blood count and serum chemistry studies are normal. Dipstick urinalysis reveals 2+ proteinuria and no blood, and microscopic analysis shows a bland urine sediment. Urinary protein–creatinine ratio is 1.2 mg/g.

Which of the following is the most appropriate next step in this patient's evaluation?

(A) Quantification of proteinuria in the upright and recumbent positions
(B) Kidney biopsy
(C) Antistreptolysin O titer
(D) Spiral CT of the abdomen
(E) Anti–glomerular basement membrane antibody assay

Item 105

A 20-year-old woman who is 37 weeks pregnant comes to the emergency department for a severe headache. She states that her blood pressure has been normal throughout her pregnancy and that she does not have a history of hypertension.

On physical examination, pulse rate is 100/min and blood pressure is 160/100 mm Hg. There is mild facial edema and 2+ lower-extremity edema.

Laboratory studies:

Hematocrit	42%
Platelet count	125,000/μL (125 × 10⁹/L)
Uric acid	6.2 mg/dL (0.37 mmol/L)
Blood urea nitrogen	16 mg/dL (5.71 mmol/L)
Creatinine	1.1 mg/dL (97.26 μmol/L)
Sodium	134 meq/L (134 mmol/L)
Potassium	3.4 meq/L (3.4 mmol/L)
Bicarbonate	23 meq /L (23 mmol/L)
Aspartate aminotransferase	65 U/L
Alanine aminotransferase	70 U/L
Urinalysis	1+ protein, trace blood

Which of the following is the most appropriate management for this patient?

(A) Labetalol; follow-up in 24 hours
(B) Home bed rest; follow-up in 48 hours
(C) Hospitalization until spontaneous delivery
(D) Emergency delivery

Answers, Critiques, and Bibliographies

Item 1   Answer: E

Sleep apnea syndrome may contribute to resistant hypertension as well as to increased cardiovascular and cerebrovascular disease risk. Affected patients may have excessive fatigue and may fall asleep while driving or working. This condition has a higher prevalence in overweight men. The pathogenesis of sleep apnea syndrome is complex and linked to obesity, insulin resistance, and increased sodium retention. Several studies have shown that patients with sleep apnea syndrome have increased activity of the sympathetic nervous system, which also occurs in obesity. Coexistent insulin resistance and impaired glucose tolerance also may be present in these patients.

Renovascular hypertension may cause resistant hypertension but is less common than sleep apnea. Atherosclerotic renovascular hypertension usually develops in older patients, whereas fibromuscular dysplasia often presents in younger patients and is more common in women. Primary aldosteronism may be present in as many as 10% of patients with resistant hypertension and is included in the differential diagnosis. However, this condition is less likely in a patient who takes hydrochlorothiazide and has a normal potassium level.

Pheochromocytoma is a rare form of hypertension mediated by excess catecholamines. This condition causes palpitations, diaphoresis, tremor, flushing, and headaches. Diagnosis of pheochromocytoma may be difficult, and the clinical manifestations vary significantly. This patient's presentation is consistent with this condition, but sleep apnea is more likely because it is more common and more likely to be associated with obesity. This patient is at risk for type 2 diabetes mellitus, but his fasting glucose level does not meet the criteria for diabetes. Diabetes is associated with hypertension but is not considered a cause of resistant hypertension.

KEY POINTS

- Sleep apnea is associated with resistant hypertension and is particularly prevalent in obese patients.
- Hypertension associated with sleep apnea may be related to insulin resistance, increased activity of the sympathetic nervous system, and increased sodium retention.

Bibliography

1. **Peppard PE, Young T, Palta M, Dempsey J, Skatrud J**. Longitudinal study of moderate weight change and sleep-disordered breathing. JAMA. 2000;284:3015-21. [PMID: 11122588]
2. **Ip MS, Lam B, Ng MM, Lam WK, Tsang KW, Lam KS**. Obstructive sleep apnea is independently associated with insulin resistance. Am J Respir Crit Care Med. 2002;165:670-6. [PMID: 11874812]
3. **Wolk R, Shamsuzzaman AS, Somers VK**. Obesity, sleep apnea, and hypertension. Hypertension. 2003;42:1067-74. [PMID: 14610096]

Item 2   Answer: E

Preemptive kidney transplantation is associated with improved mortality compared with transplantation performed after a course of dialysis. The reasons for this fact are not entirely clear, but accelerated cardiovascular disease associated with dialysis therapy most likely accounts for a portion of the excess mortality seen in patients treated with dialysis before transplantation. Timely referral of patients with chronic kidney disease to a nephrologist facilitates preemptive transplantation.

Outcomes of living donor renal transplantations are equivalent to or better than those of well-matched deceased donor transplantations. Mortality rates of patients treated with hemodialysis and peritoneal dialysis in the United States are roughly equivalent except for women with diabetes >65 years of age, in whom peritoneal dialysis has been reportedly associated with a higher mortality rate in some centers.

KEY POINT

- Referral to a nephrologist for education and evaluation for consideration of preemptive kidney transplantation is indicated for patients with chronic kidney disease when the glomerular filtration rate reaches the 30 mL/min range.

Bibliography

1. **Mange KC, Joffe MM, Feldman HI**. Effect of the use or nonuse of long-term dialysis on the subsequent survival of renal transplants from living donors. N Engl J Med. 2001;344:726-31. [PMID: 11236776]
2. **Vonesh EF, Snyder JJ, Foley RN, Collins AJ**. The differential impact of risk factors on mortality in hemodialysis and peritoneal dialysis. Kidney Int. 2004;66:2389-401. [PMID: 15569331]

Item 3   Answer: A

This patient most likely has minimal change glomerulopathy. Minimal change disease is the most common cause of the nephrotic syndrome in children and young adults. A low albumin level in the presence of proteinuria is consistent with this condition. Minimal change disease associated with the nephrotic syndrome presents with edema; hypoalbuminemia; hypercholesterolemia; urinary protein excretion >3.5 g/24 h; and numerous oval fat bodies on urinalysis, which is another hallmark of a proteinuric state.

Membranous nephropathy and focal segmental glomerulosclerosis, also forms of the nephrotic syndrome, should be included in the differential diagnosis.

This patient's symptoms are consistent with membranous nephropathy, but this condition typically presents in older individuals and develops less rapidly. Similarly, the development of focal segmental glomerulosclerosis is less drastic compared with this patient's disease course. Membranoproliferative glomerulonephritis is associated with a low C3 level, whereas both the C3 and C4 levels are low in systemic lupus erythematosus. In addition, membranoproliferative glomerulonephritis and systemic lupus erythematosus are unlikely in the absence of hematuria.

KEY POINTS
- Minimal change disease is the most common cause of the nephrotic syndrome in children and young adults.
- The presence of numerous oval fat bodies on urinalysis is a hallmark of a proteinuric state.

Bibliography
1. Minimal change disease, focal segmental glomerular sclerosis and proteinuria. Proceedings of a symposium. Manchester, United Kingdom. July 13-14, 2000. Nephrol Dial Transplant. 2003 Aug;18 Suppl 6:vi1-86. [PMID: 12953033]
2. Roth KS, Amaker BH, Chan JC. Nephrotic syndrome: pathogenesis and management. Pediatr Rev. 2002;23:237-48. [PMID: 12093934]

Item 4   Answer: D

This patient's blood pressure, pulse rate, and laboratory findings are all normal for second-trimester pregnancy. Normal pregnancy causes striking changes in renal hemodynamics and more modest changes in water metabolism. Blood pressure is decreased because of generalized vasodilation. The decreased afterload contributes to increased cardiac output and an increased heart rate. The osmotic threshold for arginine vasopressin is decreased, which causes mild hyponatremia. The antialdosterone effects of progesterone cause potassium levels to slightly decrease. Mild hyperventilation leads to lower P_{CO_2} levels and a compensatory increase in renal bicarbonate excretion, which results in slightly lower bicarbonate levels. Finally, the glomerular filtration rate and renal blood flow significantly increase, resulting in lower creatinine and blood urea nitrogen levels.

This patient's decreased blood pressure and tachycardia are normal for pregnancy. The normal leukocyte count and low-grade fever are not suggestive of sepsis, and volume depletion is unlikely in a patient with normal blood urea nitrogen and creatinine levels. Although the syndrome of inappropriate antidiuretic hormone secretion is associated with decreased sodium levels, this patient's abnormal sodium level is most likely associated with her pregnancy.

KEY POINTS
- Decreased thresholds for arginine vasopressin in normal pregnancy cause relatively lower sodium levels.
- Increased vasodilation in pregnancy is associated with a decreased blood pressure measurement and an increased heart rate.
- In normal pregnancy, increases in the glomerular filtration rate and renal blood flow result in decreased creatinine and blood urea nitrogen levels.

Bibliography
1. Davison JM, Shiells EA, Philips PR, Lindheimer MD. Serial evaluation of vasopressin release and thirst in human pregnancy. Role of human chorionic gonadotrophin in the osmoregulatory changes of gestation. J Clin Invest. 1988;81:798-806. [PMID: 3343339]
2. Chapman AB, Abraham WT, Zamudio S, Coffin C, Merouani A, Young D, et al. Temporal relationships between hormonal and hemodynamic changes in early human pregnancy. Kidney Int. 1998;54:2056-63. [PMID: 9853271]

Item 5   Answer: C

Tissue ischemia is the most likely cause of this patient's hyperkalemia. Hyperkalemia frequently develops in patients using hemodialysis therapy. However, the sudden development of hyperkalemia in an otherwise stable patient on dialysis may indicate the presence of a severe condition. In the absence of an interruption in dialysis therapy or an indication that this treatment is ineffective, hyperkalemia in this setting is caused by a potassium load. Exogenous sources of potassium are absent in this patient, but intracellular sources of this electrolyte include hemolysis, rhabdomyolysis, and tissue ischemia. Blood transfusions carry a significant potassium load; therefore, transfusion of blood off of dialysis is almost always contraindicated in patients on hemodialysis.

This patient's abdominal pain, elevated lactic acid level, and history of atrial fibrillation, as well as the presence of blood in his stool, strongly suggest a diagnosis of mesenteric ischemia. His elevated lactic acid level is characteristic of bowel infarction. Because of this patient's history of atrial fibrillation, he likely had a thromboembolic event involving the mesenteric circulation and now has an ischemic bowel.

This patient's dialysis therapy has been routine and uncomplicated, which excludes inadequate dialysis. This patient's history does not suggest insulin or catecholamine deficiency. Insulin deficiency is uncommonly associated with hyperkalemia but may develop in patients with type 1 diabetes mellitus and often is associated with diabetic ketoacidosis. Deficiency of catecholamines is not a clinically important cause of hyperkalemia. In patients using dialysis, the dialysis treatment prescription determines potassium removal and maintenance of normokalemia does not depend on urinary potassium excretion. Angiotensin-converting enzyme inhibitors decrease the renal excretion of potassium, but this complication occurs only in patients not on dialysis. Therefore, angiotensin-converting enzyme inhibitors are not contraindicated in end-stage renal disease requiring dialysis.

KEY POINTS

- **The sudden development of hyperkalemia in a patient on dialysis may be a sign of tissue necrosis.**
- **Abdominal pain, hematochezia, and lactic acidosis are suggestive of bowel infarction.**

Bibliography

1. **McKinsey JF, Gewertz BL**. Acute mesenteric ischemia. Surg Clin North Am. 1997;77:307-18. [PMID: 9146714]

Item 6   Answer: D

This patient most likely has Henoch–Schönlein purpura. This patient's intermittent episodes of mild abdominal pain are consistent with this condition and typically cause abdominal discomfort and bloating. His skin lesions are typical of cutaneous leukocytoclastic vasculitis with palpable purpuric lesions. The differential diagnosis includes other renal–dermal vasculitic syndromes such as antineutrophil cytoplasmic autoantibody–associated small-vessel vasculitis, systemic lupus erythematosus, cryoglobulinemic vasculitis, and cellulitis-associated poststreptococcal glomerulonephritis.

KEY POINT

- **Henoch–Schönlein purpura is a renal–dermal vasculitis syndrome that may present with intermittent episodes of mild abdominal pain.**

Bibliography

1. **Ballinger S**. Henoch-Schönlein purpura. Curr Opin Rheumatol. 2003;15:591-4. [PMID: 12960486]
2. **Trapani S, Micheli A, Grisolia F, Resti M, Chiappini E, Falcini F, et al**. Henoch Schönlein purpura in childhood: epidemiological and clinical analysis of 150 cases over a 5-year period and review of literature. Semin Arthritis Rheum. 2005;35:143-53. [PMID: 16325655]

Item 7   Answer: A

This patient has osmotic tubular injury due to dextran 40 use. This condition can present as oliguric or nonoliguric acute renal failure and also has been reported in patients treated with mannitol or sucrose-containing preparations of intravenous immune globulin. Patients with preexisting renal insufficiency are at increased risk for developing this disorder. There are no clearly defined diagnostic urinary or laboratory findings associated with this condition, and renal biopsy is needed for definitive diagnosis. Treatment of osmotic tubular injury generally is supportive, but patients with oliguria and sustained increases in plasma osmolality

may benefit from plasma exchange to remove retained dextran 40 and thereby limit further renal injury.

This patient's urinary sediment findings show no muddy brown casts to support a diagnosis of acute tubular necrosis. The absence of hypotension and tachycardia on physical examination and during the surgery is not consistent with prerenal azotemia. Chronic angiotensin-converting enzyme inhibitor therapy is unlikely to cause acute renal failure. Thrombotic microangiopathy is unlikely in the absence of thrombocytopenia and hemolytic anemia. However, because of this patient's recent use of clopidogrel therapy, this diagnosis should be considered. Preliminary evidence shows that IgG inhibitors of the von Willebrand factor–cleaving protease ADAMTS13 mediate clopidogrel-induced thrombotic thrombocytopenic purpura.

KEY POINT

- **Patients with chronic kidney disease have increased risk for acute renal failure because of their use of osmotic agents such as dextran 40, mannitol, and sucrose-containing preparations of intravenous immune globulin.**

Bibliography

1. **Kato A, Yonemura K, Matsushima H, Ikegaya N, Hishida A**. Complication of oliguric acute renal failure in patients treated with low-molecular weight dextran. Ren Fail. 2001;23:679-84. [PMID: 11725914]
2. **Frey L, Messmer K**. Acute oligoanuric renal failure in dextran 40 treated patients [Letter]. Ren Fail. 1998;20:543-5. [PMID: 9606743]

Item 8   Answer: C

Poorly controlled diabetes or hypertension, proteinuria, and cigarette smoking are all risk factors for chronic kidney disease progression. However, treatment of hypertension is the cornerstone in preserving renal function in patients with diabetic nephropathy. Reduction in blood pressure has been shown to influence progression of renal disease and the development of cardiovascular disease in patients with diabetes. The goal of treatment of blood pressure in both type 1 and type 2 diabetes mellitus is to maintain a blood pressure ≤130/80 mm Hg in the absence of significant proteinuria and ≤125/75 mm Hg if accompanied by >1 g/24 h of proteinuria. Angiotensin-converting enzyme inhibitors or angiotensin receptor blockers constitute first-line treatment of hypertension even in patients with advanced diabetic nephropathy.

The beneficial effect of strict metabolic control of diabetes on the progression of advanced renal disease is less established than is strict control of blood pressure. Nevertheless, metabolic control should be improved in this setting in order to minimize the risk for metabolic complications and microvascular and macrovascular complications of diabetes. Native Americans, Mexican Americans, and black patients have an increased burden of diabetic nephropathy and chronic kidney disease, and diabetic nephropathy clusters in families. Proteinuria is a well-recognized risk factor in the progression of renal disease, including diabetic nephropathy. Cigarette smoking has been shown to have significant detrimental effects on the kidney and may cause increased proteinuria and an accelerated decline in renal function.

> **KEY POINT**
>
> • Reduction in blood pressure has been shown to influence the progression of renal disease and the development of cardiovascular disease in patients with diabetes.

Bibliography

1. **Pohl MA, Blumenthal S, Cordonnier DJ, De Alvaro F, Deferrari G, Eisner G, et al.** Independent and additive impact of blood pressure control and angiotensin II receptor blockade on renal outcomes in the irbesartan diabetic nephropathy trial: clinical implications and limitations. J Am Soc Nephrol. 2005;16:3027-37. [PMID: 16120823]

2. **McCullough PA, Bakris GL, Owen WF Jr, Klassen PS, Califf RM.** Slowing the progression of diabetic nephropathy and its cardiovascular consequences. Am Heart J. 2004;148:243-51. [PMID: 15308993]

Item 9   Answer: D

The most appropriate next step in this patient's management is initiation of hemodialysis. This patient has tumor lysis syndrome. This condition may complicate chemotherapy in patients with high tumor burden but occasionally develops spontaneously.

Despite appropriate hydration, this patient developed oliguric acute renal failure associated with marked hyperuricemia and hyperphosphatemia. Failure of medical therapies to adequately control the metabolic abnormalities of tumor lysis syndrome warrants initiation of dialysis, particularly in patients with acute renal failure. Prevention of this condition includes aggressive hydration, as well as allopurinol therapy, which typically is initiated at least 2 days before starting chemotherapy.

Initial therapy for tumor lysis syndrome aims to decrease the urine uric acid, calcium, and phosphorus levels with aggressive hydration. Sodium bicarbonate traditionally has been used because an increase in urinary pH >6.5 can significantly increase the solubility of uric acid. However, an increase in the urinary pH also may promote intratubular precipitation of calcium phosphate and theoretically worsen renal function. Increasing urinary flow rates alone may be as effective as urinary alkalinization in decreasing the risk for uric acid nephropathy associated with tumor lysis syndrome. Therefore, hydration with normal saline is favored.

Recently, a recombinant urate oxidase, rasburicase, has become available for the treatment of hyperuricemia. This agent is most effective in preventing renal failure in patients with severe hyperuricemia rather than reversing established renal failure. Rasburicase is contraindicated in patients with known glucose-6-phosphate dehydrogenase deficiency.

Anaphylaxis has been reported, and rasburicase can induce hemolysis, hemoglobinuria, and methemoglobinemia even in the absence of glucose-6-phosphate dehydrogenase deficiency. Therefore, this agent should be used only in patients who are most likely to develop tumor lysis syndrome. Probenecid is a uricosuric agent and would exacerbate urate crystal formation by increasing intratubular uric acid levels.

> **KEY POINT**
>
> • Dialysis should be considered early in the course of tumor lysis syndrome in patients with oliguric acute renal failure.

Bibliography

1. **Davidson MB, Thakkar S, Hix JK, Bhandarkar ND, Wong A, Schreiber MJ.** Pathophysiology, clinical consequences, and treatment of tumor lysis syndrome. Am J Med. 2004;116:546-54. [PMID: 15063817]

Item 10   Answer: C

Measurement of urine microalbumin is the most appropriate diagnostic study for this patient. Diabetic nephropathy is characterized by abnormal kidney function and albuminuria in the setting of diabetes mellitus. Albuminuria may present as micro- or macroalbuminuria, based on the amount of albumin excreted in the urine. Microalbuminuria is characterized by a urinary albumin–creatinine ratio of 30 mg/g to 300 mg/g, whereas macroalbuminuria is characterized by a urinary albumin–creatinine ratio of >300 mg/g on two separate urine samples performed at least 6 months apart.

The development of microalbuminuria is believed to represent an early stage of diabetic nephropathy. Therefore, urine microalbumin measurement is recommended at least annually in all patients with diabetes. Dipstick urinalysis is a sensitive marker for albumin excretion, but negative results on this study do not exclude the presence of diabetic nephropathy. Because dipstick urinalysis only detects urine albumin levels >30 mg/dL (300 g/L) to 50 mg/dL (500 g/L), this diagnostic study does not detect microalbuminuria.

Inaccuracies in collection methods in 24-hour urine collections can cause underestimation or overestimation of the amount of creatinine and/or albumin excreted in the urine. Therefore, use of 24-hour urine collection to assess the glomerular filtration rate and quantify albuminuria is no longer recommended. Imaging studies such as kidney ultrasonography are useful for estimating the kidney size and revealing obstructive nephropathy in patients with chronic kidney disease but not for diagnosing and assessing risk in diabetic nephropathy.

Serum protein electrophoresis is effective for diagnosing myeloma-related kidney disorders in patients with chronic kidney disease of unknown cause. However, this patient has no symptoms or laboratory abnormalities associated with myeloma-related kidney disorders, such as anemia or hypercalcemia. Therefore, diabetic nephropathy is a more likely diagnosis. The hemoglobin A_{1c} level is useful for determining glycemic control, and poorly controlled diabetes is a risk factor for the development of diabetic nephropathy. However, results of hemoglobin A_{1c} would not confirm the diagnosis, whereas a finding of persistent albuminuria would.

KEY POINTS

- Measurement of urine microalbumin is the screening test of choice for diabetic nephropathy.
- A 24-hour urine collection is no longer recommended to assess kidney function or quantify proteinuria.

Bibliography

1. Eknoyan G, Hostetter T, Bakris GL, Hebert L, Levey AS, Parving HH, et al. Proteinuria and other markers of chronic kidney disease: a position statement of the national kidney foundation (NKF) and the national institute of diabetes and digestive and kidney diseases (NIDDK). Am J Kidney Dis. 2003;42:617-22. [PMID: 14520612]
2. Gerstein HC, Mann JF, Yi Q, Zinman B, Dinneen SF, Hoogwerf B, et al. Albuminuria and risk of cardiovascular events, death, and heart failure in diabetic and nondiabetic individuals. JAMA. 2001;286:421-6. [PMID: 11466120]
3. K/DOQI clinical practice guidelines for chronic kidney disease: evaluation, classification, and stratification. Am J Kidney Dis. 2002;39:S1-266. [PMID: 11904577]

Item 11   Answer: E

The most appropriate next step in this patient's management is adding losartan therapy to his regimen. Hypertension and proteinuria are important risk factors for progression of diabetic nephropathy to end-stage renal disease. Diabetic nephropathy and hypertension are present in 40% to 50% of patients with diabetes. The prevalence of hypertension increases with age and the duration of diabetes. At least 60% of patients who have had diabetes for 10 years have elevated blood pressure. Approximately 75% of patients with diabetes and hypertension require treatment with at least two hypertensive agents. First-line treatment in patients with diabetic nephropathy should be angiotensin-converting enzyme (ACE) inhibitors and angiotensin II receptor blockers. Combination therapy with ACE inhibitors and angiotensin receptor blockers may be more effective than single-agent therapy with either drug in reducing proteinuria and progression of chronic kidney disease. Combination therapy with these agents also may be superior to maximal ACE inhibitor therapy alone.

Dihydropyridine calcium-channel blockers may worsen proteinuria. Increasing this patient's β-blocker dose is not indicated because of his low pulse. The addition of an angiotensin II receptor blocker to this patient's regimen would be more effective than adding an α-receptor blocker. In addition, the potassium and creatinine should be monitored, particularly in patients with renal insufficiency.

KEY POINT

- Combination therapy with angiotensin-converting enzyme inhibitors and angiotensin receptor blockers may be more renoprotective than single-agent therapy with either drug in patients with diabetic nephropathy.

Bibliography

1. Jacobsen P, Andersen S, Rossing K, Jensen BR, Parving HH. Dual blockade of the renin-angiotensin system versus maximal recommended dose of ACE inhibition in diabetic nephropathy. Kidney Int. 2003 May;63(5):1874-80. [PMID: 12675866]
2. Jacobsen P, Rossing K, Parving HH. Single versus dual blockade of the renin-angiotensin system (angiotensin-converting enzyme inhibitors and/or angiotensin II receptor blockers) in diabetic nephropathy. Curr Opin Nephrol Hypertens. 2004;13:319-24. [PMID: 15073491]

Item 12   Answer: D

This patient most likely has Goodpasture's syndrome. The most useful diagnostic study for this condition is an assay for anti–glomerular basement membrane antibodies, which have been found to react with the noncollagenous portion of the α3 chain of type IV collagen in affected patients. The differential diagnosis of this patient's pulmonary–renal syndrome includes antineutrophil cytoplasmic autoantibody–associated small-vessel vasculitis, lupus nephritis, and cryoglobulinemia.

Postinfectious glomerular disease may be associated with a pulmonary–renal syndrome that is marked by pulmonary edema, but this condition is unlikely in the absence of low C3 levels. In addition, this patient has no history of pharyngitis or cellulitis to suggest that he had poststreptococcal glomerulonephritis. Therefore, antistreptolysin O and anti-DNAse B antibodies associated with this condition are likely to be negative.

This patient's condition seems limited to the lungs and kidneys and an antinuclear antibody assay is negative, which are not consistent with a diagnosis of systemic lupus erythematosus with lupus nephritis. Therefore, positive findings on anti–double-stranded DNA or antiphospholipid antibody assays are unlikely. The antiphospholipid antibody syndrome also is not associated with pulmonary hemorrhage and glomerulonephritis.

In some patients, cryoglobulinemia is associated with pulmonary bleeding and glomerulonephritis. However, this presentation is rare and would be accompanied by a very low C4 level and a normal C3 level.

KEY POINT

- An anti–glomerular basement membrane antibody assay is indicated to diagnose Goodpasture's syndrome.

Bibliography

1. Hudson BG, Tryggvason K, Sundaramoorthy M, Neilson EG. Alport's syndrome, Goodpasture's syndrome, and type IV collagen. N Engl J Med. 2003;348:2543-56. [PMID: 12815141]

Item 13   Answer: C

Ambulatory blood pressure monitoring is indicated for this patient. This patient's normal home blood pressure readings suggest a diagnosis of white coat hypertension. However, use of home blood pressure measurement to confirm a diagnosis of white coat hypertension has not been investigated and validated as extensively as ambulatory blood pressure monitoring. The Treatment of Hypertension Based on Home or Office Blood Pressure (THOP) trial suggests that home measurement is less sensitive than ambulatory monitoring. Based on this patient's history of normal blood pressure measurements at home, therapy with either hydrochlorothiazide or enalapril is not indicated and may result in side effects associated with excessive lowering of blood pressure.

KEY POINT

- **In selected patients, ambulatory blood pressure monitoring should be used to diagnose white coat hypertension.**

Bibliography

1. **Staessen JA, Den Hond E, Celis H, Fagard R, Keary L, Vandenhoven G, et al**. Antihypertensive treatment based on blood pressure measurement at home or in the physician's office: a randomized controlled trial. JAMA. 2004;291:955-64. [PMID: 14982911]
2. **Den Hond E, Celis H, Vandenhoven G, O'Brien E, Staessen JA**. Determinants of white-coat syndrome assessed by ambulatory blood pressure or self-measured home blood pressure. Blood Press Monit. 2003;8:37-40. [PMID: 12604935]
3. **Celis H, Staessen JA, Thijs L, Buntinx F, De Buyzere M, Den Hond E, et al**. Cardiovascular risk in white-coat and sustained hypertensive patients. Blood Press. 2002;11:352-6. [PMID: 12523678]

Item 14   Answer: A

This patient's laboratory findings are consistent with the syndrome of inappropriate antidiuretic hormone secretion (SIADH). This condition is characterized by hypotonic hyponatremia with a urine osmolality >100 mosm/kg H_2O in the absence of volume depletion, adrenal insufficiency, congestive heart failure, hypothyroidism, cirrhosis, and/or renal impairment. SIADH is a state in which the patient abnormally retains water despite a low serum osmolarity.

Volume depletion is unlikely in the absence of a low urinary sodium level and a history of vomiting or diarrhea. This patient's history and physical examination findings do not suggest adrenal insufficiency, although this condition may cause hyponatremia if there is a deficiency of mineralocorticoid activity. By definition, this patient has hypoosmolal hyponatremia, which excludes hyperglycemia or other causes of hyperosmolal states that cause a relative dilution of the serum sodium as well as pseudohyponatremia. In pseudohyponatremia, the patient's osmolality would be normal. In addition, trimethoprim–sulfamethoxazole is not known to cause SIADH. Psychogenic polydipsia would present with a low urine osmolality and low urine electrolyte levels. Hyponatremia due to excessive water

ingestion in the absence of renal disease is associated with a very low urine concentration (<50–100 mosm/kg H_2O). Any increase of the urine osmolality signifies an impairment of water excretion.

KEY POINT

- **The syndrome of inappropriate antidiuretic hormone secretion (SIADH) is defined as hypotonic hyponatremia with a urine osmolality >100 mosm/kg H_2O in the absence of volume depletion, adrenal insufficiency, congestive heart failure, hypothyroidism, cirrhosis, and/or renal impairment.**

Bibliography

1. **Moritz ML, Ayus JC**. The pathophysiology and treatment of hyponatraemic encephalopathy: an update [Editorial]. Nephrol Dial Transplant. 2003;18:2486-91. [PMID: 14605269]

Item 15   Answer: D

Inflammatory disorders of the kidney such as acute interstitial nephritis due to antibiotics or nonsteroidal anti-inflammatory drugs often are associated with sterile pyuria as well as eosinophiluria on Wright's or Hansel's stains. Other conditions associated with kidney inflammation such as atheroembolic disease, postinfectious glomerulonephritis, rapidly progressive glomerulonephritis, and pyelonephritis may have eosinophiluria. Therefore, the clinical presentation is essential in making an accurate diagnosis in this setting. The classic triad of acute interstitial nephritis (fever, skin rash, and arthralgias) is present in only a minority of affected patients. More commonly, patients with this condition have only a fever or skin rash in the setting of a medication exposure.

Thrombotic thrombocytopenic purpura should be considered in patients with fever, skin rash, and kidney failure. However, the absence of concomitant anemia, mental status changes, and thrombocytopenia makes this diagnosis less likely. Antineutrophil cytoplasmic autoantibody–associated small-vessel vasculitis also should be considered in patients with kidney failure and concomitant arthralgias, skin rash, and fever. However, this patient's lack of dysmorphic erythrocytes or erythrocyte casts makes this diagnosis unlikely. In addition, her exposure to medication is more suggestive of acute interstitial nephritis.

Suspicion for acute renal failure due to acute tubular necrosis from pyelonephritis should be raised in a patient with kidney failure, fever, and pyuria. However, the lack of other clinical symptoms of sepsis, such as hypotension and tachycardia, makes this condition less likely. Membranous glomerulopathy due to systemic lupus erythematosus may present with skin rash, fever, arthralgias, and kidney failure, but this patient's lack of an active urine sediment and proteinuria are uncommon in this condition and favor the diagnosis of acute interstitial nephritis from antibiotic use.

- The classical triad of acute interstitial nephritis (fever, skin rash, and arthralgias) in the setting of acute or subacute renal failure is present in only a minority of affected patients.

Bibliography

1. **Kodner CM, Kudrimoti A**. Diagnosis and management of acute interstitial nephritis. Am Fam Physician. 2003;67:2527-34. [PMID: 12825841]

2. **Michel DM, Kelly CJ**. Acute interstitial nephritis. J Am Soc Nephrol. 1998;9:506-15. [PMID: 9513915]

Item 16   Answer: C

This patient most likely has membranous nephropathy. Suspicion for this condition is raised in patients >55 years of age. The presence of a slowly progressive nephrotic syndrome suggests the possibility of solid tumor–associated membranous nephropathy. In a patient with a history of squamous cell lung cancer and a new lung nodule in the left upper lobe that may represent recurrent cancer, the association between membranous nephropathy and a solid tumor of the lung is highly likely.

Minimal change disease, focal segmental glomerulosclerosis, and membranous nephropathy are all causes of the nephrotic syndrome. However, membranous nephropathy is most frequently associated with solid tumors. IgA glomerulonephritis and antineutrophil cytoplasmic autoantibody–associated small-vessel vasculitis are unlikely in the absence of hematuria on urinalysis. Similarly, neither of these conditions would be associated with a urinary protein excretion of 15 g/24 h.

- The presence of a slowly progressive nephrotic syndrome suggests the possibility of solid tumor–associated membranous nephropathy.

Bibliography

1. **Burstein DM, Korbet SM, Schwartz MM**. Membranous glomerulonephritis and malignancy. Am J Kidney Dis. 1993;22:5-10. [PMID: 8322793]

2. **Glassock RJ**. Diagnosis and natural course of membranous nephropathy. Semin Nephrol. 2003;23:324-32. [PMID: 12923720]

Item 17   Answer: C

The most important next step in this patient's management is to discontinue ibuprofen and closely monitor renal function. This patient demonstrates many features consistent with chronic kidney disease following exposure to nonsteroidal anti-inflammatory drugs (NSAIDs). Intrarenal prostaglandin secretion is increased in patients with chronic kidney disease and maintains afferent arteriolar vasodilation. Prostaglandin secretion also may increase in hypercalcemia, heart failure, cirrhosis, and true volume depletion. Inhibition of prostaglandin synthesis with an NSAID in these settings can lead to reversible renal vasoconstriction,

decreased glomerular capillary pressure, and acute renal failure. The fractional excretion of sodium is 0.6% according to the following formula:

$$([Urine_{Na+}/Plasma_{Na+}]/[Urine_{Creatinine}/Plasma_{Creatinine}]) \times 100\%$$

This value is consistent with this effect.

Pyelonephritis, which would warrant empiric antibiotic therapy, is unlikely in the absence of fever, leukocytosis, and bacteriuria. Renal biopsy and dialysis would be helpful only if the renal failure persists despite discontinuation of ibuprofen. The presence of leukocyte casts in the urine suggests concurrent tubulointerstitial nephritis, and NSAID-induced interstitial nephritis typically does not respond to corticosteroids.

- Nonsteroidal anti-inflammatory drugs can cause acute interstitial nephritis as well as pre-renal acute renal failure through changes in local glomerular hemodynamics.

Bibliography

1. **Huerta C, Castellsague J, Varas-Lorenzo C, Garcia Rodriguez LA**. Nonsteroidal anti-inflammatory drugs and risk of ARF in the general population. Am J Kidney Dis. 2005;45:531-9. [PMID: 15754275]

2. **Bennett WM, Henrich WL, Stoff JS**. The renal effects of nonsteroidal anti-inflammatory drugs: summary and recommendations. Am J Kidney Dis. 1996;28:S56-62. [PMID: 8669431]

Item 18   Answer: B

This patient most likely has uric acid stones. The majority of kidney stones are composed of calcium, whereas uric acid, struvite, or cystine stones occur less frequently. Uric acid stones occur in 20% of patients with a history of gouty arthritis and may manifest as an acute attack of renal colic with unilateral flank pain and hematuria. Unlike calcium-containing stones, uric acid stones are radiolucent and are not visible on a plain abdominal radiograph. Therefore, spiral CT or ultrasonography of the abdomen are the imaging modalities of choice in this setting. Metabolic abnormalities such as an elevated serum uric acid level, an acidic urine with a pH <5.5, hyperuricosuria, and hypocitraturia increase the incidence of uric acid stone formation. However, crystal stone analysis definitively determines the type of kidney stone.

Although calcium oxalate stones are the most frequent type of kidney stone, uric acid stones are far more likely because of this patient's history of gout, elevated serum uric acid level, acidic urine, and lack of stone visualization on plain abdominal radiography. Calcium phosphorous stones account for 10% of all stones and typically are associated with renal tubular acidosis or primary hyperparathyroidism.

Struvite stones are more common in women and are a result of infection with urease-splitting organisms and an alkaline urine. Cystine stones are extremely uncommon and are caused by cystinuria, a heritable condition in which stones typically develop during childhood.

In patients <50 years of age with microscopic hematuria, infections and kidney diseases such as glomerulonephritis should be considered. In patients >50 years of age with microscopic hematuria and associated risk factors such as cigarette smoking, analgesic abuse, benzene exposure, or a history of voiding abnormalities, genitourinary tract malignancy is more common.

KEY POINT

- **Abdominal CT or ultrasonography are the recommended imaging modalities for uric acid stones.**

Bibliography

1. **Coe FL, Parks JH, Asplin JR.** The pathogenesis and treatment of kidney stones. N Engl J Med. 1992;327:1141-52. [PMID: 1528210]
2. **Cohen RA, Brown RS.** Clinical practice. Microscopic hematuria. N Engl J Med. 2003;348:2330-8. [PMID: 12788998]

Item 19   Answer: A

Guidelines recommend that patients with progressive chronic kidney disease should be referred for creation of a permanent vascular dialysis access when the glomerular filtration rate decreases below 30 mL/min. The best vascular access for hemodialysis is an arteriovenous fistula, which provides better dialysis clearance, longer half-life, and fewer complications compared with grafts and catheters.

Increasing this patient's protein restriction would not retard progression to end-stage renal disease. Moreover, as the glomerular filtration rate continues to decline, this patient may have increased risk for malnutrition. This patient's iron deficiency anemia should be evaluated and treated before starting erythropoietin therapy. Because this patient's blood pressure is well controlled, adding a nondihydropyridine calcium-channel blocker will not slow the progression of chronic kidney disease.

KEY POINT

- **Patients with progressive chronic kidney disease should be referred for creation of a permanent vascular dialysis access when the glomerular filtration rate decreases below 30 mL/min.**

Bibliography

1. **Kazmi WH, Obrador GT, Khan SS, Pereira BJ, Kausz AT.** Late nephrology referral and mortality among patients with end-stage renal disease: a propensity score analysis. Nephrol Dial Transplant. 2004;19:1808-14. [PMID: 15199194]
2. **Khan SS, Xue JL, Kazmi WH, Gilbertson DT, Obrador GT, Pereira BJ, et al.** Does predialysis nephrology care influence patient survival after initiation of dialysis? Kidney Int. 2005;67:1038-46. [PMID: 15698443]

Item 20   Answer: D

The most appropriate next step in this patient's management is ambulatory blood pressure monitoring. White coat hypertension due to this patient's anxiety regarding a new

physician and medication change is highly possible, and ambulatory blood pressure monitoring would confirm this diagnosis. In addition, overtreatment of hypertension in elderly patients is associated with increased adverse effects of medication, particularly symptoms associated with hypotension. Moreover, this patient's fatigue, weakness, and dizziness suggest that she is overmedicated. Although current blood pressure targets for the elderly have not been clearly defined, a systolic blood pressure ≤160 mm Hg in this population has been associated with better outcomes. Ambulatory blood pressure monitoring is useful in this setting to document the level of blood pressure control.

Performing magnetic resonance angiography would be premature in this patient. Renovascular hypertension is a possible cause of resistant hypertension in the elderly, but her symptoms are consistent with overmedication. In addition, her longstanding history of stable hypertension is consistent with primary or essential hypertension. Increasing her hydrochlorothiazide dose before excluding a white coat effect could lead to increased symptoms and worsening of her hypokalemia. Lower doses of medication are indicated for many elderly patients, and 50 mg of hydrochlorothiazide most likely will be poorly tolerated in this patient.

Discontinuation of metoprolol may be reasonable. However, because of her elevated office blood pressure measurements, this agent should be discontinued only after documenting that her blood pressure is adequately controlled. Even in the absence of a specific history of coronary artery disease, this patient's age warrants evaluation for this condition before discontinuing metoprolol.

KEY POINTS

- **Blood pressure measurements in elderly patients who tolerate medication poorly may be higher in the office than at home.**
- **In selected patients, ambulatory blood pressure monitoring can exclude white coat hypertension.**
- **Ambulatory blood pressure monitoring can detect symptoms that may be related to excessive reduction of blood pressure.**

Bibliography

1. Prevention of stroke by antihypertensive drug treatment in older persons with isolated systolic hypertension. Final results of the Systolic Hypertension in the Elderly Program (SHEP). SHEP Cooperative Research Group. JAMA. 1991;265:3255-64. [PMID: 2046107]
2. **Staessen JA, Gasowski J, Wang JG, Thijs L, Den Hond E, Boissel JP, et al.** Risks of untreated and treated isolated systolic hypertension in the elderly: meta-analysis of outcome trials. Lancet. 2000;355:865-72. [PMID: 10752701]

Item 21   Answer: C

This patient's elevated blood pressure, renal insufficiency, and proteinuria detected early in pregnancy are most consistent with chronic glomerulopathy. Preeclampsia would not present before 20 weeks gestation in the absence of a molar pregnancy. This patient's proteinuria and elevated creatinine level indicate the presence of renal disease, which is not consistent with chronic essential hypertension. In addition, signs of renal involvement, such as proteinuria or mild azotemia, are unlikely in a young patient with essential hypertension. Early hypertensive nephrosclerosis may present with these findings, but this condition is highly unlikely in a 25-year-old patient.

Gestational hypertension is characterized by normal blood pressure measurements in early pregnancy and hypertension that develops during the latter part of pregnancy. Unlike preeclampsia, this condition is not associated with proteinuria, elevated creatinine levels, or hyperuricemia. Gestational hypertension usually resolves after delivery; this presentation is known as transient hypertension in pregnancy. However, essential hypertension is the most likely diagnosis if affected patients do not become normotensive by 3 months postpartum; the decrease in blood pressure associated with early pregnancy usually masks this condition initially. Hypertension that presents in patients at <20 weeks gestation is most likely caused by a chronic condition that preceded pregnancy.

KEY POINTS
- **Elevated blood pressure in early pregnancy is most likely caused by a chronic condition.**
- **Glomerulonephritis, not preeclampsia, is the most likely diagnosis in patients with elevated creatinine levels and proteinuria early in pregnancy.**

Bibliography
1. Report of the National High Blood Pressure Education Program Working Group on High Blood Pressure in Pregnancy. Am J Obstet Gynecol. 2000;183:S1-S22. [PMID: 10920346]

Item 22   Answer: D

Abdominal magnetic resonance venography is most likely to establish a definitive diagnosis in this setting. This patient has symptoms of acute renal infarction complicating renal vein thrombosis. A high index of suspicion is needed for obstruction or a vascular event in a patient with a solitary kidney presenting with acute renal failure. Ultrasonography is the best initial screening test to evaluate for urinary tract obstruction and is indicated. However, to definitively diagnose renal vein thrombosis, detailed imaging of the renal vasculature with CT, MRI, or venography is needed.

Renal vein thrombosis occurs with greater frequency in patients with membranous nephropathy and the nephrotic syndrome, and the onset of symptoms suggesting renal infarction warrants pursuit of this condition. Magnetic resonance venography is preferred over CT or radiocontrast venography because iodinated radiocontrast is more nephrotoxic. Doppler ultrasonography can be used to diagnose renal vein thrombosis but lacks the specificity and sensitivity of the studies discussed above. The differential diagnosis includes nephrolithiasis, for which spiral CT without contrast is now the preferred study.

Treatment of renal vein thrombosis consists of anticoagulation with heparin and warfarin. Thrombolytic therapy also can be considered when acute thrombosis is documented. Concurrent pulmonary emboli occur in 10% to 30% of patients with renal vein thrombosis, and patients with renal vein thrombosis can present with symptoms solely attributable to pulmonary embolism.

KEY POINTS
- **Patients with membranous nephropathy are at increased risk for renal vein thrombosis.**
- **CT, MRI, or venography is indicated to definitively diagnose renal vein thrombosis.**

Bibliography
1. **Crew RJ, Radhakrishnan J, Appel G**. Complications of the nephrotic syndrome and their treatment. Clin Nephrol. 2004;62:245-59. [PMID: 15524054]

Item 23   Answer: B

Demeclocycline therapy is indicated to decrease this patient's urine osmolality. The most important determination to make in dealing with hyponatremia is the presence or absence of symptoms of hyponatremic encephalopathy, which include headache and nausea and correspond to cerebral edema. Seizures are the next manifestation, followed by brainstem herniation and, ultimately, respiratory arrest and death. This patient has a normal level of consciousness and does not manifest any of these signs. Demeclocycline is known to decrease urinary concentration and is indicated in this patient to prevent her water-retentive state from worsening. However, type 2 vasopressin receptor antagonists may soon replace demeclocycline in treatment of chronic hyponatremia.

Because she currently has no manifestations of hyponatremic encephalopathy, aggressive therapy is not appropriate regardless of the degree of hyponatremia. Therefore, 3% saline infusion therapy to raise the serum sodium level quickly is not warranted.

Fluid restriction would be ineffective at increasing the serum sodium level. The excretion of electrolytes (both sodium and potassium) is important for determining water balance, a fact that is formalized in the concept of electrolyte-free water clearance. Water excretory capacity can be quickly estimated by comparing the urine electrolytes (sodium + potassium) with the serum electrolytes (sodium + potassium). In this case, the urine electrolyte concentration is 144 meq/L (120 + 24), which exceeds the serum electrolyte concentration (111 + 3.6). Therefore, there is no electrolyte-free water clearance occurring. In other words, the patient is not losing any water in the urine and, as such, any degree of fluid restriction will not increase the serum sodium level.

Sodium chloride tablets are not indicated for hyponatremia. Hyponatremia is a disorder of excess water relative to the total solutes (total exchangeable sodium and potassium), but providing sodium alone does not increase the serum sodium level. Moreover, oral saline contains very little sodium. Hydrochlorothiazide impairs diluting capacity and therefore has no role in the treatment of hyponatremia.

KEY POINT

- **Hypertonic saline is not indicated for asymptomatic hyponatremia.**

Bibliography

1. **Moritz ML, Ayus JC**. The pathophysiology and treatment of hyponatraemic encephalopathy: an update [Editorial]. Nephrol Dial Transplant. 2003;18:2486-91. [PMID: 14605269]

Item 24 Answer: B

This patient most likely has focal segmental glomerulosclerosis. This condition is the most common cause of the nephrotic syndrome in black patients, particularly those of younger age.

Two other possible causes of the nephrotic syndrome, membranous nephropathy and minimal change disease, are much less likely. Minimal change disease primarily occurs in children, whereas membranous nephropathy usually affects older white patients. Membranoproliferative glomerulonephritis and focal proliferative lupus nephritis are both examples of the nephritic syndrome characterized by hypertension, hematuria, and renal insufficiency. Although this patient has hypertension and renal insufficiency, the absence of hematuria makes any form of the nephritic syndrome less likely. Moreover, membranoproliferative glomerulonephritis typically is associated with infectious diseases or systemic lupus erythematosus, of which this patient shows no signs.

KEY POINT

- **Focal segmental glomerulosclerosis is the most common cause of the nephrotic syndrome in black patients, particularly those of younger age.**

Bibliography

1. **Kitiyakara C, Eggers P, Kopp JB**. Twenty-one-year trend in ESRD due to focal segmental glomerulosclerosis in the United States. Am J Kidney Dis. 2004;44:815-25. [PMID: 15492947]

2. **Meyrier A**. Mechanisms of Disease: focal segmental glomerulosclerosis. Nature Clin Pract Nephrol. 2005;1:44-54.

Item 25 Answer: C

The most appropriate next step in this patient's management is plasmapheresis and antiretroviral therapy. This patient presents with the classic pentad of thrombocytopenia, anemia, neurologic symptoms, renal dysfunction, and fever characteristic of thrombotic thrombocytopenic purpura (TTP). The peripheral blood smear shows schistocytes that indicate an underlying thrombotic microangiopathy.

A deficiency or decreased activity of the von Willebrand factor–cleaving protease ADAMTS13 plays an important role in the pathogenesis of TTP–hemolytic uremic syndrome. Decreased cleavage of large multimers of von Willebrand factor by ADAMTS13 synthesized in endothelial cells leads to the persistence of unusually large multimers of von Willebrand factor, which results in platelet activation and endocapillary thrombosis.

Decreased ADAMTS13 activity has been demonstrated in patients with HIV who have TTP, possibly because endothelial production of ADAMTS13 by HIV-infected endothelial cells is decreased or because these patients produce an IgG inhibitor of ADAMTS13 activity. Plasmapheresis has been shown to effectively ameliorate TTP in this setting, and highly active antiretroviral therapy reduces the incidence of relapses. If plasmapheresis is not available, infusions of cryoprecipitate-free fresh frozen plasma may be helpful until plasma exchange can be performed. However, this intervention is not the preferred initial therapy.

Infusions of cryoprecipitate are contraindicated in this setting, because this fraction of plasma is enriched with von Willebrand factor. Platelet transfusions may worsen renal and neurologic complications and therefore generally are avoided. Renal biopsy is indicated for selected patients with atypical features in whom the diagnosis remains uncertain when thrombocytopenia is not a limiting factor; however, a clinical diagnosis can be established in this patient. Oral corticosteroids may be beneficial but are insufficient as the sole intervention.

KEY POINT

- **Antiretroviral therapy and plasmapheresis are indicated for patients with HIV infection and thrombotic thrombocytopenic purpura.**

Bibliography

1. **Eaton ME**. Selected rare, noninfectious syndromes associated with HIV infection. Top HIV Med. 2005;13:75-8. [PMID: 16082058]

2. **Miller RF, Scully M, Cohen H, Roedling S, Starke R, Edwards SG, et al**. Thrombotic thrombocytopaenic purpura in HIV-infected patients. Int J STD AIDS. 2005;16:538-42. [PMID: 16105187]

3. **Tsai HM**. Advances in the pathogenesis, diagnosis, and treatment of thrombotic thrombocytopenic purpura. J Am Soc Nephrol. 2003;14:1072-81. [PMID: 12660343]

Item 26 Answer: C

The presence of gram-positive bacilli on Gram stain in a renal transplant recipient strongly suggests meningitis due to *Listeria monocytogenes*. *L. monocytogenes* is one of the most common bacterial pathogens that causes meningitis in renal transplant recipients. Therapy for this condition consists of high-dose ampicillin, and gentamicin is often added for synergy during the first week of therapy or until the patient shows clinical improvement. A high index of suspicion for this pathogen should be maintained in renal transplant recipients with meningitis. *Listeria* are gram-positive rods. However, these rods also may be gram variable and therefore can be confused with *Pneumococci*, diphtheroids, or *Haemophilus* species.

Combination therapy with vancomycin and ceftriaxone constitutes appropriate empiric therapy for most patients with meningitis. However, the presence of many gram-positive bacilli on Gram stain warrants initiation of therapy for *Listeria* infection. Ceftriaxone alone would not be sufficient to treat *Listeria*.

KEY POINT

- *Listeria* is a common cause of meningitis in renal transplant recipients.

Bibliography

1. **Armstrong RW, Fung PC**. Brainstem encephalitis (rhombencephalitis) due to *Listeria monocytogenes:* case report and review. Clin Infect Dis. 1993;16:689-702. [PMID: 8507761]
2. **Singh N, Husain S**. Infections of the central nervous system in transplant recipients. Transpl Infect Dis. 2000;2:101-11. [PMID: 11429020]
3. **Mylonakis E, Hohmann EL, Calderwood SB**. Central nervous system infection with *Listeria monocytogenes*. 33 years' experience at a general hospital and review of 776 episodes from the literature. Medicine (Baltimore). 1998;77:313-36. [PMID: 9772921]

Item 27   Answer: A

The majority of kidney stones are comprised of calcium, predominantly calcium oxalate, and the most common metabolic disturbance of calcium-containing stones is hypercalciuria. This condition results from increased gastrointestinal absorption of calcium rather than a renal leakage of calcium in the urine. Less commonly, hyperoxaluria occurs in patients with increased dietary intakes of oxalate, which is contained in nuts, chocolate, rhubarb, and spinach. Hyperoxaluria also may occur in the setting of inflammatory bowel disease or malabsorption syndromes due to excessive gastrointestinal absorption of oxalate in the colon caused by a lack of intestinal calcium available for oxalate binding. The high affinity for oxalate to bind to calcium in the urine results in insoluble precipitates that form calcium oxalate stones.

Therapy to decrease the risk for stone recurrence includes increasing dietary calcium to 1 g/d to 4 g/d, restricting oxalate-rich foods, and increasing fluid intake to >2 L/d. Calcium intake has a paradoxical effect in calcium oxalate stone disease; higher amounts of dietary calcium bind to oxalate in the gastrointestinal tract, which prevents absorption.

Increased sodium intake is believed to worsen stone disease by increasing urinary excretion of calcium and uric acid. Increasing animal protein intake worsens several types of kidney stones by acidifying the urine and increasing urinary excretion of calcium, which favors crystallization of calcium stones and contributes to hyperuricosuria in patients with uric acid stone disease.

The use of thiazide diuretics such as hydrochlorothiazide or chlorthalidone decreases urinary calcium excretion and is recommended to prevent stones in patients with hypercalciuria. However, loop diuretics such as furosemide worsen hypercalciuria and increase the risk for recurrent stone formation.

KEY POINTS

- Increasing dietary calcium intake to 1 g/d to 4 g/d decreases the risk for recurrent calcium oxalate stones.
- High-protein and -sodium diets can worsen kidney stone disease by causing hypercalciuria and hyperuricosuria.

Bibliography

1. **Coe FL, Parks JH, Asplin JR**. The pathogenesis and treatment of kidney stones. N Engl J Med. 1992;327:1141-52. [PMID: 1528210]
2. **Pak CY**. Kidney stones. Lancet. 1998;351:1797-801. [PMID: 9635968]

Item 28   Answer: D

This patient most likely has a mixed anion gap metabolic acidosis with a respiratory acidosis. A decrease in the bicarbonate level accompanied by an elevated anion gap is consistent with a primary metabolic acidosis. Winter's formula can be used to estimate the expected CO_2:

$$1.5 \times [HCO_3^-] + 4 \pm 2$$

According to this formula, this patient's P_{CO_2} is significantly elevated above this level, which indicated the presence of a respiratory acidosis. In addition, this patient's P_{CO_2} is much higher than would be expected based upon the degree of acidemia, which indicates that his condition is secondary to inadequate ventilation from pneumonia.

KEY POINTS

- A decrease in the bicarbonate level accompanied by an elevated anion gap is consistent with a primary metabolic acidosis.
- In a patient with a primary metabolic acidosis, a P_{CO_2} that is much higher than would be expected based on the degree of acidemia indicates a condition that is secondary to inadequate ventilation.

Bibliography

1. **Pierce NF, Fedson DS, Brigham KL, Mitra RC, Sack RB, Mondal A**. The ventilatory response to acute base deficit in humans. Time course during development and correction of metabolic acidosis. Ann Intern Med 1970;72:633-40. [PMID: 5448093]

Item 29   Answer: C

Renal transplantation would provide this patient with the best chance of survival and the highest quality of life. Annual mortality rates are now <8% for cadaveric transplant recipients and <4% for living related transplant recipients. Renal transplantation is most beneficial in young people and in patients with diabetes mellitus.

Annual mortality rates for patients with diabetes on dialysis in recent years range from 21% to 25%. Recent evidence shows a slight increase in mortality in patients with diabetes and in elderly patients treated with peritoneal dialysis compared with hemodialysis. The best option for patients with type 1 diabetes mellitus is living related donor kidney transplantation and an insulin pump.

KEY POINTS

- **Compared with hemodialysis therapy, renal transplantation offers a survival advantage in patients with diabetic nephropathy and end-stage renal disease.**
- **Renal transplantation is most beneficial in young people and in patients with diabetes mellitus.**

Bibliography

1. **Giri M**. Choice of renal replacement therapy in patients with diabetic end stage renal disease. EDTNA ERCA J. 2004;30:138-42. [PMID: 15715116]
2. **Ganesh SK, Hulbert-Shearon T, Port FK, Eagle K, Stack AG**. Mortality differences by dialysis modality among incident ESRD patients with and without coronary artery disease. J Am Soc Nephrol. 2003;14:415-24. [PMID: 12538742]

Item 30   Answer: C

Performing an aldosterone–renin ratio (ARR) is the most appropriate next step in this patient's management. This patient's clinical presentation of hypokalemia not attributable to a diuretic, a mild metabolic alkalosis, and an elevated sodium level is consistent with primary hyperaldosteronism. Screening for this condition is indicated for all patients with early-onset, severe, or resistant hypertension, although some affected patients are persistently normokalemic. The ARR is the preferred screening test for distinguishing between essential hypertension and primary aldosteronism. Most experts recommend that an ARR between 20 and 30 warrants further diagnostic testing. However, a high ARR alone is not diagnostic of primary hyperaldosteronism, and demonstration of autonomous hypersecretion of aldosterone is needed to confirm this diagnosis. The aldosterone and renin activity are best measured after potassium levels are corrected and drugs that suppress (such as β-blockers and angiotensin-converting enzyme inhibitors) or raise (such as diuretics) renin levels have been discontinued.

Renovascular hypertension is not associated with hypokalemia in the absence of diuretic use. Renovascular hypertension may cause resistant hypertension, but this patient's presentation is more consistent with primary aldosteronism. In addition, the ARR is most likely to provide useful information and is simpler as a first screening test. Hydrochlorothiazide may improve blood pressure control but is likely to exacerbate this patient's hypokalemia and metabolic alkalosis. Benign, nonfunctioning nodules may develop in the adrenal glands that are unrelated to hypertension. Therefore, imaging of the adrenal glands is indicated in patients with suspicion for primary hyperaldosteronism only after results of biochemical and hormonal testing (such as low plasma renin activity, high aldosterone secretion, or elevated ARR) are shown to be consistent with this diagnosis.

KEY POINTS

- **Hyperaldosteronism should be considered in patients with difficult-to-control hypertension and hypokalemia in the absence of diuretic use.**
- **Hyperaldosteronism should be considered in patients with difficult-to-control hypertension even in the absence of hypokalemia.**
- **The aldosterone–renin ratio is a reasonable screening study for primary hyperaldosteronism.**

Bibliography

1. **Mulatero P, Stowasser M, Loh KC, Fardella CE, Gordon RD, Mosso L, et al**. Increased diagnosis of primary aldosteronism, including surgically correctable forms, in centers from five continents. J Clin Endocrinol Metab. 2004;89:1045-50. [PMID: 15001583]
2. **Grim CE**. Evolution of diagnostic criteria for primary aldosteronism: why is it more common in "drug-resistant" hypertension today? Curr Hypertens Rep. 2004;6:485-92. [PMID: 15527695]
3. **Plouin PF, Amar L, Chatellier G**. Trends in the prevalence of primary aldosteronism, aldosterone-producing adenomas, and surgically correctable aldosterone-dependent hypertension [Editorial]. Nephrol Dial Transplant. 2004;19:774-7. [PMID: 15031328]

Item 31   Answer: C

Statins increasingly have been recognized as a cause of acute rhabdomyolysis presenting with muscle weakness, kidney failure, and an increase in creatine kinase levels. Classically in rhabdomyolysis, release of myoglobin from skeletal muscle causes a false positive result for blood on dipstick urinalysis, but microscopic analysis of the urine sediment reveals no intact erythrocytes.

Acute glomerulonephritis may have an associated myositis such as that which presents in the vasculitic syndromes and in autoimmune disorders. However, this patient's lack of an active urine sediment with dysmorphic erythrocytes and erythrocyte casts makes this diagnosis unlikely. Hypertensive nephrosclerosis is characterized by hypertension and non-nephrotic proteinuria with a bland urine sediment and slowly progressive loss of kidney function, which is not consistent with this patient's clinical presentation. Acute interstitial nephritis presents with the classical triad of fever, skin rash, and arthralgias. This condition typically is associated with a medication exposure, and urinalysis in affected patients reveals sterile pyuria and eosinophiluria rather than hematuria.

KEY POINT

- **Rhabdomyolysis-associated acute renal failure presents with dipstick-positive hematuria but no intact erythrocytes on microscopic analysis of the urine sediment.**

Bibliography
1. **Zager RA**. Rhabdomyolysis and myohemoglobinuric acute renal failure [Editorial]. Kidney Int. 1996;49:314-26. [PMID: 8821813]
2. **Thompson PD, Clarkson P, Karas RH**. Statin-associated myopathy. JAMA. 2003;289:1681-90. [PMID: 12672737]

Item 32   Answer: C

Heparin therapy can be a cause of hyperkalemia in the hospital setting in patients with either normal renal function or renal insufficiency. This agent inhibits the synthesis of aldosterone and thus leads to impairment of renal potassium secretion in the distal tubule. Distal flow of urine to the distal nephron and aldosterone action are needed for potassium excretion to occur. This patient's glomerular filtration rate is normal, but the decreased distal secretion of potassium is associated with an impairment in potassium excretion.

Metformin is associated with lactic acidosis and is contraindicated in renal failure. However, this agent is not associated with hyperkalemia. Phenytoin and meperidine similarly are not associated with the development of hyperkalemia, although meperidine has an active metabolite, normeperidine, that can accumulate in the setting of renal insufficiency and is therefore contraindicated in patients with renal insufficiency. Atenolol blocks the uptake of potassium by the cells and therefore may theoretically cause hyperkalemia. However, this effect is β_2-adrenergic mediated and rarely occurs in β_1-receptor blockers such as atenolol. Additionally, in this case the problem developed during the hospitalization and since the patient has been on a stable dose of the medication it cannot be the primary cause of the hyperkalemia.

KEY POINT
- **Heparin therapy inhibits aldosterone synthesis and therefore may cause hyperkalemia.**

Bibliography
1. **Leehey D, Gantt C, Lim V**. Heparin-induced hypoaldosteronism. Report of a case. JAMA. 1981;246:2189-90. [PMID: 7026818]

Item 33   Answer: C

Focal segmental glomerulosclerosis is the most likely cause of this patent's proteinuria. The presence of oval fat bodies on urinalysis, proteinuria, hypoalbuminemia, and hypercholesterolemia suggests the development of the nephrotic syndrome. Focal segmental glomerulosclerosis, which may be caused by reflux nephropathy, is particularly likely in this patient.

KEY POINT
- **The development of the nephrotic syndrome in the setting of urinary reflux is most likely caused by focal segmental glomerulosclerosis.**

Bibliography
1. **Kohler JR, Tencer J, Thysell H, Forsberg L, Hellstrom M**. Long-term effects of reflux nephropathy on blood pressure and renal function in adults. Nephron Clin Pract. 2003;93:C35-46. [PMID: 12411757]

Item 34   Answer: B

The next best step in this patient's management is bolus therapy with 1000 mL of normal saline (0.9%). This patient's history of decreased intake, vomiting, and ongoing diuretic use is consistent with extracellular fluid volume contraction. Her decreased skin turgor and hypotension also support this diagnosis.

The absence of reflex tachycardia may be a result of β-blocker use. Her relatively normal to slightly elevated bicarbonate level in the setting of acute renal failure likely reflects increased proximal tubular sodium bicarbonate reabsorption, as well as a prerenal state. The fractional excretion of sodium is 6%, calculated according to the following formula:

$$([Urine_{Na+}/Plasma_{Na+}]/[Urine_{Creatinine}/Plasma_{Creatinine}]) \times 100\%$$

This finding may be associated with her use of chlorthalidone but also may reflect the transition of prerenal failure into ischemic tubular injury. The urinary sediment can be bland early in the course of ischemic tubular injury. Initial therapy should aim to correct the extracellular fluid deficit using isotonic saline. However, overzealous hydration in the setting of oliguric ischemic tubular injury, which is suspected in this patient, may cause pulmonary edema. Therefore, close monitoring of urine output and volume status is warranted.

Because this patient has asymptomatic hyponatremia in the setting of volume depletion, normal saline is preferred over hypertonic saline. Dialysis is indicated only if the renal function fails to improve after hydration. Fluid restriction would help to correct the hyponatremia but would not resolve the volume deficit and resultant impaired organ perfusion. Administration of dopamine without correcting the volume deficit could potentially exacerbate impaired renal perfusion.

KEY POINT
- **The fractional excretion of sodium may be >4% in patients with prerenal acute renal failure who use diuretics.**

Bibliography
1. **Schrier RW, Wang W, Poole B, Mitra A**. Acute renal failure: definitions, diagnosis, pathogenesis, and therapy. J Clin Invest. 2004;114:5-14. [PMID: 15232604]

Item 35   Answer: C

In the setting of the nephrotic syndrome, deteriorating renal function and a urinary protein excretion that markedly increases over the course of 6 months accompanied by worsening peripheral edema raises the suspicion for renal vein thrombosis. The loss of several inhibitors of the clotting system, such as angiotensin III, into the urine predisposes patients with the nephrotic syndrome to the development of deep venous and renal vein thrombosis.

Overaggressive diuresis can cause kidney dysfunction, but this presentation would be accompanied by findings associated with volume depletion, including elevated total bicarbonate blood urea nitrogen levels. In addition, this condition does not cause an increase in proteinuria. Renal stones can cause flank pain. However, a rise in the creatinine level indicates the presence of bilateral obstructive stones, which would present with leukocyturia, not an increase in proteinuria.

KEY POINT

- Patients with the nephrotic syndrome are predisposed to develop deep venous and renal vein thrombosis.

Bibliography

1. **Crew RJ, Radhakrishnan J, Appel G**. Complications of the nephrotic syndrome and their treatment. Clin Nephrol. 2004;62:245-59. [PMID: 15524054]
2. **Nickolas TL, Radhakrishnan J, Appel GB**. Hyperlipidemia and thrombotic complications in patients with membranous nephropathy. Semin Nephrol. 2003;23:406-11. [PMID: 12923730]

Item 36   Answer: C

The most appropriate therapy for this patient is initiation of antibiotics. Staghorn calculi are branched stones that fill all or part of the renal pelvis. These calculi most commonly are composed of struvite magnesium, ammonium phosphate, and/or calcium carbonate. Staghorn calculi form as a result of chronic infections with urease-splitting organisms such as *Proteus* and *Klebsiella* species that convert urea to ammonia, causing alkaline urine and struvite crystallization. Women are more likely to develop struvite stones, and imaging studies used to evaluate chronic urinary tract infections frequently identify these stones.

The initial treatment of struvite calculi consists of eliminating the infection with antibiotic therapy. However, this therapy rarely completely eliminates the stone, and referral for stone removal is indicated.

Further alkalinization of the urine with potassium citrate therapy is contraindicated in struvite stone disease because it is associated with increased struvite crystallization and stone growth. Allopurinol is indicated to decrease hyperuricosuria in uric acid stones but does not affect staghorn calculi. Dietary modifications such as increasing fluid and calcium intake prevent crystal formation and/or oxalate absorption in calcium-containing stones. However, these interventions do not appear to have the same benefits in struvite calculi.

KEY POINTS

- Staghorn calculi form as a result of chronic infections with urease-splitting organisms such as *Proteus* or *Klebsiella.*
- Stone removal in struvite stone disease often is indicated to prevent recurrence of infection and stone growth.

Bibliography

1. **Coe FL, Parks JH, Asplin JR**. The pathogenesis and treatment of kidney stones. N Engl J Med. 1992;327:1141-52. [PMID: 1528210]
2. **Pak CY**. Kidney stones. Lancet. 1998;351:1797-801. [PMID: 9635968]

Item 37   Answer: D

Use of angiotensin-converting enzyme inhibitors in normotensive or hypertensive patients without microalbuminuria who have type 2 diabetes mellitus has been shown to prevent the development of microalbuminuria. Microalbuminuria is the first clinical sign of diabetic nephropathy and a major risk factor for the development of clinical proteinuria, chronic kidney disease progression, and cardiovascular death.

Therapy with a nondihydropyridine calcium channel blocker or an α-blocker would not prevent the development of microalbuminuria. Dihydropiridine calcium channel blockers accelerate development of microalbuminuria and would be contraindicated in this patient.

KEY POINTS

- Angiotensin-converting enzyme inhibitor therapy has been shown to prevent the development of microalbuminuria in patients who have diabetes and normoalbuminuria.
- Microalbuminuria is the first clinical sign of diabetic nephropathy and a major risk factor for the development of clinical proteinuria, chronic kidney disease progression, and cardiovascular death.

Bibliography

1. **Ruggenenti P, Fassi A, Ilieva AP, Bruno S, Iliev IP, Brusegan V, et al**. Preventing microalbuminuria in type 2 diabetes. N Engl J Med. 2004;351:1941-51. [PMID: 15516697]
2. **Mogensen CE**. New treatment guidelines for a patient with diabetes and hypertension. J Hypertens Suppl. 2003;21:S25-30. [PMID: 12769164]

Item 38   Answer: B

The most appropriate next step in this patient's management is adrenal vein sampling for aldosterone and cortisol. This patient's suppressed plasma renin activity and high urinary aldosterone excretion are consistent with primary hyperaldosteronism. The most common causes of this condition are aldosterone-producing adenoma (Conn's syndrome) and bilateral adrenal hyperplasia.

Aldosterone-producing adenoma can be resolved surgically by removal of the involved adrenal gland, but adrenalectomy usually is associated with a cure rate of only 50% to 60%. Adrenalectomy is not curative in this setting because smaller, functioning nodules may be present in the contralateral adrenal gland that are too small to visualize on CT scanning; the nodule observed on a CT scan may not be a functional adenoma; primarily essential hypertension may be present. In older patients, coexistent essential hypertension is more likely to be present and adrenalectomy is less likely to be curative. Therefore, adrenal vein sampling to document unilateral secretion of aldosterone from the adrenal gland with the nodule and suppression of aldosterone secretion from the contralateral gland is recommended before surgery, particularly in patients >40 years of age. Simultaneous cortisol measurements document that the sample was obtained from the adrenal vein, where cortisol levels should be higher, rather than the inferior vena cava.

Laparoscopic adrenalectomy is not recommended without adrenal vein sampling in older patients with suspicion for primary aldosteronism. Iodocholesterol scanning, which distinguishes functional adrenal nodules from nonfunctional incidental masses or carcinomas, would be an appropriate alternative to this study. Even if this patient declines further testing and surgery, the appropriate medical treatment would be aldosterone blockade. Therefore, renal arteriography is not warranted. A thiazide diuretic would exacerbate her hypokalemia. An inherited chimeric gene resulting in increased aldosterone production, which is abnormally regulated by adrenocorticotropic hormone, causes glucocorticoid-remediable hyperaldosteronism. The biochemical (such as low potassium levels, high sodium levels, metabolic alkalosis) and hormonal (such as low renin activity levels, high aldosterone levels) changes associated with this condition and aldosterone-producing adenomas are similar. However, a dexamethasone suppression test is not indicated because glucocorticoid-remediable hyperaldosteronism is not associated with an adrenal adenoma.

KEY POINT

- The most common causes of primary hyperaldosteronism are aldosterone-producing adenoma (Conn's syndrome) and bilateral adrenal hyperplasia.

Bibliography

1. Nocaudie-Calzada M, Huglo D, Lambert M, Ernst O, Proye C, Wemeau JL, et al. Efficacy of iodine-131 6beta-methyl-iodo-19-norcholesterol scintigraphy and computed tomography in patients with primary aldosteronism. Eur J Nucl Med. 1999;26:1326-32. [PMID: 10541832]

2. Stowasser M, Gordon RD. Primary aldosteronism: learning from the study of familial varieties. J Hypertens. 2000;18:1165-76. [PMID: 10994747]
3. Rossi GP, Sacchetto A, Chiesura-Corona M, De Toni R, Gallina M, Feltrin GP, et al. Identification of the etiology of primary aldosteronism with adrenal vein sampling in patients with equivocal computed tomography and magnetic resonance findings: results in 104 consecutive cases. J Clin Endocrinol Metab. 2001;86:1083-90. [PMID: 11238490]

Item 39   Answer: A

The most appropriate next step in this patient's management is discontinuing 5% dextrose in 1/4 strength normal saline and initiating therapy with 3% saline via infusion pump. This patient developed iatrogenic hyponatremic encephalopathy because of hypotonic fluid use in the postoperative setting. She is at high risk for mortality or the development of permanent neurologic injury if not treated expeditiously and appropriately. Children, menstruant women, and hypoxic patients have a particularly high risk for a poor outcome in hyponatremic encephalopathy. In this setting, therapy with 3% saline would raise the serum sodium level to a mildly hyponatremic level. Early intervention is important in mild cerebral edema to prevent seizures and respiratory arrest.

Therapy with 0.9% saline would not increase this patient's serum sodium level. Because she is euvolemic, volume expansion is not indicated to correct her condition. However, this treatment would be appropriate therapy in a volume-depleted patient who is not acutely symptomatic. This patient's clinical scenario strongly suggests a diagnosis of hyponatremic encephalopathy. This condition warrants treatment with hypertonic saline, which is safe only in the setting of close monitoring. CT scanning is not likely to yield useful information and would cause a dangerous delay in therapy. Therapy with hypertonic saline is safe if proper monitoring occurs. Initiation of naloxone therapy or switching meperidine with fentanyl is not indicated because this patient's symptoms are not associated with narcotic use and would delay treatment of her condition.

KEY POINTS

- **Hypotonic fluids should not be used post-operatively.**
- **Normal saline (0.9%) is the most appropriate intravenous fluid when fluid therapy is indicated in the postoperative setting.**

Bibliography

1. Ayus JC, Krothapalli RK, Arieff AI. Treatment of symptomatic hyponatremia and its relation to brain damage. A prospective study. N Engl J Med. 1987;317:1190-5. [PMID: 3309659]
2. Ayus JC, Wheeler JM, Arieff AI. Postoperative hyponatremic encephalopathy in menstruant women. Ann Intern Med. 1992;117:891-7. [PMID: 1443949]
3. Moritz ML, Ayus JC. Prevention of hospital-acquired hyponatremia: a case for using isotonic saline. Pediatrics. 2003;111:227-30. [PMID: 12563043]

Item 40 Answer: C

This patient's symptoms are consistent with Sjögren's syndrome. Hypergammaglobulinemia is common in this condition, and anti-Ro/SSA and anti-La/SSB autoantibody assays are positive in 80% and 50% of affected patients, respectively. Renal manifestations of Sjögren's syndrome include interstitial nephritis; type I distal renal tubular acidosis; nephrogenic diabetes insipidus; and glomerular lesions, such as membranous nephropathy and membranoproliferative glomerulonephritis. Sjögren's syndrome is currently the leading cause of interstitial nephritis among white patients in the United States.

Systemic lupus erythematosus can present with interstitial nephritis. However, this condition usually is accompanied by other clinical manifestations of lupus, such as synovitis, malar rash, and hypocomplementemia. Scleroderma renal disease often presents with severe hypertension (known as scleroderma renal crisis) and typically is accompanied by the usual cutaneous manifestations associated with scleroderma, including skin thickening and hardening. Because of this patient's elevated protein level, myeloma cast nephropathy is included in the differential diagnosis. However, this diagnosis is less likely because she has symptoms of sicca syndrome, which are characteristic of Sjögren's syndrome.

KEY POINT

- Sjögren's syndrome is a common cause of interstitial nephritis.

Bibliography

1. Bossini N, Savoldi S, Franceschini F, Mombelloni S, Baronio M, Cavazzana I, et al. Clinical and morphological features of kidney involvement in primary Sjögren's syndrome. Nephrol Dial Transplant. 2001;16:2328-36. [PMID: 11733624]

Item 41 Answer: C

Collapsing focal segmental glomerulosclerosis is the most likely cause of this patient's renal dysfunction. This patient's proteinuria, low albumin level, and peripheral edema, as well as the presence of oval fat bodies on urinalysis, are consistent with the nephrotic syndrome. In black patients with HIV infection who have the nephrotic syndrome, a collapsing form of focal segmental glomerulosclerosis is the most likely diagnosis.

Crystal-induced renal failure caused by sulfamethoxazole or intravenous acyclovir is unlikely in the absence of crystals detected on urinalysis. Treatment with various medications may cause renal failure in patients with HIV infection, including highly active antiretroviral therapy, pentamidine, and ritonavir. However, these patients present with acute renal failure manifested by broad granular casts and an elevated creatinine level. Postinfectious glomerulonephritis associated with hepatitis C is a possibility but typically presents with hematuria in addition to proteinuria, as well as low C3 and C4 levels.

KEY POINTS

- A collapsing form of focal segmental glomerulosclerosis is the most likely diagnosis in black patients with HIV infection who have the nephrotic syndrome.
- Postinfectious glomerulonephritis associated with hepatitis C typically presents with hematuria, proteinuria, and low C3 and C4 levels.

Bibliography

1. Franceschini N, Napravnik S, Eron JJ Jr, Szczech LA, Finn WF. Incidence and etiology of acute renal failure among ambulatory HIV-infected patients. Kidney Int. 2005;67:1526-31. [PMID: 15780107]
2. Balow JE. Nephropathy in the context of HIV infection [Editorial]. Kidney Int. 2005;67:1632-3. [PMID: 15780122]

Item 42 Answer: D

The most appropriate next step in this patient's management is infusion of 1.5 L of normal saline over the next 24 hours. The differential diagnosis of renal failure in this patient includes prerenal azotemia, hepatorenal syndrome, ischemic tubular injury, and sepsis-induced acute renal failure. The first step in differentiating among these conditions is expansion of the plasma volume with either isotonic saline or colloid in order to exclude a prerenal cause. Evaluation for an infectious process, particularly spontaneous bacterial peritonitis, also is indicated.

Use of octreotide and midodrine, or placement of a transjugular intrahepatic portosystemic shunt (TIPS), is premature, because the diagnosis of hepatorenal syndrome has not yet been established. However, evidence suggesting that combination therapy with octreotide and midodrine is effective in improving renal function and perhaps survival in patients with hepatorenal syndrome is growing. TIPS may provide short-term improvement in renal function in patients with hepatorenal syndrome but should be used only as a last resort due to the associated increased risk for encephalopathy. Absolute contraindications to TIPS include congestive heart failure, systemic infection, and severe pulmonary hypertension.

Repeat large-volume paracentesis in a patient with moderate-volume ascites may increase the risk for further ischemic renal injury. However, a diagnostic paracentesis to evaluate for spontaneous bacterial peritonitis would be warranted, and patients with recurrent large-volume ascites frequently require repeated large-volume paracentesis. Nevertheless, removal of >5 L of ascitic fluid by paracentesis without the use of plasma expanders is associated with a derangement in circulatory function, which can cause a higher rate of recurrent ascites and renal dysfunction. Volume expansion with infusions of colloidal solutions, such as albumin, is effective in preventing these complications. The incidence of renal dysfunction also is significantly decreased in patients with spontaneous bacterial peritonitis treated with albumin infusions.

- **Albumin infusions decrease the risk for acute renal failure in patients undergoing paracentesis with >5 L of volume removed and in patients with spontaneous bacterial peritonitis.**

Bibliography

1. **Gines P, Cardenas A, Arroyo V, Rodes J**. Management of cirrhosis and ascites. N Engl J Med. 2004;350:1646-54. [PMID: 15084697]
2. **Sort P, Navasa M, Arroyo V, Aldeguer X, Planas R, Ruiz-del-Arbol L, et al.** Effect of intravenous albumin on renal impairment and mortality in patients with cirrhosis and spontaneous bacterial peritonitis. N Engl J Med. 1999;341:403-9. [PMID: 10432325]
3. **Cardenas A**. Hepatorenal syndrome: a dreaded complication of end-stage liver disease. Am J Gastroenterol. 2005;100:460-7. [PMID: 15667508]

Item 43   Answer: D

Palliative care is the most appropriate treatment for this patient. A study on outcomes of octogenarians on dialysis demonstrated poor outcomes in patients with poor functional status (defined as a Karnofsky score <40, particularly for those patients with poor nutrition and body mass indices <18). In these patients, the probability of survival at 6 months was only 50%. Therefore, palliative care and supportive measures are most appropriate in this patient.

Median survival on hemodialysis was 28.9 months in carefully selected octogenarians who were functionally independent, compared with 8.9 months in patients treated conservatively. A Karnofsky score >40, early referral, and improved nutritional status assessed by a BMI >22 correlated with improved outcomes. Outcomes on peritoneal dialysis are generally equivalent to hemodialysis in all populations except for women with diabetes >65 years of age, in whom mortality was increased. Poor nutritional status is not a contraindication to dialysis but has been demonstrated to be an independent predictor of poor survival on dialysis. Health-related quality of life is unlikely to be significantly affected by initiation of dialysis in patients with poor functional status but has been shown to improve in the first year of dialysis therapy in carefully selected octogenarians with functional independence. A low-protein diet may be useful in alleviating uremic symptoms but is relatively contraindicated in the setting of a decubitus ulcer.

- **Octogenarians with poor functional status are unlikely to experience improvement or benefit from dialysis.**

Bibliography

1. **Joly D, Anglicheau D, Alberti C, Nguyen AT, Touam M, Grunfeld JP, et al.** Octogenarians reaching end-stage renal disease: cohort study of decision-making and clinical outcomes. J Am Soc Nephrol. 2003;14:1012-21. [PMID: 12660336]
2. **Korevaar JC, Jansen MA, Dekker FW, Boeschoten EW, Bossuyt PM, Krediet RT, et al.** Evaluation of DOQI guidelines: early start of dialysis treatment is not associated with better health-related quality of life. National Kidney Foundation-Dialysis Outcomes Quality Initiative. Am J Kidney Dis. 2002;39:108-15. [PMID: 11774109]

Item 44   Answer: A

The best initial therapy for this patient is increasing his dietary calcium intake. Nephrolithiasis is a chronic, recurring condition. A total of 15% of affected patients have a stone recurrence at 1 year and 50% by 10 years after the initial stone. Several dietary modifications have been shown to decrease the recurrence rate and are recommended for patients with a history of stone disease. Unfortunately, only a minority of patients are compliant with dietary changes in the long term.

Most importantly, patients with nephrolithiasis should increase fluid intake to >2 L/d, which increases urine volume and decreases the concentration of stone promoters in the urinary tract. Calcium intake has a paradoxical effect in calcium-containing stone disease; higher amounts of dietary calcium bind to oxalate in the gastrointestinal tract and therefore prevent absorption and decrease both hyperoxaluria and calcium oxalate stone formation.

Dietary sources of citrate, such as 4 oz of lemon juice, also are recommended to increase urinary citrate levels and decrease both urinary calcium levels and the incidence of recurrent calcium oxalate stones. Increasing animal protein intake may be a factor in several types of kidney stones by acidifying the urine and increasing urinary excretion of calcium, which favors crystallization of calcium stones and contributes to hyperuricosuria in uric acid stone disease. Finally, increased sodium intake is believed to contribute to stone disease by increasing urinary excretion of calcium and uric acid and is not recommended for patients with recurrent stone disease.

- **Increasing calcium intake decreases the risk for calcium oxalate stones because calcium binds to gastrointestinal sources of oxalate and therefore prevents absorption.**
- **Dietary modifications such as decreasing animal protein intake, decreasing sodium intake, and increasing citrate can reduce the risk for recurrent kidney stones without additional medical therapy.**

Bibliography

1. **Coe FL, Parks JH, Asplin JR**. The pathogenesis and treatment of kidney stones. N Engl J Med. 1992;327:1141-52. [PMID: 1528210]
2. **Curhan GC, Willett WC, Speizer FE, Spiegelman D, Stampfer MJ**. Comparison of dietary calcium with supplemental calcium and other nutrients as factors affecting the risk for kidney stones in women. Ann Intern Med. 1997;126:497-504. [PMID: 9092314]
3. **Parks JH, Asplin JR, Coe FL**. Patient adherence to long-term medical treatment of kidney stones. J Urol. 2001;166:2057-60. [PMID: 11696706]

Item 45   Answer: C

This patient most likely has autosomal dominant polycystic kidney disease, which is the most commonly inherited kidney disease. Clinical manifestations of this condition include renal, hepatic, and pancreatic cysts; intracranial, thoracic, and abdominal aortic aneurysms; and colonic diverticulae. Hypertension also is common. Certain manifestations of autosomal dominant polycystic kidney disease, such as intracranial aneurysms, tend to cluster in families. The gene *ADPKD1* located on chromosome 16 is responsible for 85% to 90% of cases of autosomal dominant polycystic kidney disease in white patients, whereas *ADPKD2* located on chromosome 4 is responsible for the remainder of cases.

Autosomal recessive polycystic kidney disease is a rare disease caused by a gene located on chromosome 6. This condition is associated with oligohydramnios and large echogenic kidneys *in utero*, and hepatic fibrosis with biliary dysgenesis occurs in nearly all affected patients. Acquired cystic kidney disease occurs in patients with progressive, noncystic kidney disease, in up to 40% of patients who have been on dialysis for 3 years, and in up to 80% to 90% of patients on dialysis for 5 to 10 years. These patients are more prone to develop kidney neoplasms. Nephronophthisis–medullary cystic kidney disease complex is an inherited disease with two common variants, an autosomal recessive familial juvenile nephronophthisis and an autosomal dominant medullary cystic kidney disease. The clinical manifestations of this disease complex include reduced urinary concentrating ability, polyuria, polydipsia, hypovolemia, and hyponatremia early in the course of the disease.

KEY POINTS

- Clinical manifestations of autosomal dominant polycystic kidney disease include renal, hepatic, and pancreatic cysts; intracranial, thoracic, and abdominal aortic aneurysms; and colonic diverticulae.
- Certain manifestations of autosomal dominant polycystic kidney disease, such as intracranial aneurysms, tend to cluster in families.

Bibliography

1. **Wilson PD**. Polycystic kidney disease. N Engl J Med. 2004;350:151-64. [PMID: 14711914]
2. **Arnaout MA**. Molecular genetics and pathogenesis of autosomal dominant polycystic kidney disease. Annu Rev Med. 2001;52:93-123. [PMID: 11160770]

Item 46   Answer: B

Patients with pheochromocytoma should be treated with α-blockade therapy for at least 2 weeks before surgery. Phenoxybenzamine provides complete α-blockade, and dosages of this agent should be titrated to blood pressure control.

Calcium-channel blockers do not provide α-blockade and therefore are not indicated. Labetalol has been reported to effectively control hypertension in patients with pheochromocytoma. However, this agent is not a reliable α-blocker and the potential for intraoperative hypertension is greater with labetalol compared with phenoxybenzamine.

Because α-tone can exacerbate hypertension in this setting, β-blockade is not indicated for pheochromocytoma unless adequate α-blockade already has been administered. Before surgery, patients with pheochromocytoma should be euvolemic or slightly volume expanded. However, high sympathetic tone and pressure natriuresis associated with pheochromocytoma may cause volume depletion, which may result in secondary stimulation of the renin–angiotensin system and worsening hypertension. Diuretics are contraindicated because these agents may exacerbate this situation.

KEY POINTS

- Patients with pheochromocytoma should receive an α-blocker 2 weeks before surgery.
- β-Blockade in the absence of α-blockade is contraindicated in patients with pheochromocytoma and may lead to hypertensive crisis.

Bibliography

1. **Manger WM, Gifford RW**. Pheochromocytoma. J Clin Hypertens (Greenwich). 2002;4:62-72. [PMID: 11821644]
2. **Bravo EL**. Pheochromocytoma: an approach to antihypertensive management. Ann N Y Acad Sci. 2002;970:1-10. [PMID: 12381537]

Item 47   Answer: B

If present at the time of diagnosis, the combination of upper and/or lower respiratory tract disease and proteinase-3 antinuclear cytoplasmic antibody positivity is associated with the highest likelihood of a relapsing disease in antinuclear cytoplasmic antibody–associated small-vessel vasculitis. This patient has achieved clinical remission of this condition and wishes to discontinue her immunosuppressive regimen. However, she has all three of these high risk factors for relapse. Therefore, continuation of maintenance therapy is the best option in this setting.

Renal dysfunction alone or in combination with other factors is not associated with a higher risk for relapse of antinuclear cytoplasmic antibody–associated small-vessel vasculitis. However, the creatinine level at the time of diagnosis directly relates to the long-term outcome of renal dysfunction. The presence of skin vasculitis is an important predictor of better outcome in patients with small-vessel vasculitis, most likely because these patients seek medical attention for their dermatologic condition and are then diagnosed with small-vessel vasculitis early in the disease course.

KEY POINT

- The combination of upper and/or lower respiratory tract disease and proteinase-3 antinuclear cytoplasmic antibody positivity at the time of diagnosis is associated with the highest likelihood of relapsing disease in antinuclear cytoplasmic antibody–associated small-vessel vasculitis.

Bibliography

1. **Hogan SL, Falk RJ, Chin H, Cai J, Jennette CE, Jennette JC, et al**. Predictors of relapse and treatment resistance in antineutrophil cytoplasmic antibody-associated small-vessel vasculitis. Ann Intern Med. 2005;143:621-31. [PMID: 16263884]

Item 48   Answer: D

Hydrochlorothiazide is a common cause of hyponatremia in the outpatient setting. Thiazide diuretics work at the level of the cortical collecting duct. Therefore, these agents maintain urinary concentrating capacity but not diluting capacity, which makes them prone to cause hyponatremic encephalopathy. By inducing relative volume depletion, antidiuretic hormone secretion is stimulated, which leads to urinary concentration and water retention. Conversely, loop diuretics act in the ascending limb of Henle and therefore impair both urinary concentrating and diluting capacity. To prevent this complication, patients should weigh themselves before and 48 hours after initiating therapy with these agents. If a patient does not lose weight or gains weight after initiation of a thiazide diuretic, he or she has a high risk for developing hyponatremic encephalopathy.

Furosemide acts on the ascending limb of Henle on the Na-K-2Cl transporter, which causes a tremendous increase in the distal flow and brisk increase in urine output that can "wash out" the corticomedullary concentration gradient that is necessary for urinary concentrating capacity. By increasing the flow of solutes to the distal tubule, urinary diluting capacity is similarly impaired because the reabsorptive mechanisms cannot handle the tremendous flow of solutes. Theoretically, furosemide therapy would significantly increase water intake because urinary diluting capacity is impaired. Therefore, hyponatremia can result, although this presentation is rare.

Acetazolamide acts in the proximal tubule as a carbonic anhydrase IV inhibitor. Blocking this enzyme in the proximal tubule impairs bicarbonate reabsorption but not diluting capacity and is most often associated with hypokalemia and metabolic acidosis. Spironolactone is not associated with the development of hyponatremia. However, this agent acts in the kidney as a potassium-sparing diuretic and frequently is associated with hyperkalemia. Amiloride also is not associated with hyponatremia. Like spironolactone, this agent is a potassium-sparing diuretic. However, amiloride acts by blocking epithelial sodium channels important for potassium secretion in the distal tubule.

KEY POINT

- **Hydrochlorothiazide can cause severe hyponatremia.**

Bibliography

1. **Ayus JC, Arieff AI**. Chronic hyponatremic encephalopathy in postmenopausal women: association of therapies with morbidity and mortality. JAMA. 1999;281:2299-304. [PMID: 10386554]

Item 49   Answer: C

Cryoglobulinemic glomerulonephritis is most likely causing this patient's renal abnormalities. This patient's hematuria, renal insufficiency, and hypertension, as well as the presence of dysmorphic erythrocytes on urinalysis, are consistent with glomerulonephritis. In a patient with this condition, the presence of Raynaud's phenomenon, a purpuric rash, and abnormal findings on liver function studies suggest a diagnosis of cryoglobulinemia. Cryoglobulinemia typically decreases the C4 levels, which indicates activation of the classical pathway of complement activation, more than the C3 level. However, low C3 levels and normal C4 levels indicate an alternative pathway complement activation and other glomerular diseases. Finally, both an immune complex–mediated glomerulonephritis and disease processes that activate the alternative pathway are unlikely in a patient with normal C3 and C4 levels.

Henoch–Schönlein purpura, antineutrophil cytoplasmic autoantibody–associated small-vessel vasculitis, and anti–glomerular basement membrane glomerulonephritis are less likely in this patient. This patient has no manifestations of systemic lupus erythematosus. In addition, this condition is unlikely in the absence of decreased C3 and C4 levels.

KEY POINTS

- **Cryoglobulinemia is characterized by Raynaud's phenomenon, a purpuric rash, abnormal findings on liver function studies, and the presence of glomerulonephritis.**
- **Cryoglobulinemia typically decreases the C4 level, which indicates activation of the classical pathway of complement activation, more than the C3 level.**

Bibliography

1. **Trejo O, Ramos-Casals M, Garcia-Carrasco M, Yague J, Jimenez S, de la Red G, et al**. Cryoglobulinemia: study of etiologic factors and clinical and immunologic features in 443 patients from a single center. Medicine (Baltimore). 2001;80:252-62. [PMID: 11470986]
2. **Cacoub P, Costedoat-Chalumeau N, Lidove O, Alric L**. Cryoglobulinemia vasculitis. Curr Opin Rheumatol. 2002;14:29-35. [PMID: 11790993]

Item 50   Answer: B

Kidney biopsy is the most appropriate next step in the management of this patient's kidney disease. This patient has acute glomerulonephritis characterized by hypertension, edema, and findings of proteinuria and glomerular hematuria on urinalysis. Serologic studies to assess the underlying cause of glomerular disease, such as assays for antineutrophil cytoplasmic antibodies in small-vessel vasculitis, antinuclear antibodies in lupus nephritis, and hepatitis C antibodies with cryoglobulinemia, may help to narrow the differential diagnosis. However, these studies should not preclude a kidney biopsy to determine the diagnosis; indicate the cause; predict the natural history and prognosis of the injury; and, most importantly, direct treatment.

Pulmonary hemorrhage is associated with the vasculitic syndromes and Goodpasture's disease and may manifest simply as blood-streaked sputum or complete respiratory failure. Pulmonary hemorrhage with concomitant acute glomerulonephritis is associated with substantial morbidity and mortality and requires aggressive immunosuppressive therapy and possibly plasmapheresis. Although this patient is at risk for congestive heart failure based on her age, history of hypertension, and cardiac arrhythmia, her pulmonary edema and peripheral edema are attributable to hypoalbuminemia and nephrotic range proteinuria.

Presumptive treatment of the nephrotic syndrome with corticosteroids primarily is limited to the pediatric population in which minimal change disease is the most common cause of the nephrotic syndrome and who are highly responsive to this therapy. The incidence of minimal change disease declines with age, and initiation of corticosteroid therapy without a pathologic diagnosis by kidney biopsy precludes its use.

Analgesics such as nonsteroidal anti-inflammatory drugs may cause acute renal failure due to acute interstitial nephritis or the nephrotic syndrome due to membranous glomerulopathy or minimal change disease. However, narcotics such as oxycodone are not associated with acute glomerular disease. Therefore, discontinuation of these agents would be of limited value.

KEY POINTS

- **Renal biopsy is indicated for patients with acute glomerulonephritis of unknown cause.**
- **Pulmonary hemorrhage associated with acute glomerulonephritis is associated with substantial morbidity and mortality.**

Bibliography

1. Orth SR, Ritz E. The nephrotic syndrome. N Engl J Med. 1998;338:1202-11. [PMID: 9554862]
2. Jennette JC. Rapidly progressive crescentic glomerulonephritis. Kidney Int. 2003;63:1164-77. [PMID: 12631105]

Item 51   Answer: E

A recent cardiac catheterization in a patient with atherosclerosis raises the possibility of atheroembolic disease. The presence of livedo reticularis, Hollenhorst plaque, cyanotic toe, low C3 levels, and peripheral eosinophilia is consistent with this diagnosis.

Radiocontrast nephropathy also is high in the differential diagnosis. However, atheroembolic disease is more likely because of the absence of epithelial or muddy brown casts. Prerenal azotemia is unlikely in a patient with edema and abnormal urinary sediment findings with no evidence of postural hypotension or other clinical signs of left ventricular dysfunction.

Interstitial nephritis can present with eosinophilia, pyuria, and hematuria. However, peripheral cyanosis, hypocomplementemia, and clinical evidence of emboli are more suggestive of atheroembolic disease. Microscopic polyangiitis can present with abdominal pain and livedo reticularis, but this patient's history and other clinical features are more compatible with atheroemboli. In addition, complement levels are normal in microscopic polyangiitis.

KEY POINTS

- **Atheroembolic disease can mimic vasculitis.**
- **The presence of livedo reticularis, Hollenhorst plaque, cyanotic toe, low C3 levels, and peripheral eosinophilia suggests a diagnosis of atheroembolic disease.**
- **Atheroembolic disease should be suspected in patients with erosive atherosclerosis presenting with acute renal failure.**

Bibliography

1. Modi KS, Rao VK. Atheroembolic renal disease. J Am Soc Nephrol. 2001;12:1781-7. [PMID: 11461954]

Item 52   Answer: B

The most appropriate management for this patient is referral for parathyroidectomy. Approximately 20% of patients with primary hyperparathyroidism have calcium-containing stones due to hypercalciuria and hyperphosphaturia. Her clinical signs and symptoms of hyperparathyroidism include hypercalcemia, renal insufficiency, and underlying osteoporosis and warrant referral for parathyroidectomy rather than bisphosphonate or estrogen therapy or observation.

Decreasing dietary intake of calcium may temporarily affect the hypercalcemia but is contraindicated in the long term because of her osteoporosis. Stone removal is not indicated because there is no evidence of obstruction, and stones <5 mm in diameter typically can pass without surgical intervention. Alkalization of the urine with citrate therapy is recommended to decrease the solubility of uric acid or to correct hypocitraturia that predisposes patients to calcium-forming stones. However, this therapy does not prevent recurrent stone disease in primary hyperparathyroidism.

KEY POINTS

- **Asymptomatic hypercalcemia in a patient with a history of calcium stones warrants evaluation for primary hyperparathyroidism.**
- **Parathyroidectomy should be considered for patients with calcium-containing stones secondary to primary hyperparathyroidism.**

Bibliography

1. Coe FL, Parks JH, Asplin JR. The pathogenesis and treatment of kidney stones. N Engl J Med. 1992;327:1141-52. [PMID: 1528210]

Item 53   Answer: D

This patient's clinical presentation and the pattern of inheritance are consistent with Alport's syndrome. This inherited condition is caused by mutations in basement membrane collagen that result in persistent microscopic hematuria, progressive nephritis with proteinuria, and progressive decline in renal function to end-stage renal disease. Affected patients may have high-frequency sensorineural hearing loss and/or ocular abnormalities. Classic Alport's syndrome, an X-linked dominant form responsible for 80% of cases of this condition, results from a variety of mutations in the $\alpha 5$ chain of the type IV collagen gene (*COL4A5*). These mutations lead to substitution of another amino acid for a glycine residue, which alters the structure of the $\alpha 5$ collagen chain and prevents normal incorporation of $\alpha 3$ and $\alpha 4$ collagen chains into basement membranes. Mutations in the *COL4A3* and the *COL4A4* genes on chromosome 2 result in autosomal recessive (15% of cases) or autosomal dominant (5% of cases) forms.

Thin basement membrane disease, also known as benign familial hemoglobinuria, is a variant of Alport's syndrome inherited in an autosomal dominant pattern as a result of mutations in the type IV collagen gene (*COL4A3* and *COL4A4*). This condition is characterized by persistent microscopic hematuria and episodes of gross hematuria. The pathognomonic renal biopsy finding is irregular thinning of the glomerular basement membrane on electron microscopy with attenuation of the lamina densa. Unlike classic Alport's syndrome, thin basement membrane disease is rarely associated with proteinuria, loss of renal function, or extrarenal abnormalities. IgA nephropathy and membranoproliferative glomerulonephritis can cause hematuria and proteinuria but usually are not inherited.

KEY POINTS

- **Alport's syndrome causes persistent microscopic hematuria, progressive nephritis with proteinuria, and progressive decline in renal function to end-stage renal disease.**
- **Alport's syndrome is an inherited condition that may present with high-frequency sensorineural hearing loss and/or ocular abnormalities.**

Bibliography
1. Kashtan CE. The nongenetic diagnosis of thin basement membrane nephropathy. Semin Nephrol. 2005;25:159-62. [PMID: 15880326]
2. Hudson BG, Tryggvason K, Sundaramoorthy M, Neilson EG. Alport's syndrome, Goodpasture's syndrome, and type IV collagen. N Engl J Med. 2003;348:2543-56. [PMID: 12815141]

Item 54   Answer: A

The most appropriate therapeutic intervention in this patient is aggressive resuscitation with isotonic saline to optimize renal perfusion. Renal-dose dopamine has no benefit in the prevention or treatment of acute renal failure. Prophylactic fasciotomy increases the risk for sepsis in the setting of acute crush injury. Mannitol does not prevent tubular injury in rhabdomyolysis but may have a role in the treatment of acute muscle compartment syndrome. Acetazolamide can acutely raise the urinary pH, but this increase is unlikely to occur once a new steady state is achieved at a lower bicarbonate concentration. However, clinical trials have established no definitive benefit of urinary alkalinization. Urinary alkalinization can promote the precipitation of calcium phosphate within the renal tubules. Therefore, hydration with isotonic saline is preferred.

KEY POINT

- **Isotonic saline is preferred over bicarbonate-containing solutions for resuscitation of patients with rhabdomyolysis.**

Bibliography
1. Brown CV, Rhee P, Chan L, Evans K, Demetriades D, Velmahos GC. Preventing renal failure in patients with rhabdomyolysis: do bicarbonate and mannitol make a difference? J Trauma. 2004;56:1191-6. [PMID: 15211124]
2. Better OS, Rubinstein I, Reis DN. Muscle crush compartment syndrome: fulminant local edema with threatening systemic effects. Kidney Int. 2003;63:1155-7. [PMID: 12631101]

Item 55   Answer: B

Initiation of amlodipine is indicated for this patient. This patient's 30-year history of hypertension is most consistent with primary or essential hypertension. Concomitant therapy with an angiotensin-converting enzyme inhibitor and a diuretic may cause acute renal failure in the setting of bilateral renovascular hypertension. Therefore, this patient's normal creatinine level despite antihypertensive therapy with an angiotensin-converting enzyme inhibitor and a diuretic makes hemodynamically significant renal artery stenosis unlikely. In a patient whose blood pressure remains elevated on repeat measurements or ambulatory blood pressure monitoring, an increase in the antihypertensive medication is appropriate.

Before performing invasive testing in elderly patients, it is important to document high blood pressure with repeat office measurements, home measurements, or ambulatory blood pressure monitoring; therefore, renal angiography is not indicated at this time. At this time, optimization of medical therapy is indicated even in patients with renovascular hypertension. Measuring plasma renin activity can help to identify whether a primarily renin-mediated mechanism is causing hypertension. However, antihypertensive therapy can affect the accuracy of the results of this study and reduce the usefulness of this study as a screening test for hypertension. For example, β-blockers decrease renin levels, whereas diuretics and angiotensin inhibitors increase these levels.

Renovascular hypertension may be present, but essential hypertension is more likely to be the primary diagnosis. In addition, in the absence of renal failure or pulmonary edema, medical rather than invasive therapy is preferred for blood pressure control, even when renovascular hypertension is suspected. Therefore, invasive studies such as renal vein sampling and magnetic resonance angiography of the renal arteries are not indicated.

KEY POINT

- In the absence of renal failure or flash pulmonary edema, medical rather than invasive therapy is preferred for blood control, even when renovascular hypertension is suspected.

Bibliography

1. van Jaarsveld BC, Krijnen P, Pieterman H, Derkx FH, Deinum J, Postma CT, et al. The effect of balloon angioplasty on hypertension in atherosclerotic renal-artery stenosis. Dutch Renal Artery Stenosis Intervention Cooperative Study Group. N Engl J Med. 2000;342:1007-14. [PMID: 10749962]
2. Hirsch AT, Haskal ZJ, Hertzer NR, Bakal CW, Creager MA, Halperin JL, et al. ACC/AHA 2005 Practice Guidelines for the management of patients with peripheral arterial disease (lower extremity, renal, mesenteric, and abdominal aortic): a collaborative report from the American Association for Vascular Surgery/Society for Vascular Surgery, Society for Cardiovascular Angiography and Interventions, Society for Vascular Medicine and Biology, Society of Interventional Radiology, and the ACC/AHA Task Force on Practice Guidelines (Writing Committee to Develop Guidelines for the Management of Patients With Peripheral Arterial Disease): endorsed by the American Association of Cardiovascular and Pulmonary Rehabilitation; National Heart, Lung, and Blood Institute; Society for Vascular Nursing; TransAtlantic Inter-Society Consensus; and Vascular Disease Foundation. Circulation. 2006;113:e463-654. [PMID: 16549646]

Item 56   Answer: A

This patient has solute diuresis leading to hypernatremia, which commonly develops in the critical care setting. By dividing the ratio of the sodium plus potassium levels in the urine by the sodium and potassium level in the serum, urinary water losses can be assessed. The ratio of the urine sodium and potassium level in the urine is lower than that in the blood. In this patient, the ratio is 70/156, which means that 45% of his urine is "electrolyte containing" and, conversely, that 55% of the urine is electrolyte-free water. Therefore, at his current urine output, he is losing 110 mL (0.55×200 mL/h) of water per hour in the urine. Water replacement must be at least equal to this in order to replace his ongoing water losses in the urine.

This patient's high urine osmolality is caused by antidiuretic hormone secretion, which is increasing the urine concentration. His low urine sodium and potassium levels accompanied by a high urine osmolality signify the presence of a nonelectrolyte osmole in the urine that "obligates" water loss. This scenario is a classic presentation of an osmotic diuresis secondary to urea. His high urea load is most likely secondary to the hypercatabolic state secondary to critical illness, which causes an increase in protein breakdown resulting in significant urea generation, and stress. The high amount of protein in the total parenteral nutrition also is likely to exacerbate the urea load.

Central diabetes insipidus and nephrogenic diabetes insipidus are unlikely in a patient with a high urine osmo-

lality. These conditions are associated with a water diuresis and a low urine osmolality. Postobstructive diuresis usually is not associated with a concentrated urine. In addition, this patient's clinical presentation is not suggestive of this condition. Urinary tract infections do not cause hypernatremia, and polyuria is not a sequelae of a urinary tract infection. However, patients with urinary tract infection may develop urinary urgency that can be misdiagnosed as polyuria.

KEY POINT

- Solute diuresis secondary to a high urea load is a common cause of hypernatremia in the critical care setting.

Bibliography

1. Achinger SG, Moritz ML, Ayus JC. Dysnatremias: why are patients still dying? South Med J. 2006;99:353-62; quiz 363-4. [PMID: 16634244]

Item 57   Answer: C

The most appropriate management for this patient is MRI of the abdomen. Cystic lesions of the kidney are exceedingly common and increase with age and in individuals with chronic kidney disease. The majority of cystic lesions discovered by imaging studies are simple in nature and require no further investigation. Conversely, complex cysts or mass lesions in the kidney require more aggressive imaging using CT or MRI because of the associated increased risk for malignancy. Malignant cysts or mass lesions in the kidney are associated with enhancement after administration of contrast, a size >3 cm, areas of necrosis, or marginal irregularities. Nephrectomy is warranted in these patients instead of kidney biopsy, which is contraindicated because malignant tumors may metastasize via the biopsy tract. These tumors also are quite vascular, and biopsy in this setting is associated with an increased risk for bleeding.

Performing a repeat ultrasonography in 6 months or reassurance alone is not recommended in a patient in whom ultrasonography already reveals a 3.5-cm concerning lesion that is complex in nature. These management strategies may delay the diagnosis of renal cell carcinoma. Cystoscopy is the procedure of choice in a patient with persistent hematuria and risk factors for genitourinary tract malignancy, such as cigarette smoking, analgesic abuse, benzene exposure, or a history of voiding abnormalities. However, this study is not recommended as a first-line management strategy in the evaluation of a renal mass.

KEY POINTS

- Simple cysts discovered on renal imaging studies require no therapy.
- Complex renal cysts on ultrasonography require follow-up imaging with CT or MRI.
- Kidney biopsy is contraindicated in patients with complex renal masses suspicious for malignancy.

Bibliography

1. Higgins JC, Fitzgerald JM. Evaluation of incidental renal and adrenal masses. Am Fam Physician. 2001;63:288-94, 299. [PMID: 11201694]

Item 58   Answer: A

This patient most likely has light-chain nephropathy. His peripheral edema, hypoalbuminemia, hypercholesterolemia, and renal insufficiency are consistent with the nephrotic syndrome. In older patients with this condition, a paraprotein is a likely cause and is associated with such conditions as systemic amyloidosis and multiple myeloma. These conditions are in turn associated with light-chain deposition disease, hypoalbuminemia, elevated urinary protein excretion, and lipiduria on urinalysis. Therefore, pursuit of amyloid or other conditions associated with paraproteinemias, including light-chain deposition disease, with serologic studies and a bone biopsy is indicated.

Membranoproliferative glomerulonephritis is unlikely in the absence of high blood pressure and hematuria, although this patient does have a degree of renal insufficiency. Idiopathic focal segmental glomerulosclerosis is unlikely to occur in an elderly patient and would not be associated with a systemic illness. Membranous nephropathy in an older patient has an associated risk for cancer, particularly solid tumors. However, this patient's relative hypotension and systemic manifestations are not consistent with this condition.

> **KEY POINT**
>
> - A paraprotein associated with systemic amyloidosis or multiple myeloma is a likely cause of the nephrotic syndrome in older patients.

Bibliography

1. Gertz MA, Comenzo R, Falk RH, Fermand JP, Hazenberg BP, Hawkins PN, et al. Definition of organ involvement and treatment response in immunoglobulin light chain amyloidosis (AL): a consensus opinion from the 10th International Symposium on Amyloid and Amyloidosis, Tours, France, 18-22 April 2004. Am J Hematol. 2005;79:319-28. [PMID: 16044444]

2. Sezer O, Eucker J, Jakob C, Possinger K. Diagnosis and treatment of AL amyloidosis. Clin Nephrol. 2000;53:417-23. [PMID: 10879660]

3. Abraham RS, Katzmann JA, Clark RJ, Bradwell AR, Kyle RA, Gertz MA. Quantitative analysis of serum free light chains. A new marker for the diagnostic evaluation of primary systemic amyloidosis. Am J Clin Pathol. 2003;119:274-8. [PMID: 12579999]

Item 59   Answer: D

This patient most likely has angiotensin-converting enzyme (ACE) inhibitor–induced prerenal acute renal failure. Therefore, the most appropriate initial step in this patient's management is discontinuing enalapril.

Generally, an increase in the creatinine level up to 30% is acceptable after initiation of ACE inhibitors or angiotensin receptor blockers. A recent study demonstrated that continued ACE inhibitor therapy was associated with sustained renoprotective benefit in patients with stage III and IV chronic kidney disease. Therefore, continuation of ACE inhibitor therapy in patients with chronic kidney disease is indicated when possible. Once-daily administration of lower doses of these agents is initially indicated, as is measurement of the potassium and creatinine levels 7 to 10 days after initiation of therapy and then every 2 to 3 months. However, this patient demonstrated a >100% increase in the creatinine level, which should raise suspicion for bilateral renal artery stenosis or advanced intrarenal small-vessel disease.

The glomerular filtration rate (GFR) in patients with bilateral renal artery stenosis is maintained to a great extent by an angiotensin II–induced vasoconstriction at the efferent arteriole. Both ACE inhibitors and angiotensin receptor blockers cause loss of efferent arteriolar vasoconstriction with a resultant decrease in the glomerular capillary pressure and GFR.

This patient's urine sediment is not sufficiently active to warrant a renal biopsy. Discontinuation of enalapril would be favored over a dose reduction because of this patient's marked decline in GFR and the risk for subsequent ischemic renal injury. Magnetic resonance angiography of the renal arteries would document the status of the renal arteries after discontinuing enalapril. However, percutaneous angioplasty for renal artery stenosis generally is reserved for patients who remain hypertensive despite aggressive pharmacologic therapy. Prospective randomized clinical trials have yet to definitively establish indications for intervening to preserve renal function or decrease cardiovascular complications. Losartan, an angiotensin receptor antagonist, would be as likely as enalapril to cause a decrease in GFR.

> **KEY POINTS**
>
> - Angiotensin-converting enzyme inhibitor therapy is warranted in patients with stage III and stage IV chronic kidney disease unless the creatinine level rises >30% after initiation of therapy.
> - Once-daily dosing of angiotensin-converting enzyme inhibitors can decrease the risk for hyperkalemia.

Bibliography

1. Bakris GL, Weir MR. Angiotensin-converting enzyme inhibitor-associated elevations in serum creatinine: is this a cause for concern? Arch Intern Med. 2000;160:685-93. [PMID: 10724055]

2. Hou FF, Zhang X, Zhang GH, Xie D, Chen PY, Zhang WR, et al. Efficacy and safety of benazepril for advanced chronic renal insufficiency. N Engl J Med. 2006;354:131-40. [PMID: 16407508]

3. Hebert LA. Optimizing ACE-inhibitor therapy for chronic kidney disease [Editorial]. N Engl J Med. 2006;354:189-91. [PMID: 16407515]

4. Garovic VD, Textor SC. Renovascular hypertension and ischemic nephropathy. Circulation. 2005;112:1362-74. [PMID: 16129817]

Item 60   Answer: C

The most likely cause of this patient's kidney disease is interstitial nephritis from sarcoidosis. Kidney disease occurs in approximately 20% of patients with sarcoidosis. Sarcoidosis may cause various renal conditions, such as nephrolithiasis due to hypercalciuria, nephrocalcinosis, and interstitial nephritis. Tubulointerstitial nephritis and uveitis (TINU syndrome) is a rare presentation of sarcoidosis that presents more commonly in women and responds to corticosteroid treatment. Diagnosis of interstitial nephritis is based on elevations in the blood urea nitrogen and creatinine levels and a bland urine sediment that may contain occasional granular casts or leukocytes. Renal ultrasonography in affected patients typically reveals small, echogenic kidneys.

Acute glomerulonephritis would be unlikely to cause this patient's kidney disease because of the absence of glomerular hematuria and proteinuria in the urine sediment. Membranous glomerulopathy also is unlikely because the nephrotic syndrome is not present. Her anemia, renal insufficiency, and proteinuria are consistent with myeloma kidney, but this condition is unlikely in a patient with negative results on serum protein electrophoresis. In addition, her rash, osteoarthritis, uevitis, hilar lymphadenopathy, and pyuria are more consistent with sarcoidosis.

KEY POINT

- Sarcoidosis may cause nephrolithiasis, nephrocalcinosis, and interstitial nephritis.

Bibliography

1. Kadanoff R, Lipps B, Khanna A, Hou S. Tubulointerstitial nephritis with uveitis (TINU): a syndrome rheumatologists should recognize: a case report and review of the literature. J Clin Rheum. 2004;10(1):25-7.

Item 61   Answer: A

Ramipril therapy is indicated for this patient. This patient's longstanding uncontrolled hypertension; black race; bland urine sediment with non-nephrotic proteinuria; and ultrasound findings of small, echogenic kidneys are consistent with hypertensive nephrosclerosis. Treatment of this condition relies on strict blood pressure control to slow the rate of progressive kidney failure.

In the African American Study of Kidney Disease and Hypertension (AASK) trial, patients treated with the angiotensin-converting enzyme inhibitor ramipril were significantly less likely to reach the secondary outcomes of a reduction in the glomerular filtration rate, development of renal failure, or death compared with those treated with metoprolol or amlodipine. Other studies also have demonstrated the beneficial effects of medications that block the renin–angiotensin system and of slowing progression of kidney disease. Therefore, these agents are recommended for first-line therapy for both diabetic and nondiabetic kidney disease.

KEY POINT

- Angiotensin-converting enzyme inhibitors or angiotensin receptor blockers are the agents of choice for the treatment of hypertension in chronic kidney disease.

Bibliography

1. Agodoa LY, Appel L, Bakris GL, Beck G, Bourgoignie J, Briggs JP, et al. Effect of ramipril vs amlodipine on renal outcomes in hypertensive nephrosclerosis: a randomized controlled trial. JAMA. 2001;285:2719-28. [PMID: 11386927]
2. Chobanian AV, Bakris GL, Black HR, Cushman WC, Green LA, Izzo JL Jr, et al. Seventh report of the Joint National Committee on Prevention, Detection, Evaluation, and Treatment of High Blood Pressure. Hypertension. 2003;42:1206-52. [PMID: 14656957]

Item 62   Answer: D

This patient most likely has an anion gap metabolic acidosis, and suspicion is particularly raised for lactic acidosis. Although the anion gap appears normal, the degree of hypoalbuminemia should be evaluated. The negative charge on albumin is a significant component of the "normal" unmeasured anions. For every 1 g/dL (10 g/L) decrease in the albumin level, the expected anion gap decreases by 2.5 meq/L. Therefore, this patient's normal anion gap should not be greater than approximately 5 meq/L to 6 meq/L.

Mixed anion gap metabolic acidosis and respiratory alkalosis is not correct because there is no respiratory alkalosis. The P_{CO_2} in this patient is consistent with a normal compensation for the degree of acidemia, which excludes respiratory alkalosis. Similarly, neither respiratory acidosis nor an anion gap is present.

KEY POINT

- An anion gap metabolic acidosis may be present in a patient with severe hypoalbuminemia and a "normal" anion gap.

Bibliography

1. Hassan H, Joh JH, Bacon BR, Bastani B. Evaluation of serum anion gap in patients with liver cirrhosis of diverse etiologies. Mt Sinai J Med. 2004;71:281-4. [PMID: 15365595]

Item 63   Answer: D

Placement of a urinary bladder catheter is most likely to establish a diagnosis in this patient. Urinary tract obstruction is common in elderly men, and evaluation for obstruction is indicated for all patients with acute renal failure. However, this patient's limited ability to give a reliable history complicates the establishment of a diagnosis.

Acute urinary retention commonly causes abdominal pain and always should be suspected in patients with this symptom. Placement of a urinary bladder catheter is essential in the management of acute urinary retention, and drainage of a large amount of urine with concurrent relief of symptoms would support this diagnosis. The presence of hydronephrosis on renal ultrasonography also would help to establish a definitive diagnosis, but this finding may not be present in the acute setting.

Suspicion for prerenal failure would warrant a fluid challenge with normal saline. However, this patient's slightly elevated blood pressure and peripheral edema do not support this diagnosis. The blood urea nitrogen–creatinine ratio can support a diagnosis of prerenal azotemia but is not sufficiently specific to be diagnostically useful in this patient. The fractional excretion of sodium in obstructive nephropathy varies from <1% in the early phases to >2% once tubular injury has developed. Therefore, this finding will not help to establish a diagnosis of obstruction. The fractional excretion of sodium is most diagnostically useful in acute oliguric renal failure.

KEY POINTS

- Renal ultrasonography can be normal early in the course of acute urinary tract obstruction.
- Urinary tract obstruction should be suspected in elderly men with acute renal failure.

Bibliography
1. **Curtis LA, Dolan TS, Cespedes RD**. Acute urinary retention and urinary incontinence. Emerg Med Clin North Am. 2001;19:591-619. [PMID: 11554277]

Item 64   Answer: E

This patient most likely has IgA glomerulonephritis. This condition is the most common form of glomerulonephritis worldwide and typically manifests with the nephritic syndrome. IgA glomerulonephritis is associated with dysmorphic erythrocytes and erythrocyte casts and hypertension; this patient's presentation is characterized by normal renal fution. Henoch–Schönlein purpura, an IgA-dominant form of vasculitis, is unlikely in the absence of a rash.

This patient's normal complement levels exclude systemic lupus erythematosus and cryoglobulinemic glomerulonephritis, which both present with low C4 levels and possibly low C3 levels. Compared with IgA glomerulonephritis, these conditions also are less likely to develop in a 19-year-old man. Antineutrophil cytoplasmic antibody–associated small-vessel vasculitis may cause glomerulonephritis alone. However, extrarenal manifestations usually develop in this setting. In addition, this condition more commonly affects older patients, does not develop suddenly, and is not typically associated with a viral pharyngitis.

KEY POINT

- IgA glomerulonephritis is manifested by the nephritic syndrome and is associated with dysmorphic erythrocytes and erythrocyte casts.

Bibliography
1. **Haas M**. IgA nephropathy. Semin Nephrol. 2004;24:177-295.
2. **Donadio JV, Grande JP**. IgA nephropathy. N Engl J Med. 2002;347:738-48. [PMID: 12213946]

Item 65   Answer: B

This patient has a triple acid–base disorder of mixed anion gap metabolic acidosis/non–anion gap metabolic alkalosis/respiratory alkalosis. He also has diabetic ketoacidosis. The anion gap is 31, which signifies a large degree of ketoacid production. His nausea and vomiting have caused a metabolic alkalosis; therefore, the bicarbonate level is higher than would be expected in a patient with this degree of acid production. This can be formalized by calculating the Δ–Δ anion gap. Another method of conceptualizing what is occurring is to take the difference of the anion gap and a normal anion gap. Defining the normal anion gap as 12 meq/L, the difference between the patient's anion gap and the normal anion gap is 19. If this number is added to the patient's bicarbonate level, the result is 35. This value significantly exceeds the normal bicarbonate level of 24, which indicates the presence of a metabolic alkalosis. In this setting, if all of the unmeasured anions (which are potential bicarbonate) are converted back to bicarbonate, the patient would have a metabolic alkalosis.

Once mechanical ventilation is started, the P_{CO_2} is related to the minute ventilation delivered by the machine. This patient's P_{CO_2} is lower than expected for the serum bicarbonate to compensate, which establishes the presence of iatrogenic respiratory alkalosis that is increasing this patient's pH.

This patient does not have non–anion gap metabolic acidosis or respiratory acidosis, which is not consistent in a patient with an alkalemic pH. A diagnosis of mixed anion gap metabolic acidosis with respiratory alkalosis does not address this patient's metabolic alkalosis. Mixed metabolic alkalosis and respiratory acidosis would be associated with an elevated serum bicarbonate level.

KEY POINTS

- Diabetic ketoacidosis can lead to an anion gap metabolic acidosis and metabolic alkalosis simultaneously.
- Iatrogenic respiratory alkalosis may develop after initiation of mechanical ventilation.

Bibliography
1. **Pierce NF, Fedson DS, Brigham KL, Mitra RC, Sack RB, Mondal A**. The ventilatory response to acute base deficit in humans. Time course during development and correction of metabolic acidosis. Ann Intern Med. 1970;72:633-40. [PMID: 5448093]

Item 66   Answer: D

Treatment with irbesartan is indicated for this patient. The Antihypertensive and Lipid-Lowering Treatment To Prevent

Heart Attack Trial (ALLHAT) demonstrated that thiazide diuretics, angiotensin-converting enzyme inhibitors, and calcium-channel blockers were equally effective in preventing coronary artery disease in patients >55 years of age. However, patients randomized to the diuretic arm of this large clinical trial had a significantly higher incidence of new-onset diabetes during the 5-year follow-up period. This relatively young patient has several risk factors for type 2 diabetes mellitus (including a family history of this condition, obesity, and dyslipidemia) and most likely will use antihypertensive therapy for several decades. Therefore, initiation of therapy with a drug that has been associated with improved insulin resistance is prudent. Both angiotensin-converting enzyme inhibitors and angiotensin receptor antagonists have been associated with a lower incidence of new-onset diabetes compared with diuretics and β-blockers.

In the ALLHAT study, doxazosin was associated with an increased incidence of cardiovascular endpoints. Therefore, this agent is not considered appropriate first-line therapy for primary hypertension. β-Blockers have been associated with an increased risk for diabetes compared with angiotensin receptor antagonists and are therefore not the most appropriate therapy for this patient.

KEY POINT

- Antihypertensive agents such as diuretics and β-blockers have been associated with an increased risk for type 2 diabetes mellitus, whereas angiotensin-converting enzyme inhibitors and angiotensin receptor blockers may improve insulin sensitivity.

Bibliography
1. Lindholm LH, Ibsen H, Borch-Johnsen K, Olsen MH, Wachtell K, Dahlof B, et al. Risk of new-onset diabetes in the Losartan Intervention For Endpoint reduction in hypertension study. J Hypertens. 2002;20:1879-86. [PMID: 12195132]

Item 67   Answer: D

Metformin cessation is indicated for this patient. The increasing number of diagnostic imaging and cardiac procedures requiring radiocontrast has caused a parallel increase in the incidence of contrast-induced nephropathy, which accounts for >10% of hospital-acquired renal failure. Contrast nephropathy is defined as a fixed (0.5 mg/dL [44.21 µmol/L]) or proportionate (25%) rise in serum creatinine levels after exposure to the contrast medium. Risk factors for contrast nephropathy include diabetic nephropathy, dehydration, heart failure, age >70 years, impaired kidney function, and concurrent use of nephrotoxic drugs and high-osmolar or high doses of radiocontrast medium.

In patients at increased risk for this condition, the best strategy to prevent contrast nephropathy is to discontinue nephrotoxic drugs, use the lowest possible dose of low-osmolality contrast medium for the study, and administer intravenous therapy with 0.9% saline at 1 mL/kg/h for 24 hours, beginning 12 hours before administration of contrast medium. Patients given intravenous 0.9% saline before administration of contrast medium are less likely to develop contrast nephropathy than patients given the same dose of 0.45% saline.

N-acetylcysteine has been used to prevent contrast nephropathy at a dose of 600 mg or 1200 mg every 12 hours for four doses, beginning before the administration of contrast medium. However, the results from other trials regarding this therapy are inconsistent.

Because patients with diabetes are at risk for development of contrast-induced nephropathy and metformin is contraindicated in patients with renal failure, metformin therapy should be discontinued at least 2 to 3 days before use of contrast and should not be reinitiated until 3 days after contrast exposure. Metformin also increases the risk for developing lactic acidosis after exposure to radiocontrast medium.

KEY POINTS

- Risk factors for contrast nephropathy include diabetic nephropathy, dehydration, heart failure, age >70 years, impaired kidney function, and concurrent use of nephrotoxic drugs and high-osmolar or high doses of radiocontrast medium.
- Prevention of contrast nephropathy in patients at increased risk for this condition involves discontinuing nephrotoxic drugs, using the lowest possible dose of low-osmolality contrast medium for the study, and administering intravenous therapy with 0.9% saline at 1 mL/kg/h for 24 hours beginning 12 hours before administration of contrast medium.

Bibliography
1. Barrett BJ, Parfrey PS. Clinical practice. Preventing nephropathy induced by contrast medium. N Engl J Med. 2006;354:379-86. [PMID: 16436769]
2. McCartney MM, Gilbert FJ, Murchison LE, Pearson D, McHardy K, Murray AD. Metformin and contrast media—a dangerous combination? Clin Radiol. 1999;54:29-33. [PMID: 9915507]

Item 68   Answer: D

Myeloma kidney is most likely causing this patient's renal failure. Abnormalities in renal function are common in multiple myeloma, and nearly 50% of patients with this condition have an elevated creatinine level at the time of diagnosis. Myeloma kidney is characterized by an intratubular obstruction with light-chain casts that results in kidney failure. Classically, hypercalcemia, severe anemia, and a low anion gap due to an increase in unmeasured cations such as calcium and immunoglobulins in the setting of kidney disease should raise suspicion for myeloma-related kidney disease. In addition, myeloma kidney is associated with a discrepancy in proteinuria detection between the dipstick urinalysis and timed urine collection in which dipstick urinalysis reveals only albumin and not light chains. However, the addition of sulfosalicylic acid to the urine specimen precipitates all proteins, including light chains. Urine protein electrophoresis also confirms the presence and type of light chains excreted in the urine.

Chronic tubulointerstitial disease secondary to analgesic use is unlikely in a patient with no history of chronic analgesic use. Acute interstitial nephritis due to nonsteroidal anti-inflammatory drug use has developed in patients with minimal exposure to these agents. However, this condition is uncommon in the absence of skin rash, sterile pyuria, or peripheral eosinophilia. Diabetic nephropathy is the most common cause of chronic kidney disease but is unlikely to cause a discrepancy concerning the presence of proteinuria between the urinalysis and the timed urine collection. Diabetes mellitus also would not cause this patient's low anion gap or hypercalcemia.

KEY POINTS

- Myeloma-related kidney disorders should be suspected in patients with anemia, a low serum anion gap, and renal failure.
- A low serum anion gap warrants evaluation for myeloma due to an increase in unmeasured cations such as calcium and immunoglobulins.
- Myeloma kidney is associated with a discrepancy in proteinuria detection between the dipstick urinalysis and a spot urine collection.

Bibliography

1. Bataille R, Harousseau JL. Multiple myeloma. N Engl J Med. 1997;336:1657-64. [PMID: 9171069]
2. Blade J, Fernandez-Llama P, Bosch F, Montoliu J, Lens XM, Montoto S, et al. Renal failure in multiple myeloma: presenting features and predictors of outcome in 94 patients from a single institution. Arch Intern Med. 1998;158:1889-93. [PMID: 9759684]

Item 69   Answer: E

Practice guidelines from the National Kidney Foundation Kidney/Disease Outcomes Quality Initiative (K/DOQI) recommend the use of mathematical equations such as Cockcroft–Gault or Modification of Diet in Renal Disease (MDRD) to calculate the creatinine clearance to estimate the glomerular filtration rate (GFR).

Timed urine collections are cumbersome and often inaccurate due to collection of too much or too little urine; therefore, mathematical equations are preferred to estimate the GFR. Imaging studies used to estimate the GFR, such as ^{125}I-iothalamate radionuclide scanning, are considered the gold standard for an accurate measurement of the GFR. However, these studies are costly and technically difficult to perform on all patients with chronic kidney disease and are used more commonly when precise estimations of the GFR are necessary, such as research settings and for evaluation of potential kidney donors.

Cystatin C can be used to estimate the GFR independent of a patient's age, sex, muscle mass, and body weight, which are factors that limit the use of creatinine alone to estimate this value. However, widespread use of cystatin C as a marker of kidney function in the clinical setting has been sporadic and its role in the future is not known. Renal

ultrasonography is an important tool in the assessment of kidney size and anatomy in chronic kidney disease but is not helpful in the assessment of the stage of chronic kidney disease.

KEY POINT

- Mathematical equations such as Cockcroft–Gault or Modification of Diet in Renal Disease are recommended for the assessment of glomerular filtration rate rather than 24-hour urine collections or radioimaging studies.

Bibliography

1. K/DOQI clinical practice guidelines for chronic kidney disease: evaluation, classification, and stratification. Am J Kidney Dis. 2002;39:S1-266. [PMID: 11904577]
2. Levey AS, Bosch JP, Lewis JB, Greene T, Rogers N, Roth D. A more accurate method to estimate glomerular filtration rate from serum creatinine: a new prediction equation. Modification of Diet in Renal Disease Study Group. Ann Intern Med. 1999;130:461-70. [PMID: 10075613]

Item 70   Answer: B

Magnetic resonance angiography of the abdomen is the most appropriate next step in the management of this patient's hypertension. Renovascular hypertension is an increasingly common cause of uncontrolled hypertension. This condition should be suspected in elderly patients with evidence of diffuse atherosclerosis; a history of cigarette smoking; and chronic kidney disease characterized by modest elevations in creatinine levels, non-nephrotic proteinuria, and a bland urine sediment. Hyperreninemia secondary to renal ischemia often causes recurrent episodes of pulmonary edema. Evaluation in this setting warrants imaging of the renal arteries.

Renal angiography is the gold standard for the diagnosis of renal artery stenosis. However, this study should be used with caution as a screening test in those with chronic kidney disease and a glomerular filtration rate (GFR) <60 mL/min because of the risk for contrast-induced acute renal failure. Magnetic resonance angiography of the renal arteries should be used in place of renal arteriography when the GFR is <60 mL/min because gadolinium is non-nephrotoxic and therefore is not associated with a risk for contrast-induced acute renal failure.

Increasing amlodipine may be marginally beneficial in further decreasing this patient's blood pressure. However, this intervention would not identify renovascular disease, which, if treated, may prevent further episodes of congestive heart failure. Initiation of therapy with a β-blocker such as carvedilol, particularly at a high dose, may contribute to worsening congestive heart failure during an acute exacerbation. However, this patient's long-term use of carvedilol at a stable dose makes this agent an unlikely contributor to his disease. The addition of an angiotensin-converting enzyme inhibitor to a regimen including angiotensin receptor blocker therapy is recommended for patients with chronic kidney disease and proteinuria but is not recommended for patients with congestive heart failure. Use of these agents in the setting of renovascular disease may result in hyperkalemia or acute renal failure.

CT angiography involves the use of intravenous contrast and is contraindicated in patients with a GFR <60 mL/min because of the associated risks for contrast-induced acute renal failure. Angiotensin-converting enzyme inhibitor renography and duplex ultrasonography of the kidneys also have been used as screening tests for renovascular disease. However, the former is less sensitive in bilateral disease as well as when the GFR is <50 mL/min and the latter is operator dependent and may not be available at all institutions.

KEY POINTS

- **Individuals with uncontrolled hypertension and recurrent episodes of flash pulmonary edema should be screened for renovascular disease.**
- **In patients with suspected renovascular disease and a glomerular filtration rate <60 mL/min, magnetic resonance angiography is the imaging study of choice to avoid the risk for contrast-induced acute renal failure.**

Bibliography

1. **Safian RD, Textor SC**. Renal-artery stenosis. N Engl J Med. 2001;344:431-42. [PMID: 11172181]
2. **Vasbinder GB, Nelemans PJ, Kessels AG, Kroon AA, Maki JH, Leiner T, et al**. Accuracy of computed tomographic angiography and magnetic resonance angiography for diagnosing renal artery stenosis. Ann Intern Med. 2004;141:674-82; discussion 682. [PMID: 15520423]

Item 71   Answer: D

A decrease in the glomerular filtration rate (GFR) is the most likely cause of this patient's hyperphosphatemia. Primary hyperparathyroidism is characterized by hypercalcemia and hypophosphatemia. In patients with chronic kidney disease, phosphorus excretion decreases and phosphate retention occurs when the GFR declines to <60 mL/min to 80 mL/min. The increase in phosphorus levels causes a decrease in ionized calcium, and both the elevated phosphorus levels and the hypocalcemia stimulate parathyroid hormone secretion. This secondary hyperparathyroid response is a "trade-off" in which serum levels of calcium and phosphorus normalize at the expense of persistently elevated parathyroid hormone levels. As renal function worsens, deficiency of 1,25-dihydroxyvitamin D contributes to the hypocalcemia and results in further stimulation of parathyroid hormone secretion. As the GFR continues to decline, the decrease in phosphate excretion results in hyperphosphatemia.

High phosphorus intake may worsen hyperphosphatemia in patients with chronic kidney disease. Vitamin D deficiency causes hypocalcemia but not hyperphosphatemia.

KEY POINT

- **A low glomerular filtration rate is the main cause of phosphate retention and hyperphosphatemia in patients with chronic kidney disease.**

Bibliography

1. **Slatopolsky E, Brown A, Dusso A**. Role of phosphorus in the pathogenesis of secondary hyperparathyroidism. Am J Kidney Dis. 2001;37:S54-7. [PMID: 11158862]
2. **Malluche HH, Monier-Faugere MC**. Hyperphosphatemia: pharmacologic intervention yesterday, today and tomorrow. Clin Nephrol. 2000;54:309-17. [PMID: 11076107]

Item 72   Answer: D

Discontinuation of hydrochlorothiazide and the addition of spironolactone are indicated for this patient. This patient's hypokalemia and hyponatremia are most likely secondary to hydrochlorothiazide. Her low plasma renin activity level may partly be mediated by the β-blocker, although most elderly patients with hypertension have salt-sensitive hypertension and low plasma renin activity. Use of a β-blocker and/or lisinopril, as well as hypokalemia, may be causing this patient's fatigue.

Diuretic therapy is most likely to manage this patient's hypertension because of her low plasma renin activity level and the fact that elderly patients with hypertension are more likely to respond to diuretics. Because spironolactone would treat this patient's hypokalemia as well as provide blood pressure control, this agent is particularly appropriate. However, spironolactone also may contribute to hyponatremia. Therefore, her electrolyte levels should be monitored periodically.

Hydrochlorothiazide should be discontinued because it has not satisfactorily controlled this patient's blood pressure and has caused hypokalemia and hyponatremia. Increasing the hydrochlorothiazide dose would only exacerbate this patient's electrolyte abnormalities. Doubling the metoprolol dose may increase this patient's fatigue. In addition, she already has a low renin activity level, and β-blockers lower blood pressure in part by reducing renin secretion. Therefore, this intervention may not even further lower her blood pressure. Similarly, doubling the dose of lisinopril may not be effective in a patient with low-renin hypertension. Furthermore, her current dose of lisinopril is reasonable but is not particularly effective, which suggests that doubling her dose may not have a significant effect.

KEY POINTS

- **Diuretics are effective antihypertensive agents in elderly patients but may cause electrolyte abnormalities.**

Bibliography

1. Major outcomes in high-risk hypertensive patients randomized to angiotensin-converting enzyme inhibitor or calcium channel blocker vs diuretic: The Antihypertensive and Lipid-Lowering Treatment to Prevent Heart Attack Trial (ALLHAT). JAMA. 2002;288:2981-97. [PMID: 12479763]

Item 73　　Answer:　D

Salicylate toxicity typically is associated with an anion gap metabolic acidosis and respiratory alkalosis, which is present in this patient. The presence of an alkaline pH with a low serum bicarbonate level suggests either a respiratory alkalosis with an ongoing renal compensation or a metabolic acidosis with a respiratory alkalosis. His elevated anion gap indicates the presence of a metabolic acidosis. Suspicion for a mixed disorder also should be raised in a patient whose pH is above normal in the presence of a metabolic acidosis. This presentation is not consistent with a simple metabolic acidosis with respiratory compensation because the compensation would not raise the pH above normal. To confirm this suspicion, Winter's formula can be used to estimate the expected CO_2:

$$1.5 \times [HCO_3^-] + 4 \pm 2$$

According to this formula, the expected P_{CO_2} is approximately 21 mm Hg, which confirms the presence of a respiratory alkalosis.

Measurement of the serum osmolality and calculation of the osmolal gap would detect the presence of an unmeasured osmole. If present, an osmolal gap would suggest the presence of an alcohol or paraldehyde ingestion but would not establish a specific diagnosis. In addition, ingestion of these agents would cause an anion gap metabolic acidosis without respiratory alkalosis, which is not consistent with this patient's presentation.

Ethylene glycol or methanol toxicity also would cause an anion gap metabolic acidosis without respiratory alkalosis. In toluene toxicity (glue sniffing), urinary hippurate losses lead to potassium loss, which would present with an anion gap metabolic acidosis and hypokalemia.

> **KEY POINT**
> - The presentation of anion gap metabolic acidosis and respiratory alkalosis suggests salicylate toxicity.

Bibliography

1. **Krause DS, Wolf BA, Shaw LM.** Acute aspirin overdose: mechanisms of toxicity. Ther Drug Monit. 1992;14:441-51. [PMID: 1485363]

Item 74　　Answer:　D

This patient has rhabdomyolysis secondary to lumbar muscle ischemia and injury due to prolonged immobilization and compression in the exaggerated lithotomy position. The extremely elevated creatine kinase level and elevated urine myoglobin level are consistent with a diagnosis of pigment nephropathy. The initial treatment should include aggressive hydration with normal saline. Intravenous calcium therapy is indicated only for hypocalcemia with cardiac or neuromuscular manifestations.

Ischemic tubular injury is included in the differential diagnosis. However, this condition is less likely because of the absence of hemodynamic compromise intraoperatively. Urinary tract obstruction is unlikely in the absence of hydronephrosis. The time course and the absence of rash, fever, and leukocyte casts do not support a diagnosis of interstitial nephritis.

> **KEY POINTS**
> - Immobilization in the exaggerated lithotomy position can result in rhabdomyolysis.
> - An extremely elevated creatine kinase level and elevated urine myoglobin level suggest a diagnosis of pigment nephropathy.

Bibliography

1. **Melli G, Chaudhry V, Cornblath DR.** Rhabdomyolysis: an evaluation of 475 hospitalized patients. Medicine (Baltimore). 2005;84:377-85. [PMID: 16267412]
2. **Kikuno N, Urakami S, Shigeno K, Kishi H, Shiina H, Igawa M.** Traumatic rhabdomyolysis resulting from continuous compression in the exaggerated lithotomy position for radical perineal prostatectomy. Int J Urol. 2002;9:521-4. [PMID: 12410935]

Item 75　　Answer:　D

The most appropriate next step for this patient is the addition of angiotensin receptor blocker therapy. This patient's protein excretion has doubled over the course of a year, and his blood pressure is not optimally controlled at a level <130/80 mm Hg despite using a maximal dose of an angiotensin-converting enzyme inhibitor. Therefore, the addition of another antihypertensive agent is indicated. In the Combination Treatment of Angiotensin-II Receptor Blocker and Angiotensin-Converting Enzyme Inhibitor in Nondiabetic Renal Disease (COOPERATE) trial, which included many patients with IgA glomerulonephritis, combination therapy with an angiotensin-converting enzyme inhibitor and an angiotensin receptor blocker was associated with a decrease in proteinuria.

There are no prospective data showing that tonsillectomy decreases morbidity in adult patients in this setting. Corticosteroid therapy has been shown to be effective in IgA glomerulonephritis when used with pulse methylprednisolone. However, therapy with corticosteroids alone has not been shown to be useful. Finally, the addition of a calcium-channel blocker or diuretics in a patient with IgA glomerulonephritis using an angiotensin-converting enzyme inhibitor has been shown to be less useful compared with the addition of an angiotensin receptor blocker.

> **KEY POINT**
> - Combination therapy with an angiotensin-converting enzyme inhibitor and an angiotensin receptor blocker is associated with decreasing proteinuria in patients with nondiabetic renal disease.

Bibliography

1. **Nakao N, Yoshimura A, Morita H, Takada M, Kayano T, Ideura T**. Combination treatment of angiotensin-II receptor blocker and angiotensin-converting-enzyme inhibitor in non-diabetic renal disease (COOPERATE): a randomised controlled trial. Lancet. 2003;361:117-24. [PMID: 12531578]

2. **Dillon JJ**. Angiotensin-converting enzyme inhibitors and angiotensin receptor blockers for IgA nephropathy. Semin Nephrol. 2004;24:218-24. [PMID: 15156527]

3. **Pozzi C, Andrulli S, Del Vecchio L, Melis P, Fogazzi GB, Altieri P, et al**. Corticosteroid effectiveness in IgA nephropathy: long-term results of a randomized, controlled trial. J Am Soc Nephrol. 2004;15:157-63. [PMID: 14694168]

Item 76   Answer: C

This patient most likely has thin basement membrane disease, also known as benign familial hematuria. This condition presents with glomerular hematuria with dysmorphic erythrocytes on microscopic analysis of the urine without any evidence of proteinuria. Despite a 20-year history of microscopic hematuria, there is no hypertension and his physical examination is unremarkable. Therefore, his presentation is most likely a benign, long-term outcome of a glomerular disease with familial thinning of the basement membrane.

Bladder cancer would be visible on cystoscopy, and this condition is unlikely to cause microscopic hematuria of 20 years' duration. Polycystic kidney disease and renal cell carcinoma also are unlikely in a patient with a decades-long history of microscopic hematuria and two normal CT scans. Urinary tract infection is associated with pyuria, not hematuria, and is equally unlikely.

KEY POINT

- **Thin basement membrane disease (benign familial hematuria) is characterized by glomerular hematuria with dysmorphic erythrocytes on microscopic analysis of the urine and no evidence of proteinuria.**

Bibliography

1. **Gregory MC**. Alport syndrome and thin basement membrane nephropathy: unraveling the tangled strands of type IV collagen [Editorial]. Kidney Int. 2004;65:1109-10. [PMID: 14871434]

2. **Kashtan CE**. Alport syndrome and thin glomerular basement membrane disease. J Am Soc Nephrol. 1998;9:1736-50. [PMID: 9727383]

3. **Rizzoni G, Massella L**. Differential diagnosis between X-linked Alport syndrome and thin basement membrane nephropathy [Letter]. Kidney Int. 2004;66:1289-90; author reply 1290. [PMID: 15327434]

Item 77   Answer: A

The most appropriate therapy for this patient is fomepizole and hemodialysis. The presence of acute renal failure associated with an increased anion gap metabolic acidosis and an increased osmolar gap is highly suggestive of ethylene glycol poisoning. The differential diagnosis also includes methanol poisoning, but the absence of papilledema and the presence of renal failure and calcium oxalate crystals in the urine are more consistent with ethylene glycol toxicity.

The presence of an osmolar gap suggests that the ethylene glycol had not been entirely metabolized. Therefore, measures to block the metabolism of the parent alcohol to its toxic metabolites with either ethanol or fomepizole are indicated. However, use of both agents concurrently is contraindicated because fomepizole is known to prolong the half-life of ethanol. Hemodialysis also is indicated because of the severity of the acidosis and central nervous system manifestations.

Bicarbonate supplementation could be used for severe acidemia to maintain a pH >7.1 to 7.2 until definitive therapy is started but is inadequate as sole therapy. Fomepizole is considerably more costly than ethanol and is not available at many institutions. However, this agent is preferred over ethanol because it is less toxic. Hemodialysis alone is not the most appropriate treatment because this intervention would not block ethylene glycol metabolism.

KEY POINT

- **Patients with ethylene glycol poisoning presenting with both an increased anion and osmolar gap metabolic acidosis require dialysis in addition to either fomepizole or ethanol.**

Bibliography

1. **Megarbane B, Borron SW, Baud FJ**. Current recommendations for treatment of severe toxic alcohol poisonings. Intensive Care Med. 2005;31:189-95. [PMID: 15627163]

Item 78   Answer: B

The most appropriate study in this setting is serum protein electrophoresis/urine protein electrophoresis. Myeloma-related disorders such as amyloidosis are one of the most common causes of the nephrotic syndrome in older patients and should be suspected particularly in those without concomitant diabetes mellitus or hypertension. Nearly all affected patients have a positive serum or urine protein electrophoresis, and this study should be routinely performed in patients >50 years of age when evaluating kidney disease. Additionally a low anion gap due to an increase in unmeasured cations such as calcium and immunoglobulins in the setting of kidney disease should raise suspicion for myeloma-related kidney disease.

This patient clearly has had a rapid loss of his kidney function within the past 3 months. Other causes for acute renal failure, such as antineutrophil cytoplasmic antibody–associated small-vessel vasculitis or hepatitis C–associated membranoproliferative glomerulonephritis, are included in the differential diagnosis. However, these conditions are less likely in the absence of glomerular hematuria on urinalysis. Similarly, acute interstitial nephritis is a common cause of acute renal failure in adults, but this condition typically presents with a medication exposure, skin rash, sterile pyuria, eosinophiluria, and eosinophilia. Although this patient did take nonsteroidal anti-inflammatory drugs, the exposure was limited and there are no associated signs or symptoms to raise suspicion for acute interstitial nephritis.

Kidney ultrasound would be helpful in the diagnosis of obstructive uropathy in an older man with kidney failure and symptoms of benign prostatic hyperplasia. However, obstructive uropathy typically is not associated with the nephrotic syndrome or other manifestations of amyloidosis, such as carpal tunnel syndrome and cardiomyopathy.

KEY POINT
- Amyloidosis is a common cause of the nephrotic syndrome in nondiabetic patients >50 years of age.

Bibliography
1. **Blade J, Fernandez-Llama P, Bosch F, Montoliu J, Lens XM, Montoto S, et al**. Renal failure in multiple myeloma: presenting features and predictors of outcome in 94 patients from a single institution. Arch Intern Med. 1998;158:1889-93. [PMID: 9759684]

Item 79   Answer: B

Sevelamer should be added to this patient's regimen. Hyperphosphatemia contributes to renal osteodystrophy by stimulating parathyroid hormone secretion and may be an important cardiovascular risk factor in patients with chronic kidney disease. Oral calcium-free phosphate binders such as sevelamer or calcium-containing phosphate binders should be used to lower phosphorus levels and decrease parathyroid hormone secretion in chronic kidney disease.

Aluminum hydroxide is the most potent phosphate binder available. However, this agent is not recommended because its chronic use is associated with aluminum retention and erythropoietin-resistant microscopic anemia, dementia, and severe osteomalacia. With a progressive decrease in the glomerular filtration rate, 1,25-dihydroxyvitamin D synthesis (calcitriol, the active metabolite of vitamin D) decreases, which results in increased parathyroid hormone secretion by removing the direct inhibitory effect of calcitriol on the parathyroid gland and by decreasing the serum calcium level. Calcitriol or newer generations of vitamin D analogs should be considered in chronic kidney disease to prevent renal osteodystrophy but only after hyperphosphatemia is controlled.

KEY POINT
- Phosphate binders may help to treat hyperphosphatemia in patients with chronic kidney disease.

Bibliography
1. **Friedman EA**. An introduction to phosphate binders for the treatment of hyperphosphatemia in patients with chronic kidney disease. Kidney Int Suppl. 2005:S2-6. [PMID: 15954946]
2. K/DOQI clinical practice guidelines for bone metabolism and disease in chronic kidney disease. Am J Kidney Dis. 2003;42:S1-201. [PMID: 14520607]

Item 80   Answer: C

The most appropriate treatment for this patient is adding an angiotensin-converting enzyme (ACE) inhibitor. This patient has inadequately controlled hypertension, renal insufficiency, and modest proteinuria. In addition, his stage 2 chronic kidney disease may be associated with hypertensive nephrosclerosis. The African American Study of Kidney Disease and Hypertension (AASK) trial demonstrated that the ACE inhibitor ramipril has a renoprotective effect in black patients with modest renal insufficiency secondary to hypertensive nephrosclerosis.

Doubling this patient's dose of diuretic therapy may provide additional blood pressure control. However, doses >25 mg/d may be associated with increased metabolic adverse effects. In addition, according to results of the AASK trial, an ACE inhibitor should first be added to this patient's regimen for additional blood pressure control and renal protection. Adding a β-blocker may provide some additional blood pressure control, but adding an ACE inhibitor is more appropriate because this patient's renal insufficiency is mild.

The AASK trial documented a significant reduction in proteinuria and composite renal endpoints (halving of the glomerular filtration rate and the incidence of end-stage renal disease and death) with ACE inhibitor therapy compared with the dihydropyridine calcium antagonist amlodipine. The benefits of this therapy were demonstrated most conclusively in patients with urinary protein excretion >300 mg/24 h but may extend to patients with lesser degrees of proteinuria. If target blood pressure levels are not achieved after the addition of ACE inhibitor therapy, adding a dihydropyridine calcium-channel blocker or a β-blocker or increasing the dose of this patient's diuretic could be considered.

KEY POINT
- Black patients with kidney disease and hypertension have better renal outcomes after treatment with angiotensin-converting enzyme inhibitor therapy compared with amlodipine or β-blockers.

Bibliography
1. **Agodoa LY, Appel L, Bakris GL, Beck G, Bourgoignie J, Briggs JP, et al**. Effect of ramipril vs amlodipine on renal outcomes in hypertensive nephrosclerosis: a randomized controlled trial. JAMA. 2001;285:2719-28. [PMID: 11386927]

Item 81   Answer: D

The most appropriate treatment for this patient is labetalol therapy. This agent has been used extensively in pregnancy because of its combined α-and β-blocking properties. Methyldopa also has been used extensively in pregnancy and is one of the only agents in which long-term follow-up of infants exposed in utero has proved to be safe.

Diuretic agents may interfere with the normal physiologic volume expansion associated with pregnancy.

Therefore, initiation of diuretic therapy during pregnancy usually is not recommended in the absence of renal insufficiency. However, if needed, patients with hypertension treated with chronic diuretic therapy before conception may continue treatment with these agents at lower doses. Angiotensin-converting enzyme inhibitors and angiotensin receptor antagonists are contraindicated in pregnancy because of adverse effects on fetal renal function, particularly after second and third trimester exposure. There is no clear association between these drugs and teratogenic effects after first-trimester exposure. However, avoidance of these drugs is indicated during all trimesters of pregnancy because of the risk for negative fetal outcomes.

Compared with labetalol, use of pure β-blockers such as atenolol in pregnant patients has been associated with smaller birthweights. However, conditions previously associated with β-blocker use in pregnant patients, such as neonatal hypoglycemia and bradycardia, have not been clearly linked to exposure to these agents and may be attributed to underlying maternal hypertensive disease.

KEY POINTS

- **In pregnancy, labetalol is preferable to pure β-blockers, which may be associated with low birthweight.**
- **Angiotensin-converting enzyme inhibitors and angiotensin receptor blockers are contraindicated in pregnancy.**

Bibliography

1. Report of the National High Blood Pressure Education Program Working Group on High Blood Pressure in Pregnancy. Am J Obstet Gynecol. 2000;183:S1-S22. [PMID: 10920346]
2. **Podymow T, August P, Umans JG**. Antihypertensive therapy in pregnancy. Semin Nephrol. 2004;24:616-25. [PMID: 15529297]

Item 82   Answer: B

This patient's low pH and decreased serum bicarbonate level indicate the presence of metabolic acidosis. His adequate respiratory compensation excludes a complex acid–base disorder. One of the major renal responses to systemic acidosis of a nonrenal cause is to increase the excretion of ammonium. A significant amount of ammonium in the urine indicates that a nonrenal source of the acidosis is likely. The amount of ammonia in the urine can be inferred by calculating the urine anion gap using the following formula:

$$[K+] + [Na+] - [Cl-]$$

If there is an unmeasured cation such as ammonium present, then $[Cl^-]$ exceeds $[K^+] + [Na^+]$ and the urine anion gap is significantly negative. In the presence of little or no unmeasured cation, the urine anion gap will take on a positive value. In this patient, the urine anion gap is –47 (32 meq/L + 21 meq/L – 80 meq/L). This finding indicates the presence of a significant amount of ammonium in the urine, which implies a normal renal response to the systemic acidosis and, therefore, an extrarenal cause of the acidosis.

Metformin is associated with lactic acidosis, which is not consistent with this patient's lack of an elevated anion gap. This patient's calculated urine anion gap shows that the renal response to the systemic acidosis is normal, which excludes a diagnosis of type 1 or type 4 renal tubular acidosis. The renal side effects of angiotensin-converting enzyme inhibitors such as enalapril include hyperkalemia and renal insufficiency, but these agents are not associated with metabolic acidosis.

KEY POINT

- **A highly negative urine anion gap suggests that the kidney is appropriately excreting acid during metabolic acidosis.**

Bibliography

1. **Batlle DC, Hizon M, Cohen E, Gutterman C, Gupta R**. The use of the urinary anion gap in the diagnosis of hyperchloremic metabolic acidosis. N Engl J Med. 1988;318:594-9. [PMID: 3344005]

Item 83   Answer: C

This patient has a congenital glomerular disease known as Alport's syndrome, which is associated with a glomerulonephritis with dysmorphic erythrocytes, mild proteinuria of about 1.2 g/24 h, and a high-frequency hearing loss. An abnormality in type IV collagen of the glomerular basement membrane and in the ear causes this condition.

Various renal and glomerular diseases are familial, including polycystic kidney disease, Fabry's disease, and familial benign hematuria. However, the presence of hearing loss strongly suggests a diagnosis of Alport's syndrome.

KEY POINT

- **Alport's syndrome is associated with a glomerulonephritis with dysmorphic erythrocytes, mild proteinuria, and a high-frequency hearing loss.**

Bibliography

1. **Kashtan CE**. Diagnosis of Alport syndrome [Letter]. Kidney Int. 2004;66:1290-1; author reply 1291. [PMID: 15327435]
2. **Hudson BG, Tryggvason K, Sundaramoorthy M, Neilson EG**. Alport's syndrome, Goodpasture's syndrome, and type IV collagen. N Engl J Med. 2003;348:2543-56. [PMID: 12815141]

Item 84   Answer: D

This patient most likely has Wegener's granulomatosis, and positive results of a proteinase-3 antineutrophil cytoplasmic autoantibody (ANCA) assay would establish this diagnosis. This patient's older age, sinusitis, intermittent otitis media, and crusting in his right nose are consistent with this condition. His chest radiograph findings are indicative of pulmonary disease, and the presence of dysmorphic erythrocytes on microscopic analysis of the urine and peripheral edema, as well as his abnormal renal function, suggests glomerulonephritis.

This patient's age and sex, as well as his normal complement levels and the presence of upper and lower respiratory tract disease, do not suggest lupus nephritis. Therefore, the presence of antinuclear antibodies or anti–double-stranded DNA antibodies is unlikely. Anti–glomerular basement membrane disease usually affects young men; this condition also is not consistent with upper and lower respiratory tract disease. Either myeloperoxidase or proteinase-3 ANCAs may be present in this patient, but proteinase-3 ANCAs are more likely in a patient with Wegener's granulomatosis.

KEY POINT

- Wegener's granulomatosis is characterized by upper and lower airway disease, glomerulonephritis, and positive findings on a proteinase-3 antineutrophil cytoplasmic antibody assay.

Bibliography

1. Hagen EC, Daha MR, Hermans J, Andrassy K, Csernok E, Gaskin G, et al. Diagnostic value of standardized assays for antineutrophil cytoplasmic antibodies in idiopathic systemic vasculitis. EC/BCR Project for ANCA Assay Standardization. Kidney Int. 1998;53:743-53. [PMID: 9507222]

Item 85   Answer: D

This patient has multiple myeloma complicated by myeloma cast nephropathy. In a patient with hypercalcemia, trace urine dipstick proteinuria in association with approximately 3 g of daily urinary protein excretion (based on the urinary protein–creatinine ratio) strongly supports this diagnosis. The elevated globulin fraction of the protein concentration also suggests multiple myeloma. The differential diagnosis of this patient's low anion gap includes hypoalbuminemia or excess unmeasured cations, which may be associated with hypercalcemia, hyperkalemia, hypermagnesemia, lithium intoxication, or a cationic paraprotein.

Uric acid nephropathy would present with acute oliguric renal failure due to uric acid tubular precipitation caused by overproduction that typically complicates lymphoproliferative disorders or malignancies, especially after chemotherapy.

Thiazides have been shown to induce hypercalcemia, but the majority of patients in this setting have an underlying condition, such as hyperparathyroidism. AL amyloidosis may occur in patients with multiple myeloma, but these patients present with heavy albuminuria and the nephrotic syndrome. Lymphomatous infiltration of the kidneys may cause enlarged kidneys but not a discrepancy between the urine dipstick protein level and the total quantitative urinary protein excretion.

KEY POINT

- A disparity between the dipstick protein level and quantified urinary protein excretion, a low anion gap, and an increase in the globulin fraction of the total protein level suggests multiple myeloma.

Bibliography

1. Lin J, Markowitz GS, Valeri AM, Kambham N, Sherman WH, Appel GB, et al. Renal monoclonal immunoglobulin deposition disease: the disease spectrum. J Am Soc Nephrol. 2001;12:1482-92. [PMID: 11423577]

Item 86   Answer: D

This patient most likely has microscopic polyangiitis, which is associated with pulmonary infiltrates of alveolar bleeding from capillaritis. Cryoglobulinemic vasculitis and systemic lupus erythematosus are extremely rare causes of pulmonary hemorrhage and are unlikely in a patient with normal complement levels. This patient has no history of asthma or evidence of eosinophilia to suggest a diagnosis of the Churg–Strauss syndrome. This condition also usually is associated with the presence of pulmonary nodules on chest radiograph.

KEY POINT

- Microscopic polyangiitis is a nongranulomatous or small-vessel vasculitis occasionally accompanied by medium-sized vessel involvement that causes a pulmonary–renal syndrome.

Bibliography

1. Matteson EL. Small vessel vasculitis [Letter]. N Engl J Med. 1998;338:994-5. [PMID: 9527615].

Item 87   Answer: D

This patient most likely has post-transplant lymphoproliferative disorder. The presence of fever, night sweats, and lymphadenopathy; his Epstein–Barr virus–negative status and the kidney donor's Epstein–Barr virus–positive status; and his elevated lactate dehydrogenase levels are consistent with this condition. In these patients, duodenal involvement can result in ulceration. In addition, biopsies of the duodenal tissue revealed monomorphic diffuse large-cell lymphoma.

Helicobacter pylori–related disease is included in the differential diagnosis but is not likely to cause systemic symptoms. Cytomegalovirus-related disease is less likely than post-transplant lymphoproliferative disorder because of this patient's positive preoperative immune status and negative cytomegalovirus viral load. Nonsteroidal anti-inflammatory drug–induced mucosal injury also is less likely in a patient who only took a few doses of ibuprofen.

Therapy for post-transplant lymphoproliferative disease varies depending on the severity of the clinical presentation.

Polyclonal lymphoproliferative disease usually is managed with a reduction in immunosuppression and ganciclovir. However, combination therapy with anti–B-cell antibodies such as rituximab and chemotherapy such as CHOP (cyclophosphamide, doxorubicin, vincristine, prednisone) is generally indicated for patients with monoclonal lymphoma and more advanced visceral involvement. Radiation therapy is indicated for patients with central nervous system involvement, as well as those with localized disease.

KEY POINT

- Renal transplant recipients who are Epstein–Barr virus–negative are at increased risk for post-transplant lymphoproliferative disorder, especially after receiving an organ from an Epstein–Barr virus–positive donor.

Bibliography

1. **Newstead CG**. Lymphoproliferative disease post-renal transplantation [Editorial]. Nephrol Dial Transplant. 2000;15:1913-6. [PMID: 11096131]
2. **Herzig KA, Juffs HG, Norris D, Brown AM, Gill D, Hawley CM, et al**. A single-centre experience of post-renal transplant lymphoproliferative disorder. Transpl Int. 2003;16:529-36. [PMID: 12734646]

Item 88   Answer: D

Glomerulonephritis is the most likely cause of this patient's hematuria. Hematuria is a common finding that occurs in 1% to 3% of all patients and in as many as 10% of all men. One of the most important initial steps in the evaluation of microscopic hematuria is microscopic analysis of urine sediment to assess erythrocyte morphology to distinguish between glomerular and nonglomerular hematuria of the urinary tract. Monomorphic or intact erythrocytes characterize nonglomerular hematuria, whereas dysmorphic erythrocytes are associated with glomerular hematuria. The coexistence of proteinuria with hematuria and the presence of erythrocyte casts in this patient indicate a diagnosis of glomerulonephritis.

Genitourinary tract malignancy is more common in men >50 years of age who have persistent hematuria and risk factors such as cigarette smoking, analgesic abuse, benzene exposure, or a history of voiding abnormalities. Urinary tract infection is an uncommon condition in men without associated anatomic abnormalities and is not associated with glomerular hematuria and proteinuria. Nephrolithiasis is a common cause of hematuria but is unlikely in a patient without symptoms associated with this condition, such as flank pain. This patient's findings of glomerular hematuria and proteinuria on microscopic analysis of the urine sediment also do not suggest nephrolithiasis.

KEY POINTS

- One of the most important initial steps in the evaluation of microscopic hematuria is urine microscopy to assess erythrocyte morphology.
- Glomerular hematuria is associated with dysmorphic erythrocytes and erythrocyte casts on urinalysis.

Bibliography

1. **Cohen RA, Brown RS**. Clinical practice. Microscopic hematuria. N Engl J Med. 2003;348:2330-8. [PMID: 12788998]

Item 89   Answer: B

This patient most likely has glomerulopathy with secondary focal segmental glomerulosclerosis. Obesity is highly prevalent in the United States; 22% of the population is obese (BMI >30) and 55% of the population is overweight (BMI >25). Obesity is attributed to dietary habits and a sedentary lifestyle. Patients with obesity have greater risk for end-stage renal disease, hypertension, hyperlipidemia, coronary vascular disease, and diabetes. Obesity also may lead to increased renal hypertrophy, renal blood flow, and glomerular filtration rate. Renal biopsy shows glomerulomegaly, some effacement of foot processes, and few segmented sclerotic lesions.

Obesity-related glomerulopathy typically manifests with nephrotic range proteinuria but lacks other manifestations of the nephrotic syndrome seen in focal segmental glomerulosclerosis, minimal change disease, or membranous nephropathy. Compared with these conditions, obesity-related glomerulopathy is associated with a lower incidence of the nephrotic syndrome, a more benign course, and slower progression to renal failure.

KEY POINT

- Obesity may lead to proteinuria and chronic kidney disease.

Bibliography

1. **Kambham N, Markowitz GS, Valeri AM, Lin J, D'Agati VD**. Obesity-related glomerulopathy: an emerging epidemic. Kidney Int. 2001;59:1498-509. [PMID: 11260414]
2. **Hsu CY, McCulloch CE, Iribarren C, Darbinian J, Go AS**. Body mass index and risk for end-stage renal disease. Ann Intern Med. 2006;144:21-8. [PMID: 16389251]

Item 90   Answer: B

Therapy with a thiazide diuretic is indicated for this patient. This patient has type 2 diabetes mellitus, coronary artery disease, possible early diabetic nephropathy, and inadequate blood pressure control. His current regimen of a β-blocker and angiotensin-converting enzyme inhibitor is appropriate for cardiovascular disease and target organ protection. The addition of a thiazide diuretic is likely to improve blood pressure control, which is indicated to prevent further progression of target organ damage.

The addition of an angiotensin receptor blocker or potassium-sparing diuretic may provide renal protection and additional blood pressure control but would likely further exacerbate his hyperkalemia. Compared with the other options, α-blockers have not been shown to have particular advantages compared with the other agents and may not lower blood pressure sufficiently.

KEY POINTS

- Lowering blood pressure to appropriate targets is particularly important in patients with diabetes who have increased risk for cardiovascular and renal complications.
- Diuretics potentiate the blood pressure–lowering effects of angiotensin-converting enzyme inhibitors and β-blockers.

Bibliography

1. Tight blood pressure control and risk of macrovascular and microvascular complications in type 2 diabetes: UKPDS 38. UK Prospective Diabetes Study Group. BMJ. 1998;317:703-13. [PMID: 9732337]

Item 91   Answer: D

Postinfectious glomerulonephritis is the most likely diagnosis in a young woman who develops glomerular disease 3 weeks after the onset of respiratory tract infection. In addition, the presence of low serum C3 levels and normal C4 levels strongly suggests this diagnosis and raises suspicion for the significant volume expansion that accompanies this condition.

IgA glomerulonephritis, Goodpasture's syndrome, and antineutrophil cytoplasmic antibody glomerulonephritis are not associated with low complement levels. IgA glomerulonephritis would develop at the same time as pharyngitis, not 3 weeks later. Goodpasture's syndrome typically develops in young patients. However, this patient's physical examination findings do not raise suspicion for pulmonary bleeding, and the crackles in both lung bases most likely represent water, not blood. Systemic lupus erythematosus nephritis is unlikely in a patient who suddenly develops glomerulonephritis without any other previous symptoms. Similarly, this condition is associated with significantly decreased C3 and C4 levels.

KEY POINT

- Postinfectious glomerulonephritis may present 3 weeks after onset of the inciting infection and is associated with low C3 levels and normal C4 levels.

Bibliography

1. **Rodriguez-Iturbe B**. Nephritis-associated streptococcal antigens: where are we now? [Editorial]. J Am Soc Nephrol. 2004;15:1961-2. [PMID: 15213287]

2. **Tejani A, Ingulli E**. Poststreptococcal glomerulonephritis. Current clinical and pathologic concepts. Nephron. 1990;55:1-5. [PMID: 2191230]

Item 92   Answer: E

Increased minute ventilation is the most likely cause of this patient's acid–base disorder. The acid–base disturbance in this patient is a respiratory alkalosis, which commonly develops in end-stage liver disease. If the serum pH is not measured, this disturbance can be misdiagnosed as metabolic acidosis in patients with end-stage liver disease. The liver helps to metabolize circulating steroid hormones. Elevated levels of progestins in end-stage liver disease lead to stimulation of the respiratory drive, which causes a primary respiratory alkalosis. In severe liver disease, decreased clearance of lactate from the circulation can lead to lactic acidosis. However, the absence of an anion gap in this patient excludes this condition.

Renal tubular acidosis would lead to a metabolic acidosis. However, this patient's pH is alkaline, indicating that an alkalosis is the primary disorder or that another acid–base disorder is present. Reduced conversion of lactate would be associated with an anion gap metabolic acidosis (lactic acidosis), which is not present in this patient. Diarrhea would cause a metabolic acidosis, not respiratory alkalosis. Cirrhosis is not associated with a decreased buffering capacity of the blood.

KEY POINT

- Respiratory alkalosis commonly develops in end-stage liver disease.

Bibliography

1. **Lustik SJ, Chhibber AK, Kolano JW, Hilmi IA, Henson LC, Morris MC, et al**. The hyperventilation of cirrhosis: progesterone and estradiol effects. Hepatology. 1997;25:55-8. [PMID: 8985264]

Item 93   Answer: A

This patient is at high risk for the refeeding syndrome, which can be associated with rhabdomyolysis. His low blood urea nitrogen and albumin levels suggest malnutrition. In this setting, phosphate depletion also is likely despite his nearly normal phosphate level. The phosphate is sequestered in the intracellular compartment, whereas intracellular depletion of phosphate is critical. Once this patient is supplied with calories (particularly carbohydrates), oxidative phosphorylation and generation of adenosine triphosphate quickly deplete the intracellular phosphate, which leads to rhabdomyolysis. The best method of preventing this complication from occurring is recognizing patients at risk for this disorder. Phosphate levels should be monitored closely in patients in this setting to prevent the development of this complication.

Leukopenia is not associated with malnutrition or the refeeding syndrome. However, severe hypophosphatemia can rarely lead to impaired phagocytosis and granulocytic chemotaxis. Torsade des pointes is not usually associated with malnutrition. This condition usually is related to use of certain medications, a drug interaction, a prolonged QT interval, and electrolyte disturbances that typically do not include hypophosphatemia. Cerebral edema and fulminant liver failure are not typically associated with the refeeding syndrome.

KEY POINTS

- **The refeeding syndrome is a potential complication in malnourished patients who suddenly receive a large calorie load.**
- **Rhabdomyolysis is a potentially severe complication of the refeeding syndrome.**

Bibliography
1. **Marinella MA**. Refeeding syndrome and hypophosphatemia. J Intensive Care Med. 2005;20:155-9. [PMID: 15888903]

Item 94   Answer: C

The most likely diagnosis in this patient is lupus nephritis characterized by a thrombotic microangiopathy. This patient's history of spontaneous abortions and preeclampsia is consistent with the antiphospholipid antibody syndrome. Her current manifestations of acral ulcers, microangiopathic hemolytic anemia, and thrombocytopenia suggest the development of thrombotic thrombocytopenic purpura.

The thrombocytopenic microangiopathy reduces blood flow through glomerular capillaries, resulting in a bland urinary sediment with a few erythrocytes and no urinary casts. The absence of an inflammatory urinary sediment helps to exclude glomerulonephritis as a cause of the renal insufficiency.

Lupus nephritis manifested by membranous nephropathy would be associated with the nephritic syndrome, which her urinary protein–creatinine ratio excludes. Glomerular hematuria and low C3 and C4 levels would be present in a focal or diffuse proliferative lupus nephritis, whereas this patient's complement levels are normal. Similarly, postinfectious membranoproliferative glomerulonephritis is unlikely in the absence of glomerular hematuria, proteinuria, and low C3 and normal C4 levels.

KEY POINT

- **The antiphospholipid antibody syndrome is characterized by thrombosis in association with a lupus anticoagulant or persistently elevated levels of anticardiolipin antibodies.**

Bibliography
1. **Fakhouri F, Noel LH, Zuber J, Beaufils H, Martinez F, Lebon P, et al**. The expanding spectrum of renal diseases associated with antiphospholipid syndrome. Am J Kidney Dis. 2003;41:1205-11. [PMID: 12776272]

2. **Levine JS, Branch DW, Rauch J**. The antiphospholipid syndrome. N Engl J Med. 2002;346:752-63. [PMID: 11882732]

Item 95   Answer: A

Combination therapy with cefazolin and ceftazidime is indicated for this patient. The presence of abdominal pain and a peritoneal effluent cell count >100 total nucleated cells/µL establishes a diagnosis of peritoneal dialysis–related peritonitis. Patients presenting with cloudy peritoneal effluent or who fulfill the diagnostic criteria should be started on empiric gram-positive and gram-negative coverage as soon as possible; a delay in therapy by even a few hours has been associated with adverse outcomes. Cefazolin or vancomycin are the most commonly employed antibiotics for gram-positive coverage, and ceftazidime, aminoglycosides, or fluoroquinolones are alternatives for gram-negative pathogens. The severity of the clinical presentation and local antibiotic sensitivity patterns determine antibiotic choice.

Combination therapy with metronidazole and piperacillin–tazobactam afford excellent gram-negative and anaerobe coverage but would not cover *Staphylococcus* sufficiently. Vancomycin alone would not cover gram-negative pathogens. Catheter removal should be considered in patients with refractory peritonitis, relapsing peritonitis, refractory exit-site infection, concurrent exit-site or tunnel infection that progresses to peritonitis, and fungal peritonitis, as well as in patients who do not significantly improve after 48 to 96 hours of appropriate antibiotic therapy.

KEY POINTS

- **A peritoneal fluid cell count >100 total nucleated cells/µL is abnormal and consistent with the diagnosis of peritonitis.**
- **Antibiotic therapy covering both gram-negative and gram-positive pathogens should be started immediately in a patient with suspected peritoneal dialysis–related peritonitis.**

Bibliography
1. **Piraino B, Bailie GR, Bernardini J, Boeschoten E, Gupta A, Holmes C, et al**. Peritoneal dialysis-related infections recommendations: 2005 update. Perit Dial Int. 2005;25:107-31. [PMID: 15796137]

Item 96   Answer: B

This patient's urinary sediment findings and clinical presentation support a diagnosis of acute tubular necrosis. Fulminant hepatic failure related to acetaminophen overdose is known to cause ischemic tubular injury evolving from hepatorenal physiology. The relatively high urine sodium level and fractional excretion of sodium of 10% also support this diagnosis.

Hepatorenal syndrome generally is associated with a relatively unremarkable urinary sediment, 24-hour urinary protein excretion <500 mg, and urinary sodium level <20 meq/L (20 mmol/L). However, epithelial cell casts stained with bilirubin can be seen in the absence of a tubular injury because of the detergent effect of bilirubin.

KEY POINT

- Acute tubular necrosis is the most common cause of acute renal failure after acetaminophen poisoning.

Bibliography

1. **Mour G, Feinfeld DA, Caraccio T, McGuigan M**. Acute renal dysfunction in acetaminophen poisoning. Ren Fail. 2005;27:381-3. [PMID: 16060123]
2. **Alkhuja S, Aboudan M, Menkel R**. Acetaminophen toxicity induced non-oliguric acute tubular necrosis [Letter]. Nephrol Dial Transplant. 2001;16:190. [PMID: 11209028]

Item 97   Answer: C

Arteriovenous fistula is always the preferred access method for dialysis. This patient has no evidence of peripheral vascular disease, and creation of an arteriovenous fistula should be possible. This method is associated with lower mortality rates compared with other strategies, low infection rate, and high patency rates once the fistula reaches maturity. Referral to a vascular surgeon is indicated once the glomerular filtration rate reaches 30 mL/min. Assessment before fistula placement includes vein mapping to facilitate creation of a fistula with the optimal characteristics for maturation. All physicians should educate patients with chronic kidney disease to avoid venipuncture and intravenous lines above the hands in order to save veins for future creation of arteriovenous fistulas. In addition, since subclavian stenosis limits blood flow in upper-extremity dialysis sites, subclavian vein lines should be strictly avoided in patients with chronic kidney disease.

Tunneled central venous catheters have the highest mortality risk; the relative risk for death in patients using this method is 1.5 to 1.7 times higher compared with that of arteriovenous fistulas. Polytetrafluoroethylene grafts are generally easier to cannulate compared with arteriovenous fistulas. However, these grafts have a higher rate of failure over time due to thrombosis and are associated with a slightly higher mortality rate. Peritoneal dialysis would be contraindicated because of this patient's history of multiple bowel resections, which reduce the effective surface area of the peritoneal membrane and preclude effective dialysis.

KEY POINTS

- Patients with chronic kidney disease should be educated to avoid venipuncture and intravenous catheters in veins above the level of the wrist in both arms to preserve veins for future creation of arteriovenous fistulas.
- Subclavian vein lines should be strictly avoided in patients with chronic kidney disease.
- Creation of an arteriovenous fistula is indicated months before initiation of dialysis.

Bibliography

1. **Lorenzo V, Martn M, Rufino M, Hernandez D, Torres A, Ayus JC**. Predialysis nephrologic care and a functioning arteriovenous fistula at entry are associated with better survival in incident hemodialysis patients: an observational cohort study. Am J Kidney Dis. 2004;43:999-1007. [PMID: 15168379]
2. **Dhingra RK, Young EW, Hulbert-Shearon TE, Leavey SF, Port FK**. Type of vascular access and mortality in U.S. hemodialysis patients. Kidney Int. 2001;60:1443-51. [PMID: 11576358]
3. **Rodriguez JA, Armadans L, Ferrer E, Olmos A, Codina S, Bartolome J, et al**. The function of permanent vascular access. Nephrol Dial Transplant. 2000;15:402-8. [PMID: 10692528]
4. **Polkinghorne KR, McDonald SP, Atkins RC, Kerr PG**. Vascular access and all-cause mortality: a propensity score analysis. J Am Soc Nephrol. 2004;15:477-86. [PMID: 14747396]
5. III. NKF-K/DOQI Clinical Practice Guidelines for Vascular Access: update 2000. Am J Kidney Dis. 2001;37:S137-81. [PMID: 11229969]

Item 98   Answer: B

Cystoscopy is the most appropriate next step in the evaluation of this patient's hematuria. Hematuria is a common finding that occurs in 1% to 3% of all patients and in as many as 10% of all men. One of the most important initial steps in the evaluation of microscopic hematuria is microscopic analysis of urine sediment to assess erythrocyte morphology to distinguish between glomerular hematuria and nonglomerular hematuria of the urinary tract. Monomorphic or intact erythrocytes characterize nonglomerular hematuria, whereas dysmorphic erythrocytes are associated with glomerular hematuria. In men >50 years of age with persistent hematuria, genitourinary tract malignancy must be excluded by cystoscopy, especially in the setting of associated risk factors such as cigarette smoking, analgesic abuse, benzene exposure, or a history of voiding abnormalities.

Because hematuria was present in this patient 6 months ago, repeat urinalysis is not indicated, and the associated risk factors for genitourinary tract malignancy mandate further evaluation. Cystic lesions in the kidney increase with age, overwhelmingly are considered "simple," and generally do not require further evaluation. Other lesions characterized as complex cysts or mass lesions in the kidney require more aggressive evaluation, because these abnormalities carry a risk for malignancy. Urinary tract infection is commonly associated with pyuria and bacteriuria but not persistent hematuria. Moreover, a treatment course with antibiotics may delay diagnosis of urinary tract malignancy. Kidney biopsy is the procedure of choice for individuals with glomerular disease but has a low yield in identifying the cause of hematuria in the absence of demonstrable glomerular bleeding, proteinuria, or kidney insufficiency.

KEY POINT

- Patients >50 years of age with persistent hematuria should be evaluated for genitourinary tract malignancy.

Bibliography
1. **Cohen RA, Brown RS**. Clinical practice. Microscopic hematuria. N Engl J Med. 2003;348:2330-8. [PMID: 12788998]

Item 99   Answer: D

Discontinuation of ibuprofen is indicated for this patient. Nonsteroidal anti-inflammatory drugs (NSAIDs) frequently affect sodium excretion. However, these agents are routinely used by elderly patients, who are particularly vulnerable to the blood pressure–raising effects of these drugs because of this effect. Most elderly patients have musculoskeletal conditions that warrant some form of therapy, but long-term daily treatment with NSAIDs may not be necessary. Alternative treatment strategies, such as physical therapy or therapy with acetaminophen, are indicated in this setting.

Discontinuing this patient's NSAID therapy is an appropriate next step to try to decrease this patient's blood pressure. This strategy should be attempted before increasing his medications, particularly because NSAIDs may contribute to renal and electrolyte disorders when used concomitantly with angiotensin-converting enzyme inhibitors or when taken by volume-depleted patients.

KEY POINT
- **Nonsteroidal anti-inflammatory drug use is a common cause of resistance to antihypertensive therapy.**

Bibliography
1. **Morgan T, Anderson A**. The effect of nonsteroidal anti-inflammatory drugs on blood pressure in patients treated with different antihypertensive drugs. J Clin Hypertens (Greenwich). 2003;5:53-7. [PMID: 12556654]

Item 100   Answer: E

This patient has a non–anion gap metabolic acidosis with an appropriate respiratory compensation, which is most consistent with use of the carbonic anhydrase inhibitor acetazolamide. In the proximal tubule, inhibition of carbonic anhydrase impairs proximal tubular bicarbonate reabsorption, which frequently leads to a non–anion gap metabolic acidosis. This presentation is essentially the pharmacologic equivalent of a proximal (type 2) renal tubular acidosis.

Warfarin, atenolol, pioglitazone, and glipizide are not associated with the development of metabolic acidosis. However, pioglitazone causes sodium retention. This condition recently has been linked to overactivity of the epithelial sodium channel, which is present in the distal tubule. This channel is blocked by the potassium-sparing diuretic amiloride.

KEY POINT
- **Acetazolamide may cause non–anion gap metabolic acidosis.**

Bibliography
1. **Maisey DN, Brown RD**. Acetazolamide and symptomatic metabolic acidosis in mild renal failure. Br Med J (Clin Res Ed). 1981;283:1527-8. [PMID: 6799050]

Item 101   Answer: B

In addition to corticosteroids, the most appropriate treatment for this patient is intravenous cyclophosphamide followed by maintenance mycophenolate mofetil once remission is achieved. Black patients with lupus nephritis have a much poorer prognosis compared with white patients despite treatment with corticosteroids and intravenous cyclophosphamide. Therefore, maintenance therapy is indicated. Recent studies have suggested that maintenance therapy with mycophenolate mofetil or azathioprine is beneficial in lupus nephritis. In addition, a recent randomized trial compared the induction of therapy with intravenous cyclophosphamide followed by maintenance therapy with intravenous cyclophosphamide, azathioprine, or mycophenolate mofetil (Contreras). Both mycophenolate mofetil and azathioprine were shown to be less toxic and more efficacious than maintenance intravenous cyclophosphamide.

Long-term therapy with oral or intravenous cyclophosphamide is associated with much higher side effects compared with mycophenolate mofetil. In addition, maintenance therapy with cyclophosphamide results in unnecessary cyclophosphamide exposure. Therapy with corticosteroids and 6 months of oral cyclophosphamide would most likely cause a cumulative cyclophosphamide exposure two to three times higher than would 6 months of intravenous cyclophosphamide therapy. However, corticosteroids and 6 months of intravenous cyclophosphamide is insufficient therapy for this patient, for whom maintenance therapy is indicated.

KEY POINT
- **In addition to corticosteroids, the most appropriate treatment for lupus nephritis is intravenous cyclophosphamide followed by maintenance mycophenolate mofetil once remission is achieved.**

Bibliography
1. **Dooley MA, Hogan S, Jennette C, Falk R**. Cyclophosphamide therapy for lupus nephritis: poor renal survival in black Americans. Glomerular Disease Collaborative Network. Kidney Int. 1997;51:1188-95. [PMID: 9083285]
2. **Ginzler EM, Dooley MA, Aranow C, Kim MY, Buyon J, Merrill JT, et al**. Mycophenolate mofetil or intravenous cyclophosphamide for lupus nephritis. N Engl J Med. 2005;353:2219-28. [PMID: 16306519]

3. **Contreras G, Pardo V, Leclercq B, Lenz O, Tozman E, O'Nan P, et al**. Sequential therapies for proliferative lupus nephritis. N Engl J Med. 2004;350:971-80. [PMID: 14999109]

Item 102   Answer: E

Hydration with either isotonic saline or isotonic bicarbonate before and after exposure to radiocontrast has been shown to be the most beneficial intervention to decrease the incidence of radiocontrast nephropathy. According to results of a single-center study, isotonic bicarbonate may be superior to isotonic saline in this setting. However, preferential use of this agent over saline cannot be recommended until further clinical trials validate this finding. Use of minimal volumes of iso-osmolar contrast also should be considered in all patients at high risk for radiocontrast nephropathy. Whenever possible, every effort should be made to optimize renal perfusion and oxygen delivery before radiocontrast exposure. Therefore, congestive heart failure should be treated and the hemoglobin optimized, if possible, before cardiac catheterization.

Half-normal saline has been shown to be less effective in this setting than isotonic saline. *N*-acetylcysteine and theophylline have little or no impact in decreasing the development of radiocontrast nephropathy. Fenoldopam similarly has been shown to have no benefit in the prevention of radiocontrast nephropathy.

> **KEY POINT**
> - **Infusion of normal saline before and after exposure to radiocontrast is the most effective method to decrease the risk for radiocontrast nephropathy.**

Bibliography
1. **Lin J, Bonventre JV**. Prevention of radiocontrast nephropathy. Curr Opin Nephrol Hypertens. 2005;14:105-10. [PMID: 15687835]
2. **Asif A, Epstein M**. Prevention of radiocontrast-induced nephropathy. Am J Kidney Dis. 2004;44:12-24. [PMID: 15211433]

Item 103   Answer: C

The location and clinical presentation of this patient's lesions are most characteristic of calcific uremic arteriolopathy, often termed "calciphylaxis." These lesions typically present as painful violaceous nodules on the trunk, proximal extremities, and buttocks. Risk factors for development of this syndrome include use of warfarin, vitamin D analogues, and calcium-based phosphate binders; an elevated calcium–phosphorus product; protein S or C deficiency; obesity; and female sex.

Calcinosis cutis presents with painless calcified subcutaneous nodules that do not ulcerate. Necrobiosis lipoidica diabeticorum usually is asymptomatic, and the lesions associated with this condition typically appear as oval to irregularly shaped plaques on the shins of patients with diabetes. Venous stasis ulcers are shallow, red-based ulcers typically located medially in the lower leg. Warfarin-induced skin necrosis typically occurs early in the course of warfarin therapy, and lesions associated with this condition present as erythematous macules but progress to ulcers within hours.

The role of parathyroid hormone in the pathogenesis of calcific uremic arteriolopathy remains uncertain. Therapy for this condition includes avoidance of vitamin D analogues and calcium-based phosphate binders, control of the phosphorus level with non–calcium-based phosphate binders, aggressive wound care, and treatment of secondary infection. Parathyroidectomy is reserved for affected patients whose serum calcium and phosphorus levels cannot be controlled with phosphate binders and other medical interventions such as cinacalcet.

> **KEY POINT**
> - **Calcific uremic arteriolopathy typically presents with painful violaceous nodules on the trunk, proximal extremities, and buttocks in patients with chronic kidney disease.**

Bibliography
1. **Fine A, Zacharias J**. Calciphylaxis is usually non-ulcerating: risk factors, outcome and therapy. Kidney Int. 2002;61:2210-7. [PMID: 12028462]
2. **Russell R, Brookshire MA, Zekonis M, Moe SM**. Distal calcific uremic arteriolopathy in a hemodialysis patient responds to lowering of Ca x P product and aggressive wound care. Clin Nephrol. 2002;58:238-43. [PMID: 12356195]

Item 104   Answer: A

The identification and quantification of proteinuria is important in the evaluation of kidney function, as this finding is associated with the progression of chronic kidney disease. Transient proteinuria may develop in hospitalized patients with febrile illnesses or major traumatic stresses, or proteinuria may persistently be seen on repeated urinalyses. The amount of protein excreted in the urine may be helpful in determining the underlying kidney disorder; for example, proteinuria >3.5 g/24 h characterizes the nephrotic syndrome. Non-nephrotic proteinuria without hematuria or kidney disease is a common finding in adolescents and young adults. This finding indicates orthostatic proteinuria, a benign condition causing increased excretion of proteinuria during the day and normal protein excretion at night. A split 12-hour urine collection is the recommended study of choice to confirm that protein excretion is limited to the daytime. Long-term follow-up of these patients reveals no increased risk for the development of kidney disease, and no specific therapy is required.

Kidney biopsy and serologic studies such as anti-streptolysin O or anti–glomerular basement membrane antibody assays would be of low yield for glomerular disease in a patient with normal kidney function, an absence of glomerular hematuria, and non-nephrotic proteinuria. Renal ultrasonography or spiral CT of the abdomen is important in the evaluation of chronic kidney disease to assess kidney size and reveal evidence of obstructive nephropathy or in the evaluation of nephrolithiasis or genitourinary tract malignancy in patients with persistent hematuria. However, the role of these studies is limited in the evaluation of non-nephrotic proteinuria.

KEY POINTS

- Quantification of urinary protein in upright and recumbent positions to evaluate for orthostatic proteinuria is indicated for young adults with proteinuria and no other evidence of kidney disease.
- Acute glomerulonephritis is uncommon without hematuria and a bland urine sediment.

Bibliography

1. Hogg RJ, Portman RJ, Milliner D, Lemley KV, Eddy A, Ingelfinger J. Evaluation and management of proteinuria and nephrotic syndrome in children: recommendations from a pediatric nephrology panel established at the National Kidney Foundation conference on proteinuria, albuminuria, risk, assessment, detection, and elimination (PARADE). Pediatrics. 2000;105:1242-9. [PMID: 10835064]

Item 105   Answer: D

Emergency delivery is indicated for this patient. This patient's presentation of hypertension and proteinuria during the third trimester of pregnancy is consistent with preeclampsia. However, her severe headache, decreased platelet count, and increased liver enzyme levels indicate progression to more severe disease and are consistent with the HELLP (hemolysis, elevated liver enzymes, and low platelets) syndrome, which is a variant of preeclampsia. Because she is close to term and severe preeclampsia can progress to eclampsia, timely delivery is indicated. Discharging a patient with severe preeclampsia is contraindicated, and emergency delivery of patients with severe preeclampsia at or near term always is appropriate.

KEY POINTS

- Hospitalization and delivery are indicated for women with preeclampsia at term.
- The manifestations of the HELLP syndrome (hemolysis, elevated liver enzymes, and low platelets) are features of severe preeclampsia.

Bibliography

1. Haddad B, Sibai BM. Expectant management of severe preeclampsia: proper candidates and pregnancy outcome. Clin Obstet Gynecol. 2005;48:430-40. [PMID: 15805800]

Index

Hemodialysis. *See* Renal dialysis
Hemofiltration, for radiocontrast nephropathy, 45
Henoch-Schönlein purpura, 83, 84t, Q90
Hepatic disease, acute renal failure in, 47-48, 47t
Hepatitis C, membranoproliferative glomerulonephritis and, 77
Hepatorenal syndrome, 47-48, 47t
Hereditary tubulointerstitial kidney disease, 71
Human immunodeficiency virus infection, hypokalemia in, 11
Hydralazine, for hypertension, in pregnancy, 64t
Hydrochlorothiazide, for renal calculi, 68
Hyperaldosteronism
    primary, 31-32, Q101, Q99
    steroid-remediable, 29t
Hypercalcemia, 16-17, 17t
Hypercalciuria, renal calculi in, 66, 67t, 68
Hypercholesterolemia. *See* Hyperlipidemia
Hyperglycemia, hypernatremia and, 7
Hyperkalemia, 11-13, 12t, 13f, Q90
    in chronic renal disease, 52
    drug-induced, Q100
Hyperlipidemia, in glomerular disease, 73-74
Hypernatremia, 9-11, 10t, Q96-97
    causes of, 9-10, 10t
    in critical care, 9, 10t
    in diabetes insipidus, 10
    in resistant hypertension, 38
Hyperoxaluria, 70t, 72
    renal calculi in, 66, 67t, 68, Q98
Hyperparathyroidism, in chronic renal failure, 52
    dialysis and, 57
Hyperphosphatemia, in chronic renal failure, 52
Hypertension, 27-38
    adrenal, 31-32
    classification of, 28, 28t
    definition of, 28
    diastolic, 27
    epidemiology of, 27
    essential (primary), 28
    evaluation of, 30-31, Q92-93
    follow-up in, 37
    genetic factors in, 28-29, 29t
    insulin resistance and, 29-30
    outcome in, 27
    pathophysiology of, 28-30
    pheochromocytoma and, 32
    in pregnancy, 60-61, 60-62
        drug therapy for, 64t, Q116-117
        gestational, 64-65
        in HELLP syndrome, 62, Q126
        in preeclampsia, 62, 63-64
        treatment of, 63, 64, 64t, Q116-117
    in primary aldosteronism, 31-32
    in renal disease, 29, 31, 31t, 32-33, 49-50, 54
    renal dysfunction in, 29, Q107
        tubulointerstitial, 53-55
    renovascular, 32-33, Q113
    resistant, 37-38
    secondary, 31-33, 31t
    systolic, 27
    treatment of, 34-37, Q113, Q116, Q120, Q123-124
        drug therapy in, 34-37, 35t, 36t. *See also* Antihypertensives
        lifestyle modifications in, 34, 34t
    white coat, 30, Q95-96
Hypertensive nephrosclerosis, 54, Q109-110
Hyperuricemia, in acute renal failure, 42
Hyperuricosuria, renal calculi in, 66, 67t, 68
Hypocalcemia, 16, 16t
    in chronic renal disease, 52
    in nephrotic syndrome, 74
Hypochloremia, in metabolic alkalosis, 22, 23, 23t
Hypocitraturia, renal calculi in, 66, 67t, 68
Hypokalemia, 14, 14t
    in metabolic alkalosis, 23
Hyponatremia, 6-9, 8f, 9f
    in central diabetes insipidus, 10
    clinical manifestations of, 10
    diagnosis of, 6-7, 8f
    diuretic-induced, 7
    exercise-induced, 7
    hospital-acquired, 7
    mortality in, 10
    pathogenesis of, 6
    prevention of, 7-8
    risk factors for, 7
    treatment of, 10-11, Q104-105

Hyponatremic encephalopathy, 9, 9f, Q101-102
Hypophosphatemia, 15-16, 15t

I
IgA nephropathy, 3, 80-81, Q111, Q114-115
Immune globulin, nephrotoxicity of, 44t
Immunosuppression, for renal transplantation, 57-58, 58t
Indinavir, nephrotoxicity of, 44t
Insulin resistance, hypertension and, 29-30
Interstitial nephritis, acute, 46
Intravenous immune globulin, nephrotoxicity of, 44t

K
Kawasaki's disease, 84t
    renal involvement in, 84
Ketoacidosis, diabetic, 20, 20f
Kidney. *See also under* Renal
    in acid-base balance, 19, 23, 24, 25-26
        in pregnancy, 60
    biopsy of, 5
        in pregnancy, 61
    imaging of, 4-5
    medullary sponge, 70
    myeloma, 42, 79-80, Q112, Q118
    polycystic, 70, 70t, Q104
    in potassium regulation, 6
    in pregnancy, 59-65
        abnormalities of, 60-65. *See also* Renal disease, in pregnancy
        normal function in, 59-60
    in sodium regulation, 6
Kidney stones, 65-69. *See also* Nephrolithiasis

L
Labetalol, for hypertension, in pregnancy, 64t
Lactic acidosis, 20-21, 20f
Liddle's syndrome, 29t
Light-chain nephropathy, Q108
Lipid-lowering agents, for nephrotic syndrome, 74
Listeriosis, in renal transplant recipients, 58
Lithotripsy, shock wave, 68
Liver disease, acute renal failure in, 47-48, 47t
Low-phosphate diet, in chronic renal failure, 52
Low-potassium diet, in chronic renal failure, 52
Low-protein diet, in renal disease, 51
Lupus nephritis, 73t, 74, 81t, 82-83, 82t, Q121-122, Q124
    in pregnancy, 61

M
Magnesium sulfate, for preeclampsia, 63
Medullary cystic disease of kidney, 71
Medullary sponge kidney, 70
Membranoproliferative glomerulonephritis, 73t, 77
Membranous nephropathy, 76-77, Q94
Metabolic acidosis, 19-22
    anion gap, 18, 19-21, 20f, Q110
    causes of, 21-22
    in chronic renal disease, 52-53
    in diabetes, 20, 20f
    diagnosis of, 20f, Q117, Q120-121
    lactic, 20-21, 20f
    in mixed disorders, 26-27
    non–anion gap, 20f, 21-22, 21t, Q124
    in renal failure, 22
    treatment of, 19-21
Metabolic alkalosis, 22-23, 22t, 23t
    in mixed disorders, 26-27
Metabolic syndrome, hypertension and, 29-30
Metanephrines, in pheochromocytoma, 32
Methanol poisoning, osmolal gap in, 21
Methotrexate, nephrotoxicity of, 44t
Methyl tyrosine, for pheochromocytoma, 32
Methyldopa, for hypertension, in pregnancy, 64t
Methylprednisolone, for antineutrophil cytoplasmic antibody–associated vasculitis, 85
Microalbuminuria, 4, Q102
    in diabetic nephropathy, 78
Microscopic polyangiitis, 84t, Q118-119
Minimal change disease, 73t, 75, Q3
Mixed acid-base disorders, 26-27, Q98-99, Q111
Multiple myeloma, renal involvement in, 42, 79-80, Q112, Q115-116, Q118
Muscle compartment syndrome, in rhabdomyolysis, 45-46

U

Urate nephropathy, acute renal failure in, 42
Uremia. *See also* Renal disease, chronic
    management of, 52-53, 53t
Ureterointestinal diversion, metabolic acidosis in, 21
Uric acid, in renal calculi formation, 66, 67t, 68, Q95
Urinalysis, 2-4
Urinary tract infections, recurrent, in nephrolithiasis, 67
Urinary tract obstruction, acute renal failure in, 42, Q100
Urine, alkalinization of, for nephrolithiasis, 68

V

Vascular access, for hemodialysis, 56
Vasculitis. *See also* Arteritis
    antineutrophil cytoplasmic antibody–associated, 84-85, Q104
    classification of, 84t
    cryoglobulinemic, 84
    large-vessel, 84t
    medium-vessel, 84t
    renal involvement in, 83-85, Q104
    small-vessel, 84t

Vasodilators, for hypertension, in pregnancy, 64t
Vasopressin, 6
Ventilatory support, in respiratory acidosis, 25

W

Water. *See also under* Fluid
    electrolyte-free, calculation of, 6
Wegener's granulomatosis, 84, 84t, 85
    renal involvement in, 83, 84, 84t, 85
Weight reduction, for hypertension, 34
White coat hypertension, 30, Q95-96